THE WHO WORLD MENTAL HEALTH SURVEYS SERIES

Series Editors
Ronald C. Kessler, Harvard Medical School
T. Bedirhan Üstün, the World Health Organization

Ronald C. Kessler and T. Bedirhan Üstün, Eds.
The WHO World Mental Health Surveys: Global Perspectives on the Epidemiology of Mental Disorders, 2008

Michael R. Von Korff, Kate M. Scott & Oye Gureje, Eds.
Global Perspectives on Mental–Physical Comorbidity in the WHO World Mental Health Surveys, 2009

Matthew K. Nock, Guilherme Borges & Yutaka Ono, Eds.
Suicidality in the WHO World Mental Health Surveys, in preparation

Jordi Alonso, Somnath Chatterji & Yanling He, Eds.
The Burden of Mental Disorders in the WHO World Mental Health Surveys, in preparation

Global Perspectives on Mental–Physical Comorbidity in the WHO World Mental Health Surveys

Edited by

Michael R. Von Korff
Group Health Research Institute, Seattle, Washington

Kate M. Scott
University of Otago, Wellington, New Zealand

Oye Gureje
University of Ibadan, Ibadan, Nigeria

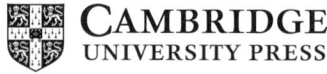

CAMBRIDGE UNIVERSITY PRESS
Cambridge, New York, Melbourne, Madrid, Cape Town, Singapore, São Paulo, Delhi

Cambridge University Press
32 Avenue of the Americas, New York, NY 10013-2473, USA

www.cambridge.org
Information on this title: www.cambridge.org/9780521199599

© World Health Organization 2009

This publication is in copyright. Subject to statutory exception
and to the provisions of relevant collective licensing agreements,
no reproduction of any part may take place without the written
permission of Cambridge University Press.

First published 2009

Printed in the United States of America

A catalog record for this publication is available from the British Library.

Library of Congress Cataloging in Publication data

Global perspectives on mental–physical comorbidity in the WHO world mental health surveys / edited by Michael R. Von Korff, Kate M. Scott, Oye Gureje.
    p. cm.
Includes index.
ISBN 978-0-521-19959-9 (hardback : alk. paper)
1. Mental health surveys.   2. Chronic diseases – Psychological aspects.   3. World health.
I. Von Korff, Michael   II. Scott, Kate M.   III. Gureje, Oye.   IV. Title.
RA790.5.G56   2009
362.2'0422–dc22   2009021483

ISBN   978-0-521-19959-9 hardback

Cambridge University Press has no responsibility for the persistence or
accuracy of URLs for external or third-party Internet Web sites referred to in
this publication and does not guarantee that any content on such Web sites is,
or will remain, accurate or appropriate. Information regarding prices, travel
timetables, and other factual information given in this work are correct at
the time of first printing, but Cambridge University Press does not guarantee
the accuracy of such information thereafter.

Every effort has been made in preparing this book to provide accurate and
up-to-date information that is in accord with accepted standards and
practice at the time of publication. Although case histories are drawn
from actual cases, every effort has been made to disguise the identities of
the individuals involved. Nevertheless, the authors, editors, and publishers
can make no warranties that the information contained herein is totally
free from error, not least because clinical standards are constantly
changing through research and regulation. The authors, editors, and
publishers therefore disclaim all liability for direct or consequential
damages resulting from the use of material contained in this book. Readers
are strongly advised to pay careful attention to information provided by
the manufacturer of any drugs or equipment that they plan to use.

Contents

Contributors		*page* xi
Foreword by David Goldberg		xiii
Acknowledgments		xvii
1	Global Perspectives on Mental–Physical Comorbidity *Michael R. Von Korff*	1

PART I. AN EPIDEMIOLOGICAL MAP OF MENTAL–PHYSICAL COMORBIDITY

2	The Global Burden of Chronic Physical Disease *Michael R. Von Korff*	15
3	The Global Burden of Chronic Pain *Adley Tsang and Sing Lee*	22
4	World Mental Health Survey Methods for Studying Mental–Physical Comorbidity *Gemma Vilagut, Kathleen Saunders, and Jordi Alonso*	29
5	The Pattern and Nature of Mental–Physical Comorbidity: Specific or General? *Oye Gureje*	51
6	The Association of Age with Depressive and Anxiety Disorders, by Physical Comorbidity Status *Kate M. Scott*	84

PART II. RISK FACTORS FOR MENTAL–PHYSICAL COMORBIDITY

7	The Development of Mental–Physical Comorbidity *Kate M. Scott*	97
8	Psychosocial Predictors of Adult-Onset Asthma *Kate M. Scott*	108
9	Childhood Adversities, Mental Disorders, and Heart Disease *Huibert Burger*	120
10	Early Child Adversity and Later Hypertension *Dan J. Stein, Kate M. Scott, and Michael R. Von Korff*	128
11	Early-Life Psychosocial Factors and Adult-Onset Diabetes *Carmen Lara*	136

12	Psychosocial Stressors in Childhood and Adult-Onset Arthritis *Michael R. Von Korff*	144
13	The Role of Childhood Adversities in Adult-Onset Spinal Pain *Ronny Bruffaerts and Koen Demyttenaere*	154
14	Childhood Adversities and Adult Obesity *Ronny Bruffaerts and Koen Demyttenaere*	165
15	Linking Depression–Anxiety Disorders and Headache in a Developmental Perspective: The Role of Childhood Family Adversities *Adley Tsang and Sing Lee*	174
16	Women, Depression, and Mental–Physical Comorbidity: Chronic Pain as a Mediating Factor *Oye Gureje and Bibilola Oladeji*	183

PART III. CONSEQUENCES OF MENTAL–PHYSICAL COMORBIDITY

17	Understanding Consequences of Mental–Physical Comorbidity *Michael R. Von Korff*	193
18	Disability and Treatment of Specific Mental and Physical Disorders *Johan Ormel, Maria V. Petukhova, Michael R. Von Korff, and Ronald C. Kessler*	210
19	The Joint Association of Mental and Physical Conditions with Disability *Kate M. Scott*	230
20	Disability in "Pure" versus "Comorbid" Mental and Physical Conditions *Paul K. Crane*	239
21	Labor Force Participation, Unemployment, and Mental–Physical Comorbidity *Michael R. Von Korff*	249
22	Perceived Stigma and Mental–Physical Comorbidity *Jordi Alonso, Andrea Buron, and Gemma Vilagut*	256
23	How Physical Comorbidity Affects Treatment of Major Depression in Developing and Developed Countries *Oye Gureje*	268
24	Mental–Physical Comorbidity and Predicted Mortality *Huibert Burger*	275

PART IV. IMPLICATIONS

25	Research Implications *Evelyn J. Bromet and Michael R. Von Korff*	287

Contents

26	Clinical Implications *Gregory E. Simon*	297
27	Policy Implications *Sergio Aguilar-Gaxiola*	302

Index   313

Contributors

Sergio Aguilar-Gaxiola, MD, PhD
University of California, Davis, School of Medicine, CA, USA

Jordi Alonso, MD, PhD
Institut Municipal d'Investigació Mèdica (IMIM-Hospital del Mar), Barcelona, Spain

Evelyn J. Bromet, PhD
State University of New York, Stony Brook, NY, USA

Ronny Bruffaerts, PhD
Department of Neurosciences and Psychiatry, University Hospital Gasthuisberg, Leuven, Belgium

Huibert Burger, MD, PhD
University Medical Center Groningen, University of Groningen, Groningen, The Netherlands

Andrea Buron, MD, MPH
Health Services Research Unit, Institut Municipal d'Investigació Mèdica (IMIM-Hospital del Mar), Barcelona, Spain; Preventive Medicine and Public Health Training Unit IMAS-UPF-ASPB, Barcelona, Spain

Paul K. Crane, MD, MPH
Department of General Internal Medicine, University of Washington, Harborview Medical Center, Seattle, WA, USA

Koen Demyttenaere, MD, PhD
Department of Neurosciences and Psychiatry, University Hospital Gasthuisberg, Leuven, Belgium

David Goldberg, Professor Emeritus
Institute of Psychiatry, King's College, London, UK

Oye Gureje, PhD, DSc
Department of Psychiatry, University of Ibadan, University College Hospital, Ibadan, Nigeria

Ronald C. Kessler, PhD
Department of Health Care Policy, Harvard Medical School, Boston, MA, USA

Carmen Lara, MD
Autonomous University of Puebla; Ramón de la Fuente National Institute of Psychiatry, Puebla, Mexico

Sing Lee, MB, BS
Department of Psychiatry, University of Hong Kong, PR China

Bibilola Oladeji, MB, BS
Department of Psychiatry, University of Ibadan, University College Hospital, Ibadan, Nigeria

Johan Ormel, PhD
Netherlands Institute of Mental Health and Addiction, Utrecht, The Netherlands

Maria V. Petukhova, PhD
Department of Health Care Policy, Harvard Medical School, Boston, MA, USA

Kathleen Saunders, JD
Group Health Research Institute, Seattle, WA, USA

Kate M. Scott, PhD
Department of Psychological Medicine, School of Medicine and Health Sciences, University of Otago, Wellington, New Zealand

Gregory E. Simon, MD, MPH
Senior Investigator, Group Health Research Institute, Seattle, WA, USA

Dan J. Stein, MD, PhD
Department of Psychiatry, University of Cape Town, Cape Town, South Africa

Adley Tsang, BSocSci
Hong Kong Mood Disorder Center, The Chinese University of Hong Kong, Hong Kong Special Administrative Region, PR China

Gemma Vilagut, BSc
Institut Municipal d'Investigació Mèdica (IMIM-Hospital del Mar), Barcelona, Spain

Michael R. Von Korff, ScD
Senior Investigator, Group Health Research Institute, Seattle, WA, USA

Foreword

This important book offers the reader a feast of new findings about common mental disorders and their relationship to physical ill health. For the first time, data on physical ill health, mental disorders, and associated disability have been carefully collected in a probability sample of the normal population drawn from 6 continents and 17 different countries. Inevitably, assessments of physical disorders had to be by self-report, as it was not possible to conduct standardized clinical examinations or to obtain medical records data from large samples in diverse countries.

The emphasis of the book is not on cross-national differences, but interesting findings are reported in comparisons between 10 developed and 7 developing countries. The message here is that the similarities are far more impressive than the differences. However, the age-standardized prevalence of chronic physical disease is somewhat higher (26.6% vs. 21.8%) in the developed countries, which might be related to greater survival in the developed countries. The other difference is in rates for asthma and chronic obstructive pulmonary disease, where rates are higher in developed countries, and heart disease, where the reverse is true.

The authors confirm that rates for either anxiety or depression ("anxious depression") are increased in all self-reported chronic physical diseases consistently across countries, as well as among persons with medically unexplained physical symptoms. But it should be emphasized that only a minority of those with chronic physical disorders were found to meet diagnostic criteria for a depressive or anxiety disorder. However, those with both anxiety and depression were more likely to have physical disorders than those with either depression or anxiety on their own. This may, of course, just reflect the greater severity of those with symptoms of both types.

The relationship of anxiety and depression in the general population is a close one. Jacob et al. (1998) analyzed data from confirmatory factor analysis of psychiatric research interviews given to subjects in four different countries and reported that a single-factor solution provided only a marginally less good solution than one with two highly correlated factors of anxiety and depression. Krueger et al. (2003) reported similar findings in general health care settings in 14 different countries. Here, a two-factor model with emotional and externalizing disorders provided the best fit for the data, a three-factor model with depression and anxiety on one "anxious misery" factor, and neurasthenia, somatization, and hypochondriasis loading on a "somatization factor" provided a reasonably good fit as well, although correlations between the various factors were substantial – around +0.70. Odds ratios for comorbidity between major depression and generalized anxiety disorder were 6.9, 8.2, and 6.4, respectively, in the Dunedin study (Moffitt et al. 2006), the U.S. National Comorbidity Survey, and the U.S. NCS – Replication Survey. As the duration requirement for symptoms of generalized anxiety is reduced, rates for this disorder rise and so do levels of comorbidity (Kessler et al. 2005, 2006). The case can therefore be made for conceptualizing a group of disorders – called variously internalizing or emotional disorders that include anxiety, depression, and somatized forms of emotional distress.

The high comorbidity between them is because the genetic causes are largely the same (Kendler et al. 1992), and early environmental disadvantages are also extremely similar (Goldberg 2008, in press). It therefore seems economical to refer to "anxious depression" rather than to assume that there is "comorbidity" between two essentially different disorders.

The features of physical disorders that are associated with either depression or anxiety are shown to include social role disability, pain, and stigma. The investigators make an important distinction between anxious depression without physical illness and anxious depression accompanying physical illness. The former is shown to decrease monotonically with increasing age, while the latter peaks in the middle years and declines thereafter. One wonders whether this last finding might be related to changes in circulating sex hormones. In contrast, physical disorders without anxious depression increase steadily with increasing age, as we would expect them to do.

Why should general physicians heed the information contained in this volume? Partly because depression is a risk factor in noncompliance with medical treatment; it has been found that depressed patients were three times as likely to be noncompliant with treatment recommendations as nondepressed patients (Di Matteo, Lepper, & Croghan 2000). Depression also predicts more reported symptoms of diabetes than either glycemic control or complications of diabetes (Ludman et al. 2004), and treatment of depression in cases of multiple sclerosis reduces both fatigue and functional outcomes (Mohr, Hart, & Vella 2007). Treatment for depression may also reduce physical symptoms in those with only diffuse, ill-defined symptoms (Kroenke 2007). Other studies reviewed, however, have failed to find positive effects on physical health status of treating depression in the physically ill, although reductions in psychological symptoms and disability have been consistently observed.

The investigators also consider why some individuals develop comorbidity, while others do not. It is possible that they share common etiology rather than one directly causing the other (Anda et al. 2006). For example, a common genetic vulnerability may underlie both depression and heart disease. Poor fetal growth resulting in low birth weight and maternal smoking are also mentioned as possible shared causes, in addition to adversities in early life that may predispose individuals to both physical and psychological disorder (Arnow 2004). Hypothalamo–pituitary–adrenal axis (HPA) dysfunction is also implicated in the etiology of both groups of disorders, and overlaps with immune axis dysfunctions (Chrousos & Kino 2007). Stress may decrease the responsivity of the HPA axis and thus lead to increased proinflammatory cytokines (Wright 2005), or HPA axis activation may trigger a counterregulatory response in white blood cells, making them more resistant to cortisol (Miller, Cohen, & Ritchey 2002).

The authors go on to argue that cumulative effects of adverse early life experience and later experience of stressful life events and adverse social conditions may account for these "comorbid" outcomes, but these arguments are not based on data presented in the present volume. In the chapters on diabetes, heart disease, arthritis, and asthma, however, they report that increasing numbers of adverse early life events do indeed increase the risk of developing these disorders, just as they are known to increase the risk of anxious depression. It is argued that these associations may be independent of one another, and may be acting on different individuals.

The investigators also present interesting findings on chronic pain. This is shown to be a major problem across the world, with the majority of cases occurring in persons who do not have co-occurring anxious depression. Female rates are higher than male rates, and prevalence increases with age. Among those with both disorders, females were more likely to have associated anxious depression than males. In the case of both frequent and severe headache and adult-onset spinal pain, hazard ratios for childhood sexual or physical abuse, parental mental disorder, and family violence are all raised, while ratios for economic adversity, parental death, or divorce are not.

As might be expected, a huge cross-sectional population survey carried out in many different countries leaves many loose ends. While females generally have higher rates than males for anxious depression, in both Nigeria and Beijing they did not. Since the WHO study (Ustun & Sartorius 1995) also showed an absence of a gender inequality in Nigeria, it would seem important to investigate the reason for this finding, although the most striking finding is that prevalence rates are very low in each gender.

These are some of the findings that interested me as I looked through the book, but others will find different things that appeal to them. The book is likely to provide a standard reference for some years to come and an invaluable resource to dip into.

David Goldberg
Professor Emeritus
Institute of Psychiatry
King's College, London

REFERENCES

Anda, R. F., Felitti, V., Bremner, J. D., Walker, J. D., Whitfield, C., Perry, D. B., & Dube, S. R. (2006). Developmental antecedents of cognitive vulnerability to depression. *Journal of Cognitive Psychotherapy*, **18**, 115–33.

Arnow, B. (2004). Relationship between childhood maltreatment, adult health and psychiatric outcomes, and medical utilization. *Journal of Clinical Psychiatry*, **65**, 10–15.

Chrousos, G. P., & Kino, T. (2007). Glucocorticoid action networks and complex psychiatric and somatic disorders. *International Journal of Psychiatry in Medicine*, **30**, 295–7.

Di Matteo, M. R., Lepper, H. S., & Croghan, T. W. (2000). Depression is a risk factor for non-compliance with medical treatment: Meta-analysis of the effects of anxiety and depression on patient adherence. *Annals of Internal Medicine*, **160**, 2101–7.

Goldberg, D. P. (2008). Towards DSM-V: The relationship between generalized anxiety disorder and major depressive episode. *Psychological Medicine*, **38**, 1–5.

Goldberg, D. P. (in press). Psychometric aspects of anxiety and depression. In *Diagnostic Issues in Depression and Generalized Anxiety Disorder: Refining the Research Agenda for DSM-V*, ed. D. Goldberg, K. S. Kendler, P. Sirovatka, & D. A. Regier. Arlington, VA: American Psychiatric Association.

Jacob, K. S., Everitt, B. S., Patel, V., Weich, S., Araya, R., & Lewis, G. H. (1998). The comparison of latent variable models of non-psychotic psychiatric morbidity in four culturally diverse populations. *Psychological Medicine*, **28**, 145–52.

Kendler, K. S., Neale, M. C., Kessler, R. C., Heath, A. C., & Eaves, L. J. (1992). Major depression and generalized anxiety disorder. Same genes (partly) different environments? *Archives of General Psychiatry*, **49**, 716–22.

Kessler, R. C., Brandenburg, N., Lane, M., Roy-Byrne, P., Stang, P. D., Stein, D. J., & Wittchen, H.-U. (2006). Rethinking the duration requirement for generalized anxiety disorder: Evidence from the National Comorbidity Survey Replication. *Psychological Medicine*, **35**, 1073–82.

Kessler, R. C., Chiu, W. T., Demler, O., & Walters, E. E. (2005). Prevalence, severity, and comorbidity of 12-month DSM-IV disorders in the National Comorbidity Survey Replication. *Archives of General Psychiatry*, **62**, 617–27.

Kroenke, K. (2007). Efficacy of treatment for somatoform disorders: A review of randomized controlled trials. *Psychosomatic Medicine*, **69**, 881–8.

Krueger, R. F., Chentsova-Dutton, Y. E., Markon, K. E., Goldberg, D., & Ormel, J. (2003). A cross-cultural study of the structure of comorbidity among common psychopathological syndromes in the general health care setting. *Journal of Abnormal Psychology*, **112**, 437–47.

Ludman, E. J., Katon, W., Russo, J., Von Korff, M., Simon, G., Ciechanowski, P., Lin, E., Bush, T., & Young, B. (2004). Depression and diabetes symptom burden. *General Hospital Psychiatry*, **26**, 430–6.

Miller, G. E., Cohen, S., & Ritchey, A. K. (2002). Chronic psychological stress and the regulation of pro-inflammatory cytokines. *Health Psychology*, **21**, 536–41.

Moffitt, T. E., Harrington, H. L., Caspi, A., Kim-Cohen, J., Goldberg, D. P., Gregory, A., & Poulton, R. (2006). Depression and generalized anxiety disorder: Cumulative and sequential comorbidity in a birth cohort followed to age 32. *Archives of General Psychiatry*, **64**, 651–60.

Mohr, D. C., Hart, S., & Vella, L. (2007). Reduction in disability in a randomized controlled trial of telephone administered CBT. *Health Psychology*, **26**, 554–63.

Ustun, T. B., & Sartorius, N. (1995). *Mental Health in General Health Care.* New York: John Wiley & Sons.

Wright, R. J. (2005). Stress and atopic disorders. *Journal of Allergy and Clinical Immunology*, **116**, 1301–6.

Acknowledgments

The editors express their gratitude to Wayne Katon and Kurt Kroenke for commenting on a near-final draft of this volume. Alison Hoffnagle played an invaluable role in facilitating communication and coordinating review of manuscripts in the World Mental Health Survey work on mental–physical comorbidity. Her efforts immeasurably strengthened collaboration among coinvestigators from many different countries. The assistance of Kari Shanahan in preparing the manuscript of this book for publication is gratefully acknowledged.

The surveys discussed in this book were carried out in conjunction with the World Health Organization (WHO) World Mental Health (WMH) Survey Initiative. We thank the WMH staff for assistance with instrumentation, fieldwork, and data analysis. These activities were supported by the U.S. National Institute of Mental Health (R01-MH070884), the John D. and Catherine T. MacArthur Foundation, the Pfizer Foundation, the U.S. Public Health Service (R13-MH066849, R01-MH069864, and R01 DA016558), the Fogarty International Center (FIRCA R03-TW006481), the Pan American Health Organization (PAHO), the Eli Lilly & Company Foundation, Ortho-McNeil Pharmaceutical, Inc., GlaxoSmithKline, and Bristol-Myers Squibb. A complete list of WMH publications can be found at http://www.hcp.med.harvard.edu/wmh/. The Chinese World Mental Health Survey Initiative is supported by the Pfizer Foundation. The Colombian National Study of Mental Health (NSMH) is supported by the Ministry of Social Protection. The ESEMeD project is funded by the European Commission (Contracts QLG5–1999-01042; SANCO 2004123), the Piedmont Region (Italy), Fondo de Investigación Sanitaria, Instituto de Salud Carlos III, Spain (FIS 00/0028), Ministerio de Ciencia y Tecnología, Spain (SAF 2000–158-CE), Departament de Salut, Generalitat de Catalunya, Spain, Instituto de Salud Carlos III (CIBER CB06/02/0046 and RETICS RD06/0011 REM-TAP), and other local agencies and by an unrestricted educational grant from GlaxoSmithKline. The Israel National Health Survey is funded by the Ministry of Health with support from the Israel National Institute for Health Policy and Health Services Research and the National Insurance Institute of Israel. The World Mental Health Japan (WMHJ) Survey is supported by the Grant for Research on Psychiatric and Neurological Diseases and Mental Health (H13-SHOGAI-023, H14-TOKUBETSU-026, and H16-KOKORO-013) from the Japan Ministry of Health, Labour, and Welfare. The Lebanese National Mental Health Survey (Lebanon) is supported by the Lebanese Ministry of Public Health, the WHO (Lebanon), Fogarty International, Act for Lebanon, anonymous private donations to IDRAAC, Lebanon, and unrestricted grants from Janssen Cilag, Eli Lilly, GlaxoSmithKline, Roche, and Novartis. The Mexican National Comorbidity Survey is supported by the National Institute of Psychiatry Ramon de la Fuente (INPRFMDIES 4280) and by the National Council on Science and Technology (CONACyT-G30544-H), with supplemental support from the

PAHO. Te Rau Hinengaro: The New Zealand Mental Health Survey is supported by the New Zealand Ministry of Health, Alcohol Advisory Council, and the Health Research Council. The Nigerian Survey of Mental Health and Well-Being is supported by the WHO (Geneva), the WHO (Nigeria), and the Federal Ministry of Health, Abuja, Nigeria. The South Africa Stress and Health Study is supported by the U.S. National Institute of Mental Health (R01-MH059575) and National Institute of Drug Abuse with supplemental funding from the South African Department of Health and the University of Michigan. The Ukraine Comorbid Mental Disorders during Periods of Social Disruption (CMDPSD) study is funded by the U.S. National Institute of Mental Health (RO1-MH61905). The U.S. National Comorbidity Survey – Replication (NCS-R) is supported by the National Institute of Mental Health (U01-MH60220), with supplemental support from the National Institute of Drug Abuse, the Substance Abuse and Mental Health Services Administration, the Robert Wood Johnson Foundation (Grant 044708), and the John W. Alden Trust.

1 Global Perspectives on Mental–Physical Comorbidity

MICHAEL R. VON KORFF

1.1. INTRODUCTION

The picture of "Earth Rising" sent back by the first lunar expedition resulted in a global change in consciousness that humans are sustained by the environment of a small planet. The contributors to this book have made a similar, albeit less dramatic, contribution. They, and their many colleagues, carried out the first population surveys able to provide a portrait of the physical and mental health of human populations worldwide. The results of the World Mental Health Surveys afford an opportunity to consider and reflect on the health and well-being of populations in both developed and developing countries. Cultural relativists may be disappointed. While cross-national differences in the frequency of specific physical and mental disorders are evident, universal features in the relationships between physical disease and mental health are more prominent.

This book presents important new information from the World Mental Health Surveys on the extent of chronic illness in general and of the co-occurrence of mental and physical morbidity in particular. Rigorous population-based surveys in Asia, Africa, the Middle East, Europe, the Americas, and the South Pacific depict a global epidemic of chronic physical disorders, often co-occurring with psychological illness.

1.2. AN EPIDEMIOLOGIC MAP

The growing burden of chronic disease, chronic pain, and mental disorders worldwide is the result of what is arguably the greatest achievement of the twentieth century: the global extension of life expectancy as the physical and social conditions of life have improved worldwide, as infant mortality has been reduced, and as death rates from infectious diseases have been lowered via socioeconomic development and public health measures (Blum 1991; McMichael et al. 2004). In 1977, Ernie Gruenberg coined the phrase "the failures of success" to refer to the increase in the prevalence of chronic diseases when mortality rates are reduced to a greater extent among persons with chronic disease than the general decline in mortality (Gruenberg 1977). Over Gruenberg's life span, from 1915 to 1991, life expectancy in the United States increased from 50 to greater than 75 years. Similar gains in life expectancy were achieved concurrently in Europe and Japan. It is less well known that most of the rest of the world was catching up during the second half of the twentieth century. In Latin America, life expectancy at birth increased from 51 years in 1950 to 70 years in 2000, while in Asia it increased from 41 to 66 years in the same time span. In Africa, gains have been less dramatic, but from 1950 to 2000 life expectancy increased from 38 to 54 years – an additional 16 years. These gains in life expectancy are resulting in older populations and increased chronic disease prevalence, both from the aging of the population and from comparatively greater reductions in mortality among those with chronic conditions.

While remarkable progress has been made in extending longevity worldwide, it is now imperative to address "the failures of success" on a global scale. The burdens of chronic disease, chronic pain, and co-occurring mental disorders experienced by growing numbers of people worldwide have an enormous impact on individuals and their families. The burdens of these disorders also have significant implications for the well-being of society at large, as larger numbers of persons depend on societal income maintenance programs due to old age or disability. With rapidly aging populations worldwide, both developed and developing countries need to maximize the ability of their adult citizens to be productive to support the growing costs of health care, old age, and disability insurance programs, as well as schools and universities to educate the next generation. These societal imperatives call attention to the need to control the major causes of chronic disease and disability in the population at large, to maximize the productivity of the adult population, and to minimize disability and dependency among the elderly.

In carrying out the World Mental Health Surveys in diverse cross-national settings, it was not possible to collect medical records data or to carry out standardized physical examinations and medical tests. For that reason, the ascertainment of physical disorders in the World Mental Health Surveys was based on self-report. In fact, the agreement of self-reported chronic physical diseases such as diabetes, heart disease, and arthritis with medical records data has generally been found to be good (Kriegsman et al. 1996; National Center for Health Statistics 1994). However, it is also likely that medically diagnosed physical diseases such as diabetes and heart disease may be under-ascertained or misclassified to some extent, particularly in developing countries where there is less adequate access to health care. Although the findings reported in this volume are in general agreement with other studies that have used medical data to diagnose comorbid physical disorders, the limitations of self-report data need to be taken into account.

1.3. MIND–BODY DUALITY RECONSIDERED

It is fitting that the first global initiative assessing physical and mental health is an opportunity to reconsider beliefs regarding the duality of physical disease and mental disorders. Plato believed that an immortal soul was imprisoned in the human body (Plato 1999). Aristotle held that the intellect was part of the soul lacking a bodily organ (Robinson 2003). Descartes viewed the body as a physical machine governed by natural laws. He believed that the mind interacted with the body, but that the mind did not exist in space and was not governed by physical laws (Descartes 1637/1968). The grand theories of the relationship between mind and body of these Western philosophers reflect a general human tendency to view mind and body as distinct and separable. Such attitudes and beliefs are manifested today in the thoughts and behaviors of physicians and patients in both developed and developing countries.

There is now a large body of research showing that beliefs in mind–body duality are neither empirically supported nor in the best interests of patients. Advances in neuroscience and medicine are inconsistent with traditional beliefs in mind–body duality (Baker, Kale, & Menken 2002; Bracken 2002; Goldberg & Goodyer 2005; Kendler 2001). Persons with mood and anxiety disorders are at increased risk of diverse physical disorders (e.g., diabetes, cardiovascular disease, arthritis, and back pain), and most physical disorders are associated with a heightened prevalence of psychological distress (Evans et al. 2005). Although it is hardly surprising that demoralization and anxiety accompany chronic physical conditions, there is considerable evidence that the presence of significant physical disease *reduces* the likelihood that physicians recognize the presence of comorbid depression (Tylee 2006). A traditional view has been that "unexplained" physical symptoms are indicative of an underlying mental disorder (Escobar, Hoyos-Nervi, & Gara 2002; Kirmayer & Sartorius 2007). Whereas cross-national research has shown that diffuse physical symptoms are associated with mood and anxiety disorders (Simon et al. 1999), unexplained physical symptoms are not invariably or even typically due to an underlying mental disorder (Burton 2003).

The first section of this book shows that mood and anxiety disorders are associated with increased risks of both well-defined chronic physical diseases and medically unexplained chronic pain conditions. It also shows that although mental and physical morbidity are related, the large majority of persons affected by chronic pain or with a well-defined chronic physical disease do *not* have a comorbid mental disorder. The second section considers risk factors that may explain the co-occurrence of chronic physical conditions and common mental disorders. New results are offered, suggesting that both early-onset mood and anxiety disorders and significant childhood adversities may increase risks of a broad spectrum of chronic physical conditions in later life, including both well-defined physical diseases and chronic pain conditions. The third section concerns the consequences of mental–physical comorbidity for people's lives, including functional disability, labor force participation, health-related stigma, use of health care services, and mortality. The World Mental Health Surveys show that the consequences of comorbid mental disorders for the health and well-being of persons with chronic physical conditions are significant in both developed and developing countries worldwide.

1.4. PHYSICAL AND PSYCHOLOGICAL MORBIDITY AS INTEGRAL

In considering the philosophical underpinnings of psychiatry, Kendler (2005) has argued that mental disorders are etiologically complex, that simple "spirochete-like" mechanisms are unlikely to be discovered, that explanatory pluralism is preferable to biological reductionism, and that we should strive for "piecemeal integration" to explain complex pathways to illness "bit by bit." These perspectives are highly relevant to understanding the relationships between physical and mental disorders as well. Current thinking holds that physical and mental disorders are associated via "bidirectional" links, in which physical disorders increase risks of mental disorders on the one hand and mental disorders increase risks of physical disease on the other (Evans et al. 2005). The findings presented in this book suggest that a more nuanced and integrated conceptualization of the relationships between physical and mental morbidity is needed.

Physical disease can occur through integrated action of the psychological and physical processes implicated in adaptation to chronic physical and psychosocial stressors. The concept of "allostasis," or the maintenance of stability through change, was initially developed to describe how the cardiovascular system adjusts to changes between arousal and resting states (Sterling & Eyer 1988). Allostasis is now viewed as having broader relevance to diverse, interrelated homeostatic systems. "Allostatic load" refers to the burdens placed on homeostatic systems repeatedly activated and deactivated in response to chronic psychosocial, psychological, and physical stressors (McEwen 1998a, 1998b). Chronic effects of allostatic load on neural, endocrine, and immune stress mediators are believed to have adverse effects on diverse organ systems. These adverse effects increase risks of physical disease as effects of allostatic load accumulate over time (McEwen & Stellar 1993). Individual differences in genetics, development, and prior experience modify effects of such stressors on allostatic load and downstream effects on physical disease and psychological illness risks (Goldberg & Goodyer 2005; Korte et al. 2005). The integrated action of the central nervous system, the neuroendocrine system, and the immune system influences risks of both physical disease (Kopps & Rethelyi 2004) and psychological illness (Goldberg & Goodyer 2005). From this perspective, the effects of psychological processes on physical health and of physiological processes on psychological health are integral and concurrent, rather than mental disorders acting on physical health status and physical disorders acting on mental health status as if mind and body were distinct entities.

Chronic pain mechanisms exemplify the integrated action of physical and psychological processes in producing both physical and psychological morbidity. Pain is a sensory and emotional experience that results from the integrated action of peripheral and central nervous systems (Schaible 2007). The peripheral nervous system is activated by mechanical, chemical, thermal, or electrical stimulation. The central nervous system transmits and regulates transmission of pain signals from the peripheral nerves to the central projection neurons and then to those parts of the brain responsible for perception and evaluation of painful stimuli. Tissue damage, degenerative disease (e.g., arthritis), and life stress inducing allostatic load can each cause inflammatory changes that produce substances such as bradykinins, prostaglandins, cytokines, and chemokines (Millan 1999). These substances mediate tissue repair and healing, but they are also irritants that result in peripheral sensitization of sensory neurons (Rittner, Brack & Stein 2003). Sustained stimulation of peripheral and central pain pathways, accompanied by inflammatory changes, can result in sensitization. Thresholds for transmission of pain signals are temporarily or permanently lowered and the area of peripheral sensitization expands beyond the original site of injury (Melzack et al. 2001). In effect, pain pathways and neurotransmitters are modified so that the neurons develop a "memory" that facilitates responding to pain signals. In the development of persistent pain states, psychological factors are implicated in many ways. Depression and anxiety amplify physical sensations so that noxious stimuli are perceived as more severe (Barsky et al. 1988). This may occur via interrelated psychological processes such as hypervigilance, and neurophysiological processes, such as centrally mediated neurotransmitter changes that facilitate transmission of pain signals (Ren & Dubner 1999). At the same time, pain itself is a significant physical and psychological stressor that may induce or increase psychological distress (Von Korff & Simon 1996). Depression and anxiety may, in turn, alter the meaning attached to pain so that the same pain inputs are regarded as more severe and more threatening when the person is psychologically distressed (Edwards et al. 2006). Depression and anxiety also influence behavioral responses to painful stimuli, resulting in a person being more likely to rest and limit activities, more fearful and vigilant about actions that may cause pain, and less likely to engage in pleasant or productive activities that distract attention from pain (Grotle et al. 2004; Pincus et al. 2002). Physical and psychological processes act in concert in producing chronic pain and associated activity limitations in a highly integrated fashion.

1.5. A LIFE-SPAN PERSPECTIVE

Relationships between physical and mental disorders are multifaceted and develop over the life span. For example, emotional distress and sleep disturbance are integral features of physical pain, whether the physical pain is medically explained or not (deBock et al. 1995; Von Korff & Simon 1996). Persons who are depressed or anxious are more likely to amplify physical symptoms and develop catastrophic ideas about the causes and consequences of their symptoms, whether the physical symptoms are medically explained or not (Barsky 1979; Edwards et al. 2006). Childhood adversities may increase risks of early-onset mental disorders (Goldberg & Goodyer 2005), while both childhood adversities and early-onset mental disorders may increase risks of a range of physical diseases in later life (Felitti et al. 1998; Gluckman & Hanson 2004). Mood and anxiety disorders present in adolescence may increase risks of tobacco use, obesity, and sedentary lifestyle; the presence of both affective disorder and behavioral risk factors may have independent effects on risks of cardiovascular disease and diabetes in later life (Lett et al. 2004). Among persons with medically diagnosed chronic disease, both disease severity and emotional distress contribute to functional disability (Ormel et al. 1993; Von Korff et al. 1992, 2005). Mood and anxiety disorders increase the likelihood of poor self-management of physical disease, less positive disease control, and less favorable physical disease outcomes (DiMatteo, Lepper, & Croghan 2000; Katon et al. 2004; Lin et al. 2004). These observations suggest that we need to think about the relationships between mental and physical factors in illness as multifaceted and developmental rather than as distinct. Rather than trying to identify causal pathways from mental to physical disorder and from physical to mental disorder, the empirical results of the World Mental Health Surveys suggest that "piecemeal integration" of multifaceted, life-span developmental pathways, in which boundaries between physical disease and mental disorder are inherently blurred, is more likely to be productive.

1.6. ECOLOGICAL AND POPULATION PERSPECTIVES

In the nineteenth century, explanations of disease focused on the role of microorganisms. Koch's famous postulates (e.g., that a cultured microorganism should reliably cause disease when introduced into a healthy organism) are now recognized as overly simplistic (Evans 1976). In the wake of the Darwinian revolution, ecological and systems models of disease espoused by Rene Dubos (1959/1987) and others came to the fore, in which host, agent, and environmental factors were viewed as interacting to cause disease. The ecological perspective and the host–agent–environment model served as the foundations for revolutionary advances in public health that increased longevity. These included more sanitary and healthful water and food supplies, mass immunization to prevent infectious diseases, compulsory public education for boys and girls, and improved prenatal and postnatal care. Ecological approaches, and the host–agent–environment model, are equally applicable to the control of chronic physical disease and mental disorders, but new approaches are needed. In developing new approaches to control the burden of chronic physical and mental disorders, population-based data on the extent and distribution of physical and mental disorders are critically important.

1.7. INTEGRATION OF LIFE-SPAN, ECOLOGICAL, AND POPULATION PERSPECTIVES

In applying epidemiologic methods to study comorbidity of chronic physical disease, chronic pain, and mental disorders, the ecological (host–agent–environment) model goes hand in hand with population and life-span (developmental) perspectives (Von Korff 1999). The population perspective implies that efforts to control chronic conditions must be grounded in an understanding of the distribution and determinants of illness on a population basis, not only among cases seen in clinical settings. The life-span or developmental perspective views the development and course of disease as changing and dynamic rather than fixed and static (Goldberg & Goodyer 2005). In combination with the ecological model, the life-span perspective calls attention to the potential for diverse factors to influence the development and expression of disease in human populations. There is a natural affinity between the ecological model of epidemiology and the biopsychosocial model (Engel 1960) of the behavioral sciences. Both models are multifactorial systems perspectives that view disease as occurring within a complex web of factors operating both within and external to the affected individual (Dworkin, Von Korff, & Le Resche 1992).

Chronic conditions develop and run their course over time spans measured in decades. The ecological, life-span, and population perspectives suggest very different approaches to controlling disease than when a single disease is considered in isolation. For chronic recurrent conditions, the prevalence of the disease in a population is the product of its incidence rate, the average episode duration, and the average number of recurrences of the condition over a life span (Von Korff & Parker 1980). This means that from a life-span perspective, a chronic condition can be controlled by preventing onset, by shortening episode duration, and by reducing the likelihood of recurrence. Even though this volume reports data from cross-sectional surveys, the interpretation of results is informed by a life-span perspective that may offer clues to new strategies for reducing the burden of chronic physical disease and of mental disorders on a population basis, by preventing onset, by shortening episode duration, or by preventing recurrence. In addition, the burden of disease can be reduced on a population basis by improving adaptation to disease, by reducing disability, by enhancing self-management of disease, and by increasing participation in life activities among persons affected by mental or physical disorder.

1.8. THE SEARCH FOR BROAD-SPECTRUM RISK FACTORS

The findings of the World Mental Health Surveys reported in this volume are consistent with three significant generalizations: (1) diverse chronic physical diseases, chronic pain conditions, and mental disorders frequently occur together; (2) these diverse conditions may have common risk factors that influence onset, duration, recurrence, and adaptation to illness; and (3) risk factors for disease expression may also be important determinants of adaptation to disease (disability and chronic disease self-management). These findings, when viewed from ecological, life-span, and population perspectives, suggest that it may be productive to search for broad-spectrum risk factors. Broad-spectrum risk factors refer to (1) common causes of multiple disorders and (2) risk factors whose effects are realized over different developmental stages of those disorders, including onset, duration, and recurrence, as well as adaptation to disease. Examples of broad-spectrum risk factors include educational attainment, childhood adversities that result in chronic stress and less-than-optimal development, socioeconomic adversities that induce physical and psychological hardships, and health behaviors such as tobacco use, sedentary lifestyle, and poor diet that result in malnutrition or obesity.

The value of identifying broad-spectrum risk factors is that they are at play across conditions and at different phases in the natural history of specific conditions and comorbidities. Control of broad-spectrum risk factors may yield benefits across diverse conditions and over the full developmental cycle of those disorders. While the results of cross-sectional population surveys, such as the World Mental Health Surveys, are limited in their ability to identify causal pathways, the results reported in this volume provide intriguing observations regarding possible broad-spectrum risk factors relevant to strategies for preventing and controlling mental–physical comorbidity and associated disability. In particular, the findings regarding the association of childhood adversities and early-onset mood and anxiety disorders with a broad range of chronic physical conditions merit further investigation. This research may suggest avenues for controlling chronic disease in human populations with potential for larger population benefit than do traditional efforts to recognize and treat prevalent cases. Case finding and treatment programs in health care settings are only one tool for controlling physical disease and psychological illness on a population basis, a tool that has significant limitations and considerable costs. The findings reported in this volume may provide a launching pad for consideration of broader and ultimately more cost-effective strategies to control chronic physical disease and psychological illness, such as programs to enhance the developmental circumstances of children and adolescents (Goldberg & Goodyer 2005).

1.9. HEALTH CARE IMPLICATIONS

Even casual perusal of the findings reported in this volume suggests that the co-occurrence of physical disease and mental disorders is a common phenomenon in both developed and developing countries. An obvious implication of these findings, often commented on by mental health professionals, is that physicians and other health care providers treating persons with physical conditions need to be adequately trained to recognize and treat common mental disorders. An equally important implication, less often noted, is that mental health professionals now need to be adequately trained to treat mental disorders in patients who are afflicted by co-occurring physical diseases and chronic pain conditions. In fact, many primary care physicians are now well trained in the recognition and management of major depression, and most treatment of depression worldwide occurs in general medical settings. In contrast, the mental health professional adequately trained to treat patients with comorbid diabetes, heart disease, respiratory disease, neurological disorders, or chronic pain is the exception rather than the rule. If mental health professionals aspire to offer holistic treatment of their patients, not treatment of mental disorder in isolation from the broader health status of their patients, then they will need to pay increased attention to addressing co-occurring physical diseases and chronic pain conditions as part of adequate treatment of mental disorders.

A second implication is that health care may need to develop new strategies of protecting population health beyond traditional efforts to identify and treat prevalent cases of chronic physical and psychological disorders, including efforts that address broad-spectrum risk factors.

1.10. POLICY IMPLICATIONS

Countries spending far less on health care now have mortality rates approaching those of Europe and the United States. For example, Costa Rica, whose annual per capita health care expenditures at the turn of the millennium were around $500 per year, had achieved life expectancy among its citizens equal to that of the United States, whose per capita health care expenditures exceeded $5,000 per year. On the one hand, this means that developing countries face significant health care challenges with limited resources currently allocated to health care, as the extent of chronic disease in their populations grows. On the other hand, these countries have unique opportunities to devise more innovative and less costly approaches to managing the growing burden of chronic physical diseases and mental disorders. They have opportunities to develop more effective and efficient health care systems than the legacy systems of developed countries now staggering under the burden of rapidly inflating health care costs.

The results reported in this volume suggest that both developed and developing countries face tremendous burdens in caring for rapidly growing populations with chronic conditions, including those with multiple physical conditions and mental health problems. However, leaving aside mortality rate differences that may be largely due to factors other than health services, it is not evident from the results of the World Mental Health Surveys that countries spending far more on health care have consistently achieved notably better population health than those countries spending less. An important question, one not addressed by the World Mental Health Surveys, is the relative health benefit of investment in educational programs and socioeconomic development versus traditional health care services in terms of benefits for health outcomes of common chronic physical and psychological disorders. Perhaps the developed world will have an opportunity to learn from the developing world in finding better ways of addressing population health in the coming decades.

1.11. RESEARCH IMPLICATIONS

This volume provides an epidemiologic map of the occurrence of common chronic physical diseases, common chronic pain conditions, and common mental disorders on a global basis. The focus of this volume is on the universals of the occurrence and co-occurrence of physical and mental morbidity, not on cross-national or cross-cultural differences. The many authors who have contributed to this volume share a common perspective that it is time to reconsider traditional and deeply ingrained beliefs in the duality of physical disease and mental disorders. Although the work presented in this volume is empirical and descriptive, the view that physical and mental morbidity are integral permeates the work reported here. In particular, the results of the World Mental Health Surveys invite future researchers to investigate the role of early-onset mental disorders and childhood adversities as broad-spectrum risk factors for a wide range of adverse health outcomes. The results reported in this volume also suggest the need for future research that seeks to understand the role of mood and anxiety disorders in increasing risks of physical disease and in impairing the abilities of persons affected by chronic disease to adapt to their health conditions, thus minimizing disability and optimizing self-management. In reporting data from cross-national population surveys, ecological, life-span, and population-based perspectives can be brought to bear on the vexing and complex problems of understanding whether and why specific physical and mental disorders tend to co-occur in human populations.

The collective efforts of the research teams that carried out the World Mental Health Surveys provide an unprecedented view of the health and mental health status of the world population at the dawn of a new millennium. The results presented in this volume provide a basis for new ideas and fresh perspectives concerning how the growing burden of chronic physical and psychological disorders in aging populations can be effectively addressed so that the worldwide gains in life expectancy achieved in the twentieth century can be matched by comparable gains in health and quality of life of the world population in the twenty-first century.

REFERENCES

Baker, M. G., Kale, R., & Menken, M. (2002). The wall between neurology and psychiatry: Advances in neuroscience indicate it's time to tear it down. *British Medical Journal*, **324**, 1468–9.

Barsky, A. J. (1979). Patients who amplify bodily sensations. *Annals of Internal Medicine*, **91**, 63–70.

Barsky, A. J., Goodson, J. D., Lane, R. S., & Cleary, P. D. (1988). The amplification of somatic symptoms. *Psychosomatic Medicine*, **5**, 510–19.

Blum, R. W. (1991). Global trends in adolescent health. *The Journal of the American Medical Association*, **265**, 2711–19.

Bracken, P. (2002). Time to move beyond the mind-body split. *British Medical Journal*, **325**, 1433–4.

Burton, C. (2003). Beyond somatization: A review of the understanding and treatment of medically unexplained physical symptoms (MUPS). *The British Journal of General Practice*, **53**, 231–9.

deBock, G. H., Kaptein, A. A., Touw-Otten, F., & Mulder, J. D. (1995). Health-related quality of life in patients with osteoarthritis in a family practice setting. *Arthritis Care and Research*, **8**, 88–93.

Descartes, R. (1637/1968). *Discourse on Method and the Meditations*, trans. (with introduction) F. E. Sutcliffe. London: Penguin Books Ltd.

DiMatteo, M. R., Lepper, H. S., & Croghan, T. W. (2000). Depression is a risk-factor for noncompliance with medical treatment: Meta-analysis of the effects of anxiety and depression on patient adherence. *Archives of Internal Medicine*, **160**, 2101–7.

Dubos, R. (1959/1987). *Mirage of Health: Utopias, Progress & Biological Change*. Reprint, New Jersey: Rutgers University Press.

Dworkin, S. F., Von Korff, M., & Le Resche, L. (1992). Epidemiologic studies of chronic pain: A dynamic-ecologic perspective. *Annals of Behavioral Medicine*, **14**, 3–11.

Edwards, R. R., Bingham, C. O., III, Bathon, J., & Haythornewaite, J. A. (2006). Catastrophizing and pain in arthritis, fibromyalgia and other rheumatic diseases. *Arthritis and Rheumatism*, **55**, 325–32.

Engel, G. L. (1960). A unified concept of health and disease. *Perspectives in Biology and Medicine*, **3**, 459–85.

Escobar, J. I., Hoyos-Nervi, C., & Gara, M. (2002). Medically unexplained physical symptoms in medical practice: A psychiatric perspective. *Environmental Health Perspectives*, **110**, 631–6.

Evans, A. S. (1976). Causation and disease: The Henle-Koch postulates revisited. *The Yale Journal of Biology and Medicine*, **49**, 175–95.

Evans, D. L., Charney, D. S., Lewis, L., Golden, R. N., Gorman, J. M., Krishnan, K. R., Nemeroff, C. B., Bremner, J. D., Carney, R. M., Coyne, J. C., Delong, M. R., Frasure-Smith, N., Glassman, A. H., Gold, P. W., Grant, I., Gwyther, L., Ironson, G., Johnson, R. L., Kanner, A. M., Katon, W. J., Kaufmann, P. G., Keefe, F. J., Ketter, T., Laughren, T. P., Leserman, J., Lyketsos, C. G., McDonald, W. M., McEwen, B. S., Miller, A. H., Musselman, D., O'Connor, C., Petitto, J. M., Pollock, B. G., Robinson, R. G., Roose, S. P., Rowland, J., Sheline, Y., Sheps, D. S., Simon, G., Spiegel, D., Stunkard, A., Sunderland, T., Tibbits, P., Jr., & Valvo, W. J. (2005). Mood disorders in the medically ill: Scientific review and recommendations. *Biological Psychiatry*, **58**, 175–89.

Felitti, V. J., Anda, R. F., Nordenberg, D., Williamson, D. F., Spitz, A. M., Edwards, V., Koss, M. P., & Marks, J. S. (1998). Relationship of childhood abuse and household dysfunction to many of the leading causes of death in adults. *American Journal of Preventive Medicine*, **14**, 245–58.

Gluckman, P. D., & Hanson, M. A. (2004). Living with the past: Evolution, development, and patterns of disease. *Science*, **305**, 1733–6.

Goldberg, D., & Goodyer, I. (2005). *The Origins and Course of Common Mental Disorders*. London: Routledge.

Grotle, M., Vollestad, N. K., Veirod, M. B., & Brox, J. I. (2004). Fear-avoidance beliefs and distress in relation to disability and chronic low back pain. *Pain*, **112**, 343–52.

Gruenberg, E. M. (1977). The failures of success. *Milbank Memorial Fund Quarterly. Health and Society*, **55**, 3–24.

Katon, W., Von Korff, M., Ciechanowski, P., Russo, J., Lin, E. H. B., Simon, G., Ludman, E., Walker, E., Bush, T., & Young, B. (2004). Behavioral and clinical factors associated with depression among individuals with diabetes. *Diabetes Care*, **27**, 914–20.

Kendler, K. S. (2001). A psychiatric dialogue on the mind-body problem. *The American Journal of Psychiatry*, **158**, 989–1000.

Kendler, K. S. (2005). Toward a philosophical structure for psychiatry. *The American Journal of Psychiatry*, **162**, 433–40.

Kirmayer, L. J., & Sartorius, N. (2007). Cultural models and somatic syndromes. *Psychosomatic Medicine*, **69**, 832–40.

Kopps, M. S., & Rethelyi, J. (2004). Where psychology meets physiology: Chronic stress and premature mortality – The Central-Eastern European health paradox. *Brain Research Bulletin*, **62**, 351–67.

Korte, S. M., Koolhaas, J. M., Wingfield, J. C., & McEwen, B. S. (2005). The Darwinian concept of stress: Benefits of allostasis and costs of allostatic load and the trade-offs in health and disease. *Neuroscience and Biobehavioral Reviews*, **29**, 3–38.

Kriegsman, D. M., Penninx, B. W., van Eijk, J. T., Boeke, A. J., & Deeg, D. J. (1996). Self-reports and general practitioner information on the presence of chronic diseases in community dwelling elderly. A study on the accuracy of patients' self-reports and on determinants of inaccuracy. *Journal of Clinical Epidemiology*, **49**, 1407–17.

Lett, H. S., Blumenthal, J. A., Babyak, M. A., Sherwood, A., Strauman, T., Robins, C., & Newman, M. F. (2004). Depression as a risk factor for coronary artery disease: Evidence, mechanisms and treatment. *Psychosomatic Medicine*, **66**, 305–15.

Lin, E. H. B., Katon, W., Von Korff, M., Rutter, C., Simon, G. E., Oliver, M., Ciechanowski, P., Ludman, E., Bush, T., & Young, B. (2004). Relationship of depression and diabetes self-care, medication adherence and preventive care. *Diabetes Care*, **27**, 2154–60.

McEwen, B. S. (1998a). Stress, adaptation, and disease: Allostasis and allostatic load. *Annals of the New York Academy of Sciences*, **840**, 33–44.

McEwen, B. S. (1998b). Protective and damaging effects of stress mediators. *The New England Journal of Medicine*, **338**, 171–9.

McEwen, B. S., & Stellar, E. (1993). Stress and the individual: Mechanisms leading to disease. *Archives of Internal Medicine*, **153**, 2093–101.

McMichael, A. J., McKee, M., Shkolnikov, V., & Valkonen, T. (2004). Mortality trends and setbacks: Global convergence or divergence. *Lancet*, **363**, 1155–9.

Melzack, R., Coderre, T. J., Katz, J., & Vaccarino, A. L. (2001). Central neuroplasticity and pathological pain. *Annals of the New York Academy of Sciences*, **933**, 157–74.

Millan, M. J. (1999). The induction of pain: An integrative review. *Progress in Neurobiology*, **57**, 1–164.

National Center for Health Statistics. (1994). Evaluation of National Health Interview Survey diagnostic reporting. *Vital and Health Statistics 2*, **120**, 1–116.

Ormel, J., Von Korff, M., Van Den Brink, W., Katon, W., Brilman, E., & Oldehinkel, T. (1993). Depression, anxiety and social disability show synchrony of change in primary care patients. *American Journal of Public Health*, **83**, 385–90.

Pincus, T., Burton, A. K., Vogel, S., & Field, A. P. (2002). A systematic review of psychological factors as predictors of chronicity/disability in prospective cohorts of low back pain. *Spine*, **27**, 109–20.

Plato. (1999). *Pheado*, trans. & ed. D. Gallop. Oxford: Oxford University Press.

Ren, K., & Dubner, R. (1999). Central nervous system plasticity and persistent pain. *Journal of Orofacial Pain*, **13**, 155–63.

Rittner, H. L., Brack, A., & Stein, C. (2003). Pro-algesic and analgesic actions of immune cells. *Current Opinion in Anaesthesiology*, **16**, 527–33.

Robinson, H. (2003). Dualism. In *The Blackwell Guide to Philosophy of Mind*, ed. S. Stich & T. Warfield, pp. 85–101. Oxford: Blackwell.

Schaible, H. G. (2007). Peripheral and central mechanisms of pain generation. *Handbook of Experimental Pharmacology*, **177**, 3–28.

Simon, G. E., Von Korff, M., Piccinelli, M., Fullerton, C., & Ormel, J. (1999). An international study of the relation between somatic symptoms and depression. *The New England Journal of Medicine*, **341**, 1329–35.

Sterling, P., & Eyer, J. (1988). Allostasis: A new paradigm to explain arousal and pathology. In *Handbook of Life Stress, Cognition and Health*, ed. S. Fisher & J. Reason, pp. 629–49. New York: John Wiley & Sons.

Tylee, A. (2006). Identifying and managing depression in primary care in the United Kingdom. *The Journal of Clinical Psychiatry*, **67**, 41–45.

Von Korff, M. (1999). Epidemiologic methods. In *Epidemiology of Pain*, ed. I. K. Crombie, P. R. Croft, S. J. Linton, L. Le Resche & M. Von Korff, pp. 7–15. Seattle, WA: IASP Press.

Von Korff, M., Katon, W., Lin, E. H. B., Simon, G., Ludman, E., Oliver, M., Ciechanowski, P., Rutter, C., & Bush, T. (2005). Potentially modifiable factors associated with disability among persons with diabetes. *Psychosomatic Medicine*, **67**, 233–40.

Von Korff, M., Ormel, J., Katon, W., & Lin, E. H. B. (1992). Disability and depression among high utilizers of health care: A longitudinal analysis. *Archives of General Psychiatry*, **49**, 91–100.

Von Korff, M., & Parker, R. D. (1980). The dynamics of the prevalence of chronic episodic disease. *Journal of Chronic Diseases*, **33**, 79–85.

Von Korff, M., & Simon, G. E. (1996). The relationship between pain and depression. *The British Journal of Psychiatry*, **30**, 101–8.

PART ONE

An Epidemiological Map of Mental–Physical Comorbidity

2 The Global Burden of Chronic Physical Disease

MICHAEL R. VON KORFF

2.1. INTRODUCTION

In the twenty-first century, the health challenges facing developed and developing countries are converging. On a global basis, infant mortality has declined and life expectancy has increased. In fact, life expectancy in many developing countries is now approaching that achieved in developed countries in the 1970s. While many developing countries continue to face significant challenges in controlling infectious disease, the prevalence rates of chronic physical diseases are rapidly increasing worldwide. The Oxford Health Alliance found that although "chronic diseases have traditionally been considered 'diseases of affluence' that affect only the elderly and wealthy," chronic disease now accounts for the largest share of mortality in all regions of the world except sub-Saharan Africa and that chronic diseases are a major problem among working-age and elderly persons, and among all economic groups, in both developed and developing countries (Suhrcke et al. 2006). Yach et al. (2004) observed that "chronic diseases are the largest cause of death in the world – cardiovascular disease, cancer, chronic respiratory disease, and diabetes – caused 29 million deaths worldwide. Despite growing evidence of epidemiological and economic impact, the global response remains inadequate.... A more concerted, strategic and multi-sector policy approach, underpinned by solid research, is essential to help reverse the negative trends in the incidence of chronic disease." Daar et al. (2007) have identified the "grand challenges" of the twenty-first century for controlling chronic, noncommunicable diseases. These include raising public awareness; enhancing economic, legal, and environmental policies; modifying risk factors; engaging community institutions and business; mitigating the impacts of poverty and urbanization; and reorienting health care systems.

As the world population ages, both developed and developing countries will grapple with major dilemmas of the demographic transition. How will society provide and pay for health care for elderly citizens and for those with major chronic conditions? How will the economic security of the retired and disabled be ensured? How will long-term care be provided for persons with severe physical and mental impairments unable to care for themselves? The developed countries furthest along in the demographic transition have higher dependency ratios as persons live longer after they retire. The dependency ratio is the number of persons younger than 20 or older than 65 years divided by the population aged 20–64 years (OECD 2007). These challenges of the demographic transition mean that it will be essential to maximize the productivity of working-age citizens so that the educational, health care, retirement, and income maintenance for the disabled and long-term care needs of society can be met. Maximizing the productivity of working-age citizens who have significant chronic physical and psychological disorders will be especially important as the well-being of society at large will hinge,

Table 2.1. Per capita income, sustainable access to improved sanitation, and physicians per thousand population in the countries participating in the WMH Surveys

Countries	Per capita income (in international dollars), purchase-parity adjusted – 2005	Percent of urban population with sustained access to improved sanitation (%)	Life expectancy at birth in 2004	Life expectancy at age 65 in in 2004
Developing countries				
China	6,600	69	71.9	14.8
Colombia	7,420	96	72.6	17.0
Lebanon	5,740	100	70.1	14.2
Mexico	10,030	91	74.4	17.3
Nigeria	1,040	53	45.5	11.6
South Africa	12,120	79	48.1	12.4
Ukraine	6,720	98	67.5	13.9
Developed countries				
Belgium	32,640	100	78.5	18.2
France	30,540	NA	79.7	19.6
Germany	29,210	100	79.2	18.5
Israel	25,280	100	80.1	19.0
Italy	28,840	NA	80.7	19.5
Japan	31,410	100	82.3	21.1
The Netherlands	32,480	100	79.3	18.2
New Zealand	23,030	NA	79.7	19.0
Spain	25,820	100	80.1	19.3
United States	41,950	100	77.6	18.3

Source: World Health Organization. WHOSIS (WHO Statistical Information System). Retrieved January 25, 2008, from http://www.who.int/whosis/.

in part, on the productivity of persons living with chronic physical and psychological disorders.

Although economic development in many parts of the developing world has been accelerating in recent years, there remains a large gap in per capita income between developed and developing countries. Among the countries participating in the World Mental Health (WMH) Surveys, the seven developing countries had purchase-parity adjusted per capita incomes of $1,040–$12,120 in 2005 (see Table 2.1). In contrast, the 10 developed countries had per capita incomes of $25,280–$41,950. These developed countries participating in the WMH Surveys had achieved essentially universal sustained access to improved sanitation, whereas this was highly variable in the developing countries (Table 2.1). These disparities in economic wealth and environmental protection correspond to notable differences in life expectancy between developed and developing countries, both at birth and at age 65 (Table 2.1). Life expectancy at age 65 ranged from 18 to 21 years in the developed countries and from 12 to 17 years in the developing countries.

There are also marked differences between developed and developing countries in health care costs as a percent of gross domestic product (GDP), purchase-parity adjusted per capita health care costs, and physicians per thousand population (Table 2.2). With the exception of the United States, per capita

Table 2.2. Health care costs and physicians per thousand population in the countries participating in the WMH Surveys

Countries	Health care costs in 2004 (% of GDP)	Purchase-parity adjusted per capita health care costs in 2004 (in international dollars)	Physicians per thousand population
Developing countries			
China	4.7	277	1.06
Colombia	7.8	570	1.35
Lebanon	11.6	817	3.25
Mexico	6.5	655	1.98
Nigeria	4.6	53	0.28
South Africa	8.6	748	0.77
Ukraine	6.5	427	2.95
Developed countries			
Belgium	9.7	3,133	4.49
France	10.5	3,040	3.37
Germany	10.6	3,171	3.37
Israel	8.7	1,972	3.82
Italy	8.7	2,414	4.20
Japan	7.8	2,292	1.98
The Netherlands	9.2	3,092	3.15
New Zealand	8.4	2,082	2.37
Spain	8.1	2,099	3.30
United States	15.4	6,096	2.56

Source: World Health Organization. WHOSIS (WHO Statistical Information System). Retrieved January 9, 2008, from http://www.who.int/whosis/.

health care costs in developed countries ranged from $2,000 to $3,200, with spending amounting to 8–11% of GDP. Developed countries had between 2.0 and 4.5 physicians per thousand population. In contrast, the developing countries participating in the WMH Surveys generally had fewer than two physicians per thousand population (except for Lebanon and Ukraine), with per capita expenditures substantially lower than those in the developed countries. The United States, with its unique approach to insuring health care that leaves 16% of the population without health insurance coverage, managed to spend 15% of its GDP on health care at an average cost of more than $6,000 per person. Despite extraordinary expenditures on health care in the United States, the number of physicians per thousand population was lower than that in most other developed countries. However, it is important to note that the country with the longest life expectancy, Japan, had the lowest physician staffing ratio and among the lowest per capita health care costs of any of the developed countries. Thus, there is not a simple relationship between resources devoted to health care and a country's health status.

2.2. APPROACH

This chapter provides a brief overview of the prevalence of common chronic physical diseases in developed and developing countries

Table 2.3. Crude and age-standardized prevalence of chronic physical disease

Countries	Crude prevalence of chronic physical disease (%)	Age-standardized prevalence of chronic physical disease (%)
Developing countries		
Beijing	17.6	19.9
Shanghai	26.7	26.4
Colombia	19.6	17.5
Lebanon	11.4	12.9
Mexico	11.5	11.0
Nigeria	7.6	9.0
South Africa	22.5	26.0
Ukraine	34.4	31.3
Any developing country	18.9	21.8
Developed countries		
Belgium	24.5	21.6
France	23.7	22.3
Germany	23.6	19.7
Israel	29.1	28.1
Italy	16.9	13.9
Japan	29.5	25.8
The Netherlands	25.2	23.5
New Zealand	31.5	31.0
Spain	20.4	18.7
United States	32.5	31.4
Any developed country	28.1	26.6

Note: Prevalence rates were standardized to the age distribution of the pooled survey populations. Chronic physical diseases included in these prevalence rates are asthma/chronic obstructive pulmonary disease, heart disease, diabetes, ulcers, tuberculosis, epilepsy, cancer, and HIV/AIDS.

based on self-reported chronic conditions ascertained in the WMH Surveys Initiative. The chronic physical diseases reported include asthma/chronic obstructive pulmonary disease, heart disease, diabetes, ulcers, tuberculosis, epilepsy, cancer, stroke, and HIV/AIDS. Information on the prevalence of depressive or anxiety disorders among persons with and without one of these chronic physical diseases is also presented. The depressive and anxiety disorders assessed include major depression, dysthymia, generalized anxiety disorder, posttraumatic stress disorder, panic disorder, agoraphobia, and social phobia. More extensive information on how these physical and mental disorders were assessed is presented in Chapter 4.

2.3. FINDINGS

The prevalence of chronic physical disease in the adult populations of developed countries was somewhat higher than that of the developing countries (Table 2.3). However, differences in the age distributions of the populations in developed and developing countries explained about half of this difference. The developing countries have age-standardized prevalence rates of chronic physical diseases that approach those in developed countries,

The Global Burden of Chronic Physical Disease

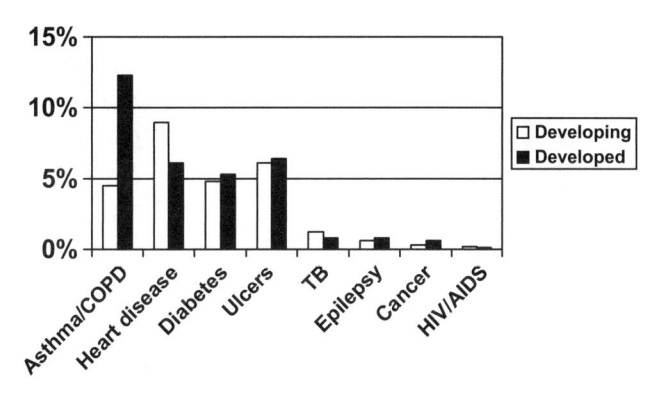

Figure 2.1. Age-standardized prevalence of chronic physical diseases in developed and developing countries.

while they typically have fewer physicians and substantially lower health care expenditures per capita. The challenge of addressing the health care needs of the increasing prevalence of chronic disease in developing countries may foster innovative approaches to more efficient care of chronically ill populations. Innovation to increase the effectiveness and efficiency of chronic illness care is also needed in developed countries struggling with the twin challenges of rapidly increasing health care costs (Anderson & Poullier 1999) and major deficiencies in the quality of chronic disease care (Wagner, Austin, & Von Korff 1996).

The similarities of the age-specific prevalence rates of chronic physical disease in the developing and developed countries participating in the WMH Surveys are surprising. Figure 2.2 shows the age-specific prevalence rates of chronic physical diseases (including asthma/chronic obstructive pulmonary disease, heart disease, diabetes, ulcers, tuberculosis, epilepsy, cancer, and HIV/AIDS) in the adult populations of the developed and developing countries participating in the WMH Surveys. If the greater expenditures on health care in developed countries were markedly reducing mortality among persons with these chronic diseases, then age-specific prevalence rates of these chronic physical diseases might be expected to be substantially higher in developed than developing countries. Research comparing health care and outcomes for common chronic diseases in developed and developing countries is needed to better understand the contributions of health care services to differences in longevity of persons with chronic conditions.

The profile of the most common chronic diseases in developed and developing countries (Figure 2.1) is more similar than different. Asthma/chronic obstructive pulmonary disease was substantially more common in the developed countries participating in the WMH Surveys, while heart disease was reported more frequently in developing countries. Overall, the relative frequency of the major chronic diseases was similar. Respiratory disease, heart disease, and ulcers were the most common chronic diseases in both developed and developing countries.

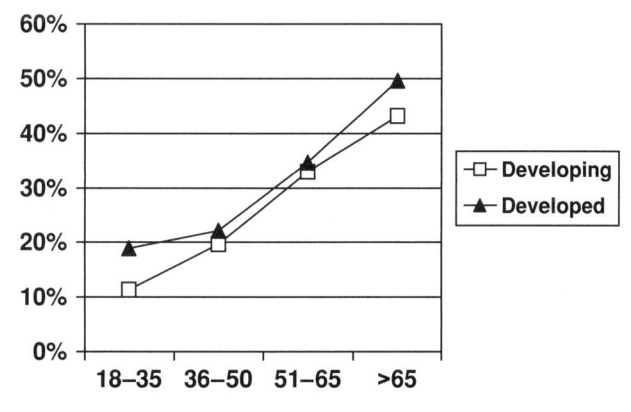

Figure 2.2 Age-specific prevalence of chronic physical diseases.

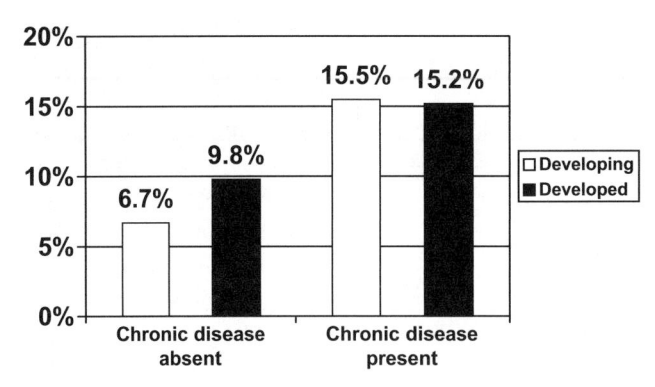

Figure 2.3. Percent with mood or anxiety disorder by chronic physical disease status.

Turning to the primary focus of this volume, the co-occurrence of mood and/or anxiety disorders with chronic physical disease is also similar in developed and developing countries (Figure 2.3). In both developed and developing countries, the prevalence of mood or anxiety disorder present in the prior 12 months was substantially higher among persons with chronic physical disease than among persons without. At the same time, the large majority (85%) of persons with a chronic physical disease do not meet diagnostic criteria for either depressive or anxiety disorders in the prior 12 months. Subsequent chapters provide greater insight into the relationships between specific mental disorders and specific chronic physical diseases, risk factors for these associations, and the health consequences of the co-occurrence of mental and physical morbidity.

2.4. DISCUSSION

In considering the occurrence of chronic physical disease, the health problems of developed and developing countries are converging in the twenty-first century. As mortality rates of developing countries have improved to levels achieved in developed countries as recently as the 1970s, the age-specific prevalence rates of chronic physical diseases are converging in developing and developed countries. The challenges of the pandemic of chronic physical disease in developed and developing countries differ. In developed countries, substantial and rapidly increasing economic resources are devoted to health care, but improving the effectiveness and controlling the costs of health care for chronic disease are major societal challenges. In developing countries, the economic resources devoted to health care are substantially less than those in the developed world, but the prevalence of chronic disease is rapidly approaching that in developed countries. How developed and developing countries meet the challenges of caring for chronic disease will play a significant role in determining if the miraculous improvements in population health achieved worldwide in the twentieth century can be replicated in the twenty-first century. In facing these challenges, developed countries may have an opportunity to learn about effective care of chronic disease from innovations borne of necessity in the developing world.

REFERENCES

Anderson, G. F., & Poullier, J. P. (1999). Health spending, access, and outcomes: Trends in industrialized countries. *Health Affairs*, **18**, 178–92.

Daar, A. S., Singer, P. A., Persad, D. L., Pramming, S. K., Matthews, D. R., Beaglehole, R., Bernstein, A., Borysiewicz, L. K., Colagiuri, S., Ganguly, N., Glass, R. I., Finegood, D. T., Koplan, J., Nabel, E. G., Sarna, G., Sarrafzadegan, N., Smith, R., Yach, D., & Bell, J. (2007). Grand challenges in chronic non-communicable diseases: The 20 top policy and research priorities for conditions such as diabetes, stroke and heart disease. *Nature*, **450**, 494–6.

OECD. (2007). Definition and measurement: Age-dependency ratio. In *Society at a Glance: OECD*

Social Indicators – 2006 Edition. Paris: OECD Publishing.

Suhrcke, M., Nugent, R. A., Stuckler, D., & Rocco, L. (2006). Chronic disease: An economic perspective. London: Oxford Health Alliance. Retrieved April 4, 2008, from http://www.oxha.org/knowledge/publications/oxha-chronic-disease-an-economic-perspective.pdf.

Wagner, E. H., Austin, B. T., & Von Korff, M. (1996). Organizing care for patients with chronic illness. *The Milbank Quarterly, 74,* 511–44.

Yach, D., Hawkes, C., Gould, C. L., & Hofman, K. J. (2004). The global burden of chronic diseases: Overcoming impediments to prevention and control. *The Journal of the American Medical Association,* **291,** 2616–22.

3 The Global Burden of Chronic Pain

ADLEY TSANG AND SING LEE

3.1. INTRODUCTION

Chronic pain affects people's well-being and their ability to sustain daily activities, to be productive at work, and to fully engage in social relationships (Breivik et al. 2006; Elliott et al. 2002). Surveys in developed countries, using different definitions of chronic pain, have typically found that 20–30% of the population is affected by chronic pain (Breivik et al. 2006; Demyttenaere et al. 2006; Ohayon & Schatzberg 2003; Verhaak et al. 1998). Even though chronic pain is believed to be common worldwide, most studies of the prevalence of chronic pain have been conducted in Western developed countries (Kleinman 1982; Lee 1998). Little is known about the relative prevalence of different chronic pain conditions in developed versus developing countries (Gureje et al. 2008).

Chronic pain varies not only in duration but also in its severity and impact on affected individuals. Among researchers and clinicians, there is no clear consensus on how chronic pain should be defined operationally. The International Association for the Study of Pain defines chronic pain as "pain which persists past the normal time of healing." With nonmalignant pain, 3 months is a convenient point of division between acute and chronic pain, but for research purposes 6 months is often employed to define chronicity (Merskey & Bogduk 1994). The lack of severity criteria for identifying clinically significant pain conditions and a lack of clarity about how to define chronic pain among persons with recurrent pain (Von Korff & Dunn 2008) may explain some of the variability in the prevalence of chronic pain found in different surveys.

Chronic pain has features of both physical and psychological illness. Pain is an unpleasant sensory *and* emotional experience associated with actual or potential tissue damage (Mersky & Bogduk 1994). In both developed and developing countries, mood and anxiety disorders are associated with chronic pain among medical patients (Gureje et al. 1998; Lepine & Briley 2004). However, Bair et al. (2003) observed that the prevalence of concurrent major depression in patients with pain ranged widely across studies, from 13 to 85%. Apart from reflecting methodological differences, not all people distressed by chronic pain suffer from mental disorders, but it remains unclear to what extent psychological disorders occur among persons reporting typical chronic pain problems in the general populations of developing and developed countries.

The World Mental Health Surveys provide comparable estimates of the prevalence of common chronic pain problems in developed and developing countries. This chapter presents an overview of how the prevalence of chronic pain differs by age and gender in developed and developing countries. It also compares the co-occurrence of depression and anxiety disorders with chronic pain in developing and developed countries.

The Global Burden of Chronic Pain

Table 3.1. Crude and age-standardized prevalence of chronic pain in the prior 12 months

Countries	Crude prevalence of chronic pain (%)	Age-standardized prevalence of chronic pain (%)
Developing countries		
Beijing	37.0	38.0
Shanghai	34.5	34.7
Colombia	27.3	–
Lebanon	26.4	28.4
Mexico	24.1	–
Nigeria	30.4	37.4
South Africa	48.3	51.8
Ukraine	60.4	58.2
Any developing country	37.7	41.1
Developed countries		
Belgium	40.5	38.9
France	49.6	47.8
Germany	32.4	30.4
Israel	33.5	33.3
Italy	45.5	42.8
Japan	28.1	27.4
The Netherlands	33.3	32.4
New Zealand	39.1	38.5
Spain	34.9	33.4
United States	43.9	43.0
Any developed country	38.9	37.3

Note: Prevalence rates were standardized to the age distribution of the pooled survey populations. Chronic pain conditions included in these prevalence rates are back pain, headache, joint pain/arthritis, and other chronic pain.

3.2. APPROACH

Pain conditions were assessed with a standard chronic condition checklist adapted from the questions in the U.S. Health Interview Survey. Respondents were asked if they ever had "arthritis or rheumatism" in their lifetime and if it was present in the prior 12 months. They were also asked if they ever had "chronic back or neck problems," "frequent or severe headaches," and "other chronic pain" in the prior 12 months.

Age-standardized prevalence rates for any chronic pain condition were estimated for each survey, for developing and developed countries, and for all countries combined. Since Colombia and Mexico did not include persons older than the age of 65, it was not possible to estimate age-standardized estimates for those two surveys. The prevalence of any chronic pain condition by gender and age group (18–35, 36–50, 51–65, >66) and the prevalence of comorbid depression–anxiety disorders by chronic pain status were estimated for developed and developing countries and for all countries combined.

3.3. FINDINGS

The prevalence rate of any chronic pain problem estimated by each survey ranged from 24% in Mexico to 60% in Ukraine (Table 3.1). The age-standardized prevalence of chronic pain was somewhat higher in developing

Table 3.2. Age-standardized prevalence of chronic pain conditions in the prior 12 months for developing and developed countries in the World Mental Health Surveys

	% (95% CI)		
	All countries	Developing countries	Developed countries
Headache	14.4 (13.9, 14.9)	20.7 (20.0, 21.4)	11.7 (11.4, 12.1)
Back pain	20.0 (19.4, 20.5)	24.3 (23.6, 25.1)	18.5 (18.0, 18.9)
Arthritis	16.5 (16.0, 17.1)	14.1 (13.5, 4.7)	17.5 (17.1, 17.9)
Others	6.9 (6.5, 7.2)	9.0 (8.5, 9.6)	6.2 (5.9, 6.4)
Overall chronic pain	38.4 (37.7, 39.2)	41.1 (40.3, 41.9)	37.3 (36.7, 37.8)

countries (41.1%) than in developed countries (37.3%), but the country-specific estimates for developed and developing countries showed considerable overlap (Table 3.1). In both developed and developing countries, chronic pain was a common health problem among adults.

The age-standardized prevalence estimates of headache and back pain were notably higher in developing countries than in developed countries (Table 3.2). In contrast, the age-standardized prevalence of arthritis was slightly higher in developed countries than in developing countries.

The prevalence of any chronic pain condition was markedly higher among females than males in both developed and developing countries (Figure 3.1). The gender-specific prevalence rates for any chronic pain condition were similar for males and females between developed and developing countries.

The age-standardized population prevalence rates of persons with both a depression–anxiety disorder and a chronic pain condition are shown in Figure 3.2. Whereas about 40% of adults reported a chronic pain problem (as shown in Figure 3.1), only 3–8% of adults had both a chronic pain condition and a depression–anxiety disorder (Figure 3.2). Thus, while chronic pain is relatively common among adults in both developed and

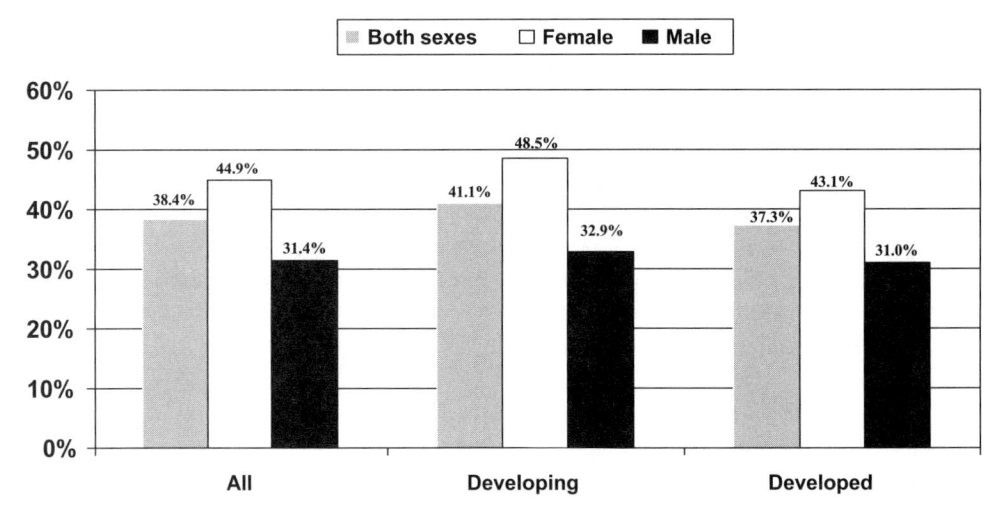

Figure 3.1. Age-standardized prevalence rate of any chronic pain condition in the prior 12 months by gender.

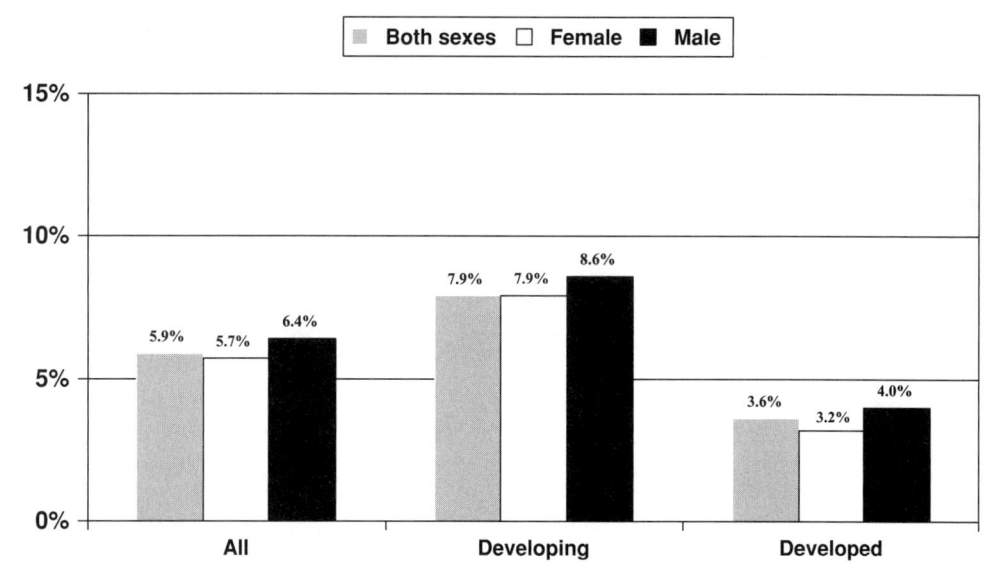

Figure 3.2. Age-standardized prevalence rate of persons with both a chronic pain condition and a depression–anxiety disorder in the prior 12 months by gender.

developing countries, the co-occurrence of both a psychological disorder meeting diagnostic criteria and chronic pain is substantially less common.

The proportion of persons with chronic pain who also had a depression–anxiety disorder by gender is shown in Table 3.3. Overall, 15.4% of those reporting a chronic pain condition also met criteria for a depression–anxiety disorder. In both developed and developing countries, females with chronic pain were more likely to have a depression–anxiety disorder than were males with chronic pain. However, even among females, more than 80% of persons with chronic pain did not meet diagnostic criteria for any of the depression–anxiety disorders assessed (major depression, dysthymia, generalized anxiety disorder, posttraumatic stress disorder, panic disorder/agoraphobia, and social phobia).

The prevalence of any chronic pain condition increased with age in both developing and developed countries (Figure 3.3). Across all ages, more females than males reported any chronic pain condition. The difference in age-specific chronic pain prevalence rates between developing and developed countries was small among both males and females, except for the oldest age group (66 years or older). In the oldest age group, the prevalence of chronic pain was higher among both males and females in developing countries.

3.4. DISCUSSION

Despite wide variation in socioeconomic, demographic, and cultural characteristics across

Table 3.3. Percent of persons with chronic pain in the prior 12 months who also had a comorbid depression–anxiety disorder in the prior 12 months

	Developed countries (%)	Developing countries (%)	All countries (%)
Females	19.7	16.3	17.6
Males	12.9	9.7	11.5
Both sexes	17.2	13.9	15.4

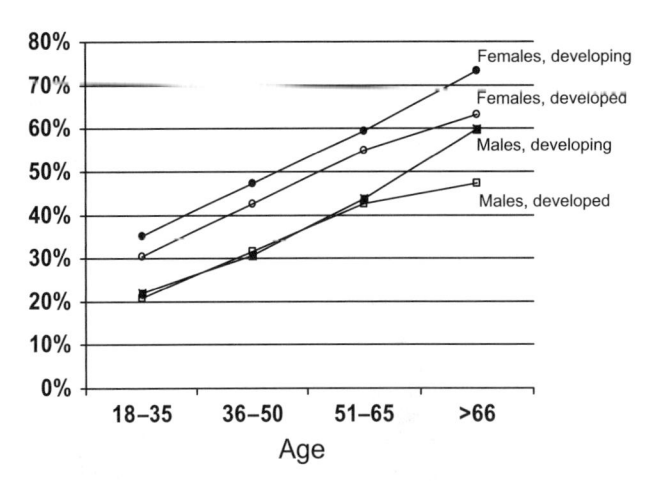

Figure 3.3. Age-specific prevalence rates of any chronic pain condition in the prior 12 months by gender for developed and developing countries.

the participating countries, and in the country-specific prevalence rates of chronic pain conditions, several findings were cross-nationally consistent. Females were more likely to report chronic pain than were males, a finding in line with prior research (Demyttenaere et al. 2006, 2007; Ohayon & Schatzberg 2003; Unruh 1996). Gender differences in the prevalence of chronic pain may be due to hormonal and other physiological differences as well as psychosocial differences between males and females (Berkley 1997). The increasing prevalence of chronic pain with age is also consistent with prior research, largely due to marked increases in the prevalence of arthritis with age (Bair et al. 2003; Currie & Wang 2004; Ohayon & Schatzberg 2003). It should be noted that the age–sex distribution of pain differs across specific pain conditions, so the age–sex differences in chronic pain prevalence overall do not reflect age–sex differences in the prevalence of each specific pain condition. For example, back pain is not consistently more common among females than males, and headache does not increase in prevalence with older age.

The large majority of persons with a chronic pain condition in these general population samples did not meet diagnostic criteria for a depression–anxiety disorder. This suggests that chronic pain in the community should be viewed as a unique illness rather than typically a somatic presentation of a comorbid depression–anxiety disorder (Kleinman 1982). Depression–anxiety disorders were more likely to be comorbid with chronic pain among females than males, reflecting gender differences in the occurrence of mood and anxiety disorders generally. In some prior studies, the proportion of persons with chronic pain who have a comorbid depression–anxiety disorder has been much higher. There may be several explanations for the lower percentage of persons with chronic pain who were found to have a comorbid psychological disorder in the World Mental Health Surveys. First, these are community samples rather than pain patients ascertained in health care settings. Depression–anxiety disorders are associated with higher rates of treatment seeking, which may elevate rates of comorbid psychological disorder. A broad spectrum of chronic pain severity was represented in the cases identified in the World Mental Health Surveys. Some prior studies have focused on chronic pain patients with more severe pain conditions, tending to increase rates of comorbid psychological disorder. Finally, the mental disorders in the World Mental Health Surveys were diagnosed with a highly specific diagnostic interview, whereas some prior studies have employed psychological screening scales that identify a larger percentage of the population as psychologically distressed.

As mentioned previously, the assessment of pain conditions in the World Mental Health Surveys did not include explicit assessment of the severity or the duration of pain. Since respondents subjectively defined chronicity in response to interview questions that asked about "frequent," "severe," and "chronic" pain, their responses likely reflect a broad spectrum of pain conditions varying in both severity and duration. Responses could also reflect their differences in understanding of specific pain conditions as well.

Since chronic pain often accompanies mental disorders, and can increase their duration and severity, mental health professionals should be prepared to address comorbid chronic pain conditions among their patients (Kathol & Clarke 2005; Lepine & Briley 2004; Ohayon, 2004; Peveler et al. 2006; Stahl 2002). Similarly, health professionals managing chronic pain conditions need to be cognizant of the increased risk of depression–anxiety disorders among their patients (Evans et al. 2005; Gureje et al. 2008). The management of comorbid chronic pain and mental disorders may be particularly problematic in developing countries where mental health literacy of both patients and health care practitioners is low and the divisions between physical health and mental health services are marked (Lee, Chan, & Berven 2007). Among elderly people in both developing and developed countries, the present study suggests that clinical sensitivity to comorbid mental disorders and chronic pain (including arthritis) is needed.

In conclusion, chronic pain was common in both developed and developing countries. It was more common among females than males, and increased with age. Depression–anxiety disorders were more often comorbid with chronic pain among females than males, but more than 80% of persons with chronic pain in the general population did not meet criteria for a depression–anxiety disorder.

ACKNOWLEDGMENT

Some material in this chapter appeared in Tsang et al. (2008). This material is reprinted with the permission of the *Journal of Pain*.

REFERENCES

Bair, M. J., Robinson, R. L., Katon, W., & Kroenke, K. (2003). Depression and pain comorbidity: A literature review. *Archives of Internal Medicine*, **163**, 2433–45.

Berkley, K. J. (1997). Sex differences in pain. *The Behavioral and Brain Sciences*, **20**, 371–80.

Breivik, H., Collett, B., Ventafridda, V., Cohen, R., & Gallacher, D. (2006). Survey of chronic pain in Europe: Prevalence, impact on daily life, and treatment. *European Journal of Pain*, **10**, 287–333.

Currie, S. R., & Wang, J. (2004). Chronic back pain and major depression in the general Canadian population. *Pain*, **107**, 54–60.

Demyttenaere, K., Bonnewyn, A., Bruffaerts, R., Brugha, T., De Graaf, R., & Alonso, J. (2006). Comorbid painful physical symptoms and depression: Prevalence, work loss, and help seeking. *Journal of Affective Disorders*, **92**, 185–93.

Demyttenaere, K., Bruffaerts, R., Lee, S., Posada-Villa, J., Kovess, V., Angermeyer, M. C., Levinson, D., de Girolamo, G., Nakane, H., Mneimneh, Z., Lara, C., de Graaf, R., Scott, K. M., Gureje, O., Stein, D. J., Haro, J. M., Bromet, E. J., Kessler, R. C., Alonso, J., & Von Korff, M. (2007). Mental disorders among persons with chronic back or neck pain: Results from the World Mental Health Surveys. *Pain*, **129**, 332–42.

Elliott, A. M., Smith, B. H., Hannafold, P. C., Smith, W. C., & Chambers, W. A. (2002). The course of chronic pain in the community: Results of a 4-year follow-up study. *Pain*, **99**, 299–307.

Evans, D. L., Charney, D. S., Lewis, L., Golden, J. M., Ranga Rama Krishnan, K., & Nemeroff, C. B. (2005). Mood disorders in the medically ill: Scientific review and recommendations. *Biological Psychiatry*, **58**, 175–89.

Gureje, O., Von Korff, M., Kola, L., Demyttenaere, K., He, Y., Posada-Villa, J., Lepine, J. P., Angermeyer, M., Levinson, D., de Girolamo, G., Iwata, N., Karam, A., Borges, G., de Graaf, R., Oakley Browne, M., Stein, D., Bromet, E., Kessler, R. C., & Alonso, J. (2008) The relation between multiple pains and mental disorders: Results from the World Mental Health Surveys. *Pain*, **135**, 82–91.

Gureje, O., Von Korff, M., Simon, G. E., & Gater, R. (1998). Persistent pain and well-being: A World Health Organization study in primary care. *The Journal of the American Medical Association*, **280**, 147–51.

Kathol, R., & Clarke, D. (2005). Rethinking the place of the psyche in health: Toward the integration of health care systems. *The Australian and New Zealand Journal of Psychiatry*, **39**, 816–25.

Kleinman, A. (1982). Neurasthenia and depression: A study of somatization and culture in China. *Culture, Medicine and Psychiatry*, **6**, 117–90.

Lee, G. K., Chan, F., & Berven, N. L. (2007). Factors affecting depression among people with chronic musculoskeletal pain: A structural equation model. *Rehabilitation Psychology*, **52**, 33–43.

Lee, S. (1998). Estranged bodies, simulated harmony, and misplaced cultures: Neurasthenia in contemporary Chinese society. *Psychosomatic Medicine*, **60**, 448–57.

Lepine, J. P., & Briley, M. (2004). The epidemiology of pain in depression. *Human Psychopharmacology*, **19**, S3–7.

Merskey, H., & Bogduk, N. (1994). *Classification of Chronic Pain: Descriptions of Chronic Pain Syndromes and Definitions of Pain Terms.* Seattle, WA: IASP Press.

Ohayon, M. M. (2004). Specific characteristics of the pain/depression association in the general population. *Journal of Clinical Psychiatry*, **65**, 5–9.

Ohayon, M. M., & Schatzberg, A. F. (2003). Using chronic pain to predict depressive morbidity in the general population. *Archives of General Psychiatry*, **60**, 39–47.

Peveler, R., Katona, C., Wessley, S., & Dowrick, C. (2006). Painful symptoms in depression: Under-recognised and under-treated? *British Journal of Psychiatry*, **188**, 202–3.

Stahl, S. M. (2002). Does depression hurt? *Journal of Clinical Psychiatry*, **63**, 273–4.

Tsang, A., Von Korff, M., Lee, S., Alonso, J., Karam, E., Angermeyer, M. C., Borges, G. L., Bromet, E. J., de Girolamo, G., de Graaf, R., Gureje, O., Lepine, J. P., Haro, J. M., Levinson, D., Oakley Browne, M. A., Posada-Villa, J., Seedat, S., & Watanabe, M. (2008). Common chronic pain conditions in developed and developing countries: Gender and age differences and comorbidity with depression–anxiety disorders. *The Journal of Pain*, **9**(10), 883–91.

Unruh, A. M. (1996). Gender variations in clinical pain experience. *Pain*, **65**, 123–67.

Verhaak, P. F. M., Kerssens, J. J., Dekker, J., Sorbi, M. J., & Bensing, J. M. (1998). Prevalence of chronic benign pain disorder among adults: A review of the literature. *Pain*, **77**, 231–9.

Von Korff, M., & Dunn, K. (2008). Chronic pain reconsidered. *Pain*, **38**, 267–76.

4 World Mental Health Survey Methods for Studying Mental–Physical Comorbidity

GEMMA VILAGUT, KATHLEEN SAUNDERS, AND JORDI ALONSO

4.1. INTRODUCTION

When considering the empirical findings of the World Mental Health (WMH) Surveys, it is easy to overlook the toil and effort that lie behind each percentage and odds ratio (OR). The deceptively simple numbers reported in this book result from almost a decade of work on the WMH Survey Initiative by literally thousands of researchers and staff from many different countries of six different continents. Each figure and table reflects careful consideration of, and decisions regarding, issues such as sampling, measurement, and questionnaire design. This chapter seeks to make these methodological considerations and decisions transparent, to reflect the underpinnings behind the numbers – details related to study implementation, sampling, and measurement that can have a profound effect on the final results.

Anyone who has been involved in survey research will immediately understand the challenges involved in an effort such as the WMH Surveys. One need to consider only some of the key features of the survey – *nationally representative, face-to-face interviews, mental health, worldwide scope* – to grasp the complexity of the tasks faced by participating countries. The methodological challenges were compounded in difficulty by the defining feature of the WMH Survey Initiative – a coordinated effort of international scope. Instead of individual countries relying on local best practices to implement their surveys, the initiative sought to standardize methodologies related to all aspects of the project, from sampling to data preparation. The goal was to achieve consistent data of the highest-possible quality across a wide range of developed and developing countries, thus making future cross-national comparisons more meaningful than studies relying on post hoc comparisons.

The up-front data coordination and planning was undertaken by the World Mental Health Data Collection Coordination Center at the University of Michigan. The challenge for the center was to strike a balance between country autonomy, on the one hand, and rigid standardization, on the other. To that end, the center worked closely with representatives from the participating countries to develop guidelines that imposed minimum standards but allowed for adaptations to local circumstances.

WMH Survey guidelines covered the following areas: study design, questionnaire development, interviewer recruitment and training, research ethics, field structure, data collection procedures and quality control, and data preparation. The specific issues covered under each topic are beyond the scope of this chapter; indeed, five chapters in the first volume in this series (Kessler & Ustun 2008) dealt solely with research methods. This chapter provides an overview of the methods of the WMH Survey Initiative that illustrate the initiative's overarching goal of consistent data quality across countries while allowing for country-specific customization and deviations in consistency sometimes necessitated by budgetary and personnel constraints, as well as local considerations (Pennell et al. 2008). Then, consideration of study design, measurement methods, and analytic methods that are most pertinent to the research presented in this volume are presented in greater detail.

4.2. OVERVIEW OF WMH SURVEY METHODS

4.2.1. Sampling

While guidelines set goals such as a probability sample and minimum response rate (65%), countries varied in sampling frames, stages of selection, age of majority, and response rate. For example, New Zealand used a special screening procedure to oversample two ethnic groups (Heeringa et al., 2008).

4.2.2. Pretesting

Recognizing that pretest results do not necessarily generalize across countries because of variations in language, social conventions, and response styles, each country was required to conduct a pretest of the interview schedule and field procedures with at least 40 respondents.

4.2.3. Survey Administration

The WMH Data Collection Center received feedback from survey organizations across the participating countries that the WMH Survey was one of the most complex they had ever administered. Primarily due to this complexity, face-to-face interviews were required in all participating countries.

4.2.4. Mode of Data Collection

After weighing the pros and cons of paper-and-pencil interviews (PAPI) versus computer-assisted personal interviews (CAPI); the majority of WMH countries chose CAPI administration. However, due to logistical issues, several developing countries had no choice but to use paper-and-pencil surveys. Thus, the Data Collection Coordination Center had to decide at the outset whether all countries should use the same form of data collection – in this case it would have to be PAPI. The center decided that concerns about mixed modes of data collection were outweighed by the fact that for the majority of countries, CAPI represented the best approach to collecting high-quality data.

4.2.5. Survey Content

Certain core modules were required, but countries were also free to introduce country-specific content. For example, New Zealand developed health services and demographic items specifically for their Maori population.

4.2.6. Interviewer Training

The survey was conducted by trained lay interviewers. Each country sent at least two interviewer supervisors to a "train-the-trainer" session conducted by the Data Collection Coordination Center at the University of Michigan. Through these trainings, lasting an average of 6 days, the supervisors gained the information to train their own staff using consistent procedures.

4.2.7. Interviewer Payment

Guidelines strongly recommended paying interviewers by the hour rather than by the interview in order to prevent shortcuts. But the research tradition in most countries was to pay by the interview and in some cases the contract with the interviewers could not be modified.

4.2.8. Informed Consent

The WMH protocol allowed for variation in how interviewers obtained informed consent, with the countries almost evenly divided among those requiring written versus oral informed consent. This inconsistency reflected the diverse cultural traditions and norms regarding individual decision making and signing of official documents.

4.2.9. Interview Verification

Guidelines required that 10% of an interviewer's work be verified. Most countries adhered to this guideline, but uniform enforcement was difficult, given factors such as geographic dispersion, structure of the field operation, cultural and behavioral norms, and funding.

4.2.10. Translation

An entire chapter in a previous volume (Harkness et al. 2008) was devoted to the methods for translating the WMH interview schedule. Briefly, almost all countries translated from the source English to the target language, relying partly on preexisting translations. The ultimate goal of the WMH translation protocol was to achieve equivalence in meaning and consistency in measurement across countries.

4.2.11. Overview of Detailed Information on Research Methods

The remainder of this chapter provides details of WMH Survey Initiative methods most pertinent to studies of mental–physical comorbidity. In the interests of brevity, detailed descriptions of these measures are not included in each relevant chapter. Instead, this methods chapter is intended to be used as a reference for later chapters. The chapter is divided into three parts:

1. *Study design and sampling:* This section describes the core design and sampling methods of the WMH Survey Initiative.
2. *Measurement methods:* This section describes key measures used in later chapters, including

World Health Organization (WHO) Composite International Diagnostic Interview (CIDI),
chronic physical conditions,
social role disability measures, and
measurement of childhood adversities.

3. *Analytic methods:* This section provides brief descriptions of some analytic methods that are used widely throughout the book.

4.3. STUDY DESIGN AND SAMPLING

4.3.1. Study Design

The WMH Survey Initiative includes 29 participating countries. However, this chapter focuses on the 17 countries that have completed the data collection and processing so far (see Table 4.1 for WMH Survey sample design, stages, and selection unit). The 17 surveys are distributed across five WHO regions: African Region (Nigeria and South Africa); Region of the Americas (PAHO) (Colombia, Mexico, and the United States); European Region (Belgium, France, Germany, Israel, Italy, the Netherlands, Spain, and Ukraine); Eastern Mediterranean Region (EMRO) (Lebanon); and Western Pacific Region (WPRO) (China,

Table 4.1. WMH surveys sample design, stages, and selection units

WMH country	Design stages	Primary sampling stage Stratification	Units	Additional stages of selection Second	Third	Fourth
Belgium	3	Provinces	Municipality	Household (registry)	Adult	–
Colombia	4	Urban area size	Community: cities, towns	Area segment	Household	Random adult
France	2	Region, municipality size	Household	Random adult	–	–
Germany	2	Urbanicity, population size	Municipality	Adult (registry)	–	–
Italy	3	Geographic region, municipality size	Municipality	Electoral districts	Adult (registry)	–
Israel	1	Gender, age, ethnicity, geographic region	Adult (registry)	–	–	–
Japan	1	City, prefecture	Adult (registry)	–	–	–
Lebanon	3	Geographic region, urban/rural status	Area segment ("sectors")	Household	Random adult	–
Mexico	4	Geographic region, urban/rural status	Census ED	Household	Random adult	–
The Netherlands	2	Region, county, urban/rural status	Household (postal list)	Random adult	–	–
New Zealand	3	Ethnicity, geographic region	Census ED (mesh blocks)	Household	Random adult	–
Nigeria	4	Geographic region, urban/rural	Municipality (MSAs)	Census ED	Household	Random adult
People's Republic of China	3	None	Neighborhood community	Household	Random adult	–
South Africa	3	Regions, ethnic composition of ED	Census ED	Household	Random adult	–
Spain	4	Region and municipality size	Municipality	Census ED (tracts)	Household	Random adult
Ukraine	3	Region (oblast), urban/rural status	Municipality	Postal districts	Household cluster	Adult (listing)
United States	4	Census region, urban/rural status, pop demography	Counties, MSAs	Area segments	Household	Random adult

ED, enumeration district; MSA, metropolitan statistical area.

Japan, and New Zealand). Seven of these countries were classified by the World Bank as less developed (China, Colombia, Lebanon, Mexico, Nigeria, South Africa, and Ukraine).

All surveys were conducted face to face by trained lay interviewers using either PAPI or CAPI. Belgium, Colombia, France, Germany, Israel, Italy, Japan, Mexico, the Netherlands, New Zealand, Spain, and the United States used the CAPI version of the survey; China, Lebanon, Nigeria, South Africa, and Ukraine used the PAPI version of the survey. The CAPI version of the questionnaire was implemented with Blaise (Blaise for Windows, version 4.7), a software package developed by Statistics Netherlands (1999).

4.3.2. Sampling Methods

The WMH Survey Initiative established guidelines that set minimum standards for the sampling procedures but allowed for country-specific adaptations. For example, probability methods were required at all stages of sample selection, but country-specific implementation of these methods varied due to differences in the types of sampling frames available (e.g., individual, address, and voter registries) or the geographical areas that could be feasibly surveyed.

Within certain constraints, countries were allowed to define their own target populations that were eligible for sampling under the survey design. For example, countries could vary in the following: age range of the sample, geographic scope limitations, language restrictions, citizenship requirements, and inclusion of special populations such as institutionalized persons. For instance, while the WMH Survey was designed to focus on adults, the age of majority varied across participating countries. Most countries had a minimum age of 18 years, while the minimum ages for New Zealand, Japan, and Israel were 16, 20, and 21 years, respectively. On the other hand, Colombia and Mexico fixed a maximum age limit of 65 years, while China used 70 years as the maximum age limit. Regarding geographic scope, most countries conducted national surveys, but Mexico restricted the survey populations to urban areas nationwide, and China, Nigeria, and Japan restricted the survey populations to specific areas of the country (e.g., cities, major regions, or some urban areas).

The final sampling frames (i.e., the list or enumeration procedure that identifies all population elements and enables the sampler to assign nonzero selection probabilities to each element (Kish 1965)) for the WMH Surveys were mainly of three types: (1) a list of individual contact information provided in the form of national population registries, voter registration lists, postal address lists, or household telephone directories; (2) a multistage area probability sampling; or (3) combined uses of area probability methods in the initial stages and a registry or population list in the penultimate and/or final stages of sample selection.

Most countries applied multistage probability sampling methods. The number of sampling stages used to obtain the final sample differed across countries, but in all countries the first primary sampling unit was selected after stratification. In Israel and Japan, individuals were randomly selected from population registries. Germany, France, and the Netherlands used a two-stage survey. In France and the Netherlands, households were selected at the first stage and at the second stage an adult was randomly selected from the household. In the Netherlands, the household addresses at the first stage were selected from postal registries. In Germany, the first primary sampling unit consisted of municipalities and the second sampling unit consisted of individuals randomly selected from the registry. Belgium, Italy, and New Zealand required an additional stage before the selection of the individuals to be interviewed. In Belgium and Italy, individuals were selected from the registry at the third stage. Spain and Ukraine used four sampling stages and in both countries, the units selected at the first stage were municipalities, and the third stage consisted of the selection of the households from which the individuals were selected at the final stage.

It is important to note that none of the WMH Surveys used a nonprobability method of sample selection, such as a convenience sample or an interviewer-managed quota sampling. A more detailed description of the implementation and the sampling of the WMH Surveys can be found elsewhere (Heeringa et al. 2008; Pennell et al. 2008).

4.3.3. Two-Part Sampling

In all but two countries, Israel and South Africa, internal subsampling was used to reduce respondent burden by dividing the interview into two parts: Part One included the core diagnostic assessment, while Part Two consisted of information about correlates and disorders of secondary interest. All respondents completed Part One. Individuals who presented a number of symptoms of specific mood and anxiety disorders and a random percentage of those who did not were administered Part Two.

4.4. MEASUREMENT METHODS

4.4.1. The World Mental Health Survey Version of the WHO Composite Diagnostic Interview

Both the PAPI and CAPI versions of the questionnaire were based on an updated version of the WHO Composite International Diagnostic Interview (CIDI v. 3.0) that was designed specifically for the WMH Survey Initiative (Kessler & Ustun 2004). The CIDI v. 3.0 is a fully structured interview that is designed to be administered by trained lay interviewers and is used to generate diagnoses of commonly occurring mental disorders according to the definitions and criteria of the *Diagnostic and Statistical Manual of Mental Disorders*, Fourth Edition (DSM-IV) (American Psychiatric Association 1994), and the WHO International Classification of Mental and Behavioural Disorders (ICD-10) (World Health Organization 1993). The CIDI v. 3.0 included 41 sections. The first section is an introductory screening and lifetime review section that is administered to all respondents, and includes diagnostic stem questions for all core diagnoses. The survey instrument includes 22 diagnostic sections that assess mood disorders, anxiety disorders, substance-use disorders, childhood disorders, eating disorders, and other disorders. Four additional sections assess various kinds of functioning and physical conditions. Two other sections assess treatment of mental disorders. Four sections assess risk factors; six assess sociodemographic characteristics; and the final two sections collect methodological information. Kessler and Ustun (2004) provide additional information about the CIDI v. 3.0 instrument. Several of the sections were optional and not administered in all countries, or were completed by a subsample of the respondents. The questionnaire was first produced in English, and it underwent a rigorous process of adaptation in order to obtain conceptually and cross-culturally comparable versions in each of the target countries and languages.

As compared with the previous versions of the CIDI, some of the modifications implemented in the CIDI v. 3.0 are as follows:

a. In the previous versions of the CIDI, a set of diagnostic stem questions was located at the beginning of each diagnostic section to determine whether a lifetime syndrome of a particular sort might have ever occurred. If so, additional questions assessed the specifics of the syndrome. If not, the remaining questions about this syndrome were skipped. In the CIDI v. 3.0, all the diagnostic stem questions were asked near the beginning of the interview because it became clear that respondents quickly learned the logic of the stem–branch structure and realized they could shorten the interview considerably by saying "no" to the stem questions. Moreover, in debriefing interviews, respondents said that their energy flagged as the interview progressed, making it much more difficult to carry out a serious memory search later in the interview than at the beginning.

b. The diagnostic sections of the CIDI were made more operational by expanding questions to break down critical criteria, including the clinical significance criteria required in the DSM-IV system.

c. The diagnostic sections were expanded to include dimensional information along with the categorical information that existed in previous CIDI versions.

d. The number of disorders included was increased.

Lifetime and 12-month mental disorder diagnoses according to the ICD-10 (World Health Organization 1993) and the DSM-IV (American Psychiatric Association 1994) were obtained by means of computerized algorithms. For this book, disorders were assessed using the definitions and criteria of the DSM-IV. Core diagnoses used in this book include anxiety disorders (panic disorder, agoraphobia without panic disorders, social phobia, generalized anxiety disorder, and posttraumatic stress disorder), mood disorders (major depressive disorder and dysthymic disorder), and substance-use disorders (alcohol and drug disorder with or without dependence). Simple phobias were not included in the analyses reported in this volume due to their uncertain clinical significance for some persons affected. Bipolar disorder was not included as a mood disorder because the Western European countries and Ukraine did not assess this disorder. Several other disorders such as separation anxiety were not asked in all countries or were administered to a subset of respondents, so they were not included in the broad categories of anxiety disorders. It should be noted that Israel did not include the social phobia section and that the Western European countries did not assess drug dependence.

For the analyses of mental–physical comorbidity reported in this volume, mental disorders were assessed without diagnostic hierarchies because of the interest in the overlap of mental disorder syndromes with physical conditions. CIDI organic exclusion rules were applied for diagnoses of major depressive disorder and panic disorder (see Chapter 6, section 6.2.1 for details). Clinical calibration studies (Haro et al. 2006; Kessler et al. 2004) found the CIDI to assess mood and anxiety disorders with generally good validity in comparison to blinded clinical reappraisal interviews using the Structured Clinical Interview for DSM-IV (SCID) (First et al. 2002).

4.4.2. Physical Conditions

Physical disorders were assessed with a standard chronic disorders checklist that was included in the WMH-CIDI. This checklist was modified from the list used in the National Health Interview Survey (NHIS) (Schoenborn, Adams, & Schiller 2003) to ask about the lifetime occurrence, age of onset (for CAPI countries only), and recency of commonly occurring chronic conditions that are thought to be associated with substantial role impairment. The complete chronic conditions checklist assessed in each WMH country is presented in Table 4.2.

Table 4.2. Chronic conditions checklist assessed in each of the WMH countries

Chronic conditions	ESEMeD[a]	PRC[b]	Colombia	Israel	Japan	Lebanon	Mexico	New Zealand	Nigeria	South Africa	Ukraine	United States
Chronic pain conditions												
Arthritis or rheumatism	LT[c]/12m[d]	12m	LT	LT	LT	12m	LT	LT	12m	12m	12m	LT
Chronic back or neck problems	LT/12m	12m	LT/12m	LT/12m	LT/12m	12m	LT/12m	LT/12m	12m	12m	12m	LT/12m
Frequent or severe headaches	LT/12m	12m	LT/12m	LT/12m	LT/12m	12m	LT/12m	LT/12m	12m	12m	12m	LT/12m
Any other chronic pain	LT/12m	12m	LT/12m	LT/12m	LT/12m	12m	LT/12m	LT/12m	12m	12m	12m	LT/12m
Chronic physical conditions												
Seasonal allergies, such as hay fever	LT/12m	12m	LT/12m	LT/12m	LT/12m	12m	LT/12m	LT/12m	12m	12m	12m	LT/12m
A stroke	LT/12m	12m	LT	LT	LT	12m	LT	LT	12m	12m	12m	LT
A heart attack	LT/12m	12m	LT	LT	LT	12m	LT	LT	12m	12m	12m	LT
Heart disease	LT/12m	LT	LT	LT	LT	LT	LT	LT	LT	LT	LT	LT
High blood pressure	LT/12m	LT	LT/12m	LT/12m	LT/12m	LT	LT/12m	LT/12m	LT	LT	LT	LT/12m
Asthma	LT/12m	LT	LT	LT	LT	LT	LT	LT/12m	LT	LT	LT	LT
Tuberculosis	LT/12m	LT	LT/12m	LT/12m	LT/12m	LT	LT/12m	LT/12m	LT	LT	LT	LT/12m
Any other chronic lung disease, such as COPD[e] or emphysema	LT/12m	LT	LT	LT	LT	LT	LT	LT	LT	LT	LT	LT
Malaria or some other parasitic disease	LT/12m	LT	–[f]	–	–	LT	–	–	LT	LT	LT	–
Diabetes or high blood sugar	LT/12m	LT	LT/12m	LT/12m	LT/12m	LT	LT/12m	LT/12m	LT	LT	LT	LT/12m
An ulcer in your stomach or intestine	LT/12m	LT	LT/12m	LT/12m	LT/12m	LT	LT/12m	LT/12m	LT	LT	LT	LT/12m
Thyroid disease	LT/12m	LT	–	LT/12m	–	LT	–	–	LT	LT	LT	–
A neurological problem, such as multiple sclerosis, Parkinson's (or seizures)	LT/12m	LT	–	LT/12m	–	LT	–	–	LT	LT	LT	–
HIV infection or AIDS	LT/12m	LT	LT	–	LT	LT	LT	LT	LT	LT	LT	LT
Epilepsy or seizures	–	LT	LT	–	LT	LT	LT	LT	LT	LT	LT	LT
Cancer	LT/12m	LT	LT	LT	LT	LT	LT	LT	LT	LT	LT	LT

[a] ESEMeD study includes Belgium, France, Germany, Italy, the Netherlands, and Spain.
[b] People's Republic of China.
[c] LT means lifetime.
[d] 12m means 12 months.
[e] COPD stand for chronic obstructive pulmonary disease.
[f] Disorder not assessed.

The checklist asked whether the respondent had experienced chronic pain conditions, including arthritis, chronic back or neck pain, frequent or severe headaches, and other chronic pain in their lifetime, in the last 12 months, or in both time periods, depending on the type of survey (CAPI or PAPI). The analyses in this book use a 12-month time frame for all the chronic pain conditions except for arthritis, for which inconsistent time frames were assessed. The six Western European countries (Belgium, France, Germany, Italy, the Netherlands, and Spain) asked about the lifetime and 12-month presence of arthritis; the remaining CAPI countries asked only about lifetime history of arthritis; and the PAPI surveys asked only about the presence of arthritis in the last 12 months. This meant that any measure of arthritis used in cross-national analyses would be based on inconsistent time frames. Because of the chronic nature of arthritis, the lifetime time frame was used when possible (CAPI countries). This mixture of time frames, while not optimal, was of less concern because of analyses showing good agreement between the 12-month and lifetime measures. In the six Western European countries that assessed both the 12-month and lifetime time frames for arthritis, the kappa statistic measuring agreement of the two classifications ranged from 0.61 to 0.88, indicating a high level of agreement between the lifetime and 12-month classifications.

The checklist also included a list of chronic physical conditions. Respondents were asked whether they had had a heart attack or stroke – PAPI countries used a 12-month time frame for these items; the six Western European countries asked about lifetime and the last 12 months; and the remaining CAPI countries used a lifetime time frame. The remaining questions about chronic conditions (e.g., heart disease, asthma, and diabetes) were prefaced by the phrase "have you *ever* been told by a doctor or health professional that you had any of these conditions." Some countries followed up with questions about the presence of the condition in the last 12 months. Focusing on the chronic nature of these conditions, analyses in this book use a lifetime time frame for these chronic physical conditions (except for heart attack and stroke that were assessed only in the last 12 months in PAPI countries). Some analyses in this book combine the categories of heart disease and heart attack, and the categories of asthma and other lung disease. Cancer was counted as a chronic condition only if the respondent reported that it was under treatment. It should be noted that the six Western European countries and Israel included a question about diverse neurological problems, including seizures, but did not ask a question specific to epilepsy or seizures. Israel's survey did not assess HIV/AIDS. See Table 4.2 for a list of the chronic conditions assessed in each of the surveys, and the time frame employed.

The chronic pain and physical conditions were assessed through self-report based on a chronic disorders checklist. These types of checklists have been found to yield more complete and accurate reports about chronic conditions than estimates derived from responses to open-ended questions (Knight, Stewart-Brown, & Fletcher 2001). Prior methodological studies have documented moderate-to-good concordance between checklist reports and medical records in developed countries (Baker, Stabile, & Deri 2001; Bergmann et al. 1998; Kriegsman et al. 1996; National Center for Health Statistics 1994). Information collected from physical disorder checklists has been shown to predict outpatient health care use, hospitalization, and mortality (Fan et al. 2002).

An evaluation of self-report of chronic conditions in the U.S. National Health Interview Survey found that self-report of diabetes showed very high agreement with medical records data (kappa = 0.82) (National Center for Health Statistics 1994). Data from Taiwan also showed that self-report of diabetes yielded high agreement (kappa = 0.86) when compared with physical examination and glycosylated hemoglobin (Goldman et al. 2003). Not all validity studies of diabetes self-report have yielded completely positive results. In one study, diabetes self-report consistently underestimated diabetes prevalence when compared to medical or laboratory records (National Center for Health Statistics 1994). This underestimation is likely to be increased among persons from developing countries with less access to medical services (Aguilar-Salinas et al. 2003; Alberts et al. 2005; Bautista et al. 2006; Nyenwe et al. 2003).

Self-reports of medically diagnosed heart disease have been shown to have acceptable validity, with some underreporting but little overreporting (Kehoe et al. 1994; Kriegsman et al. 1996; National Center for Health Statistics 1994; Tretli, Lund-Larsen, & Foss 1982). Self-report measures of heart disease have been used previously in research on heart disease and psychopathology (Ormel et al. 1997; Penninx et al. 1996; Stansfeld et al. 2002; Yates et al. 2004). Similarly, self-report measures of asthma have been used in international asthma prevalence surveys such as the European Community Respiratory Health Survey (Burney et al. 1996; Pearce, Douwes, & Beasley 2000). An investigation of U.S. National Health Interview Survey data found that self-reported asthma was in fairly good agreement with medical records data, though underreported by 20–30% (National Center for Health Statistics 1994).

Several studies of the validity of self-report of arthritis have been reported. Lin et al. (2003) compared arthritis self-report to receiving a diagnosis or treatment for arthritis in the prior 3 years and found that more than 90% of self-reported cases were confirmed by information in the medical record. In another study, self-report of arthritis showed moderate agreement with medical records data (kappa = 0.40), but it was noted that many persons reporting arthritis had not received medical care for their condition (National Center for Health Statistics 1994). A lower agreement (kappa = 0.3) of self-report arthritis with general practitioner information among community elderly in the Netherlands was reported by Kriegsman et al. (1996). The Framingham study evaluated the degree of discrepancy between radiographic evidence of osteoarthritis and self-reported symptoms related to the severity of the disease (Felson et al. 1987). Neither the medical record nor radiographic examination is considered a gold standard for assessing validity of ascertainment of arthritis in a community survey.

These results suggest that self-report information on the presence of chronic physical conditions has variable agreement with validating diagnostic data. Overall, the level of agreement is sufficient to support use of these data in the context of analyses of cross-national survey data. Of course, the limitations and potential biases of self-report of medically recognized chronic conditions need to be carefully considered in interpreting the results of the WMH Surveys.

4.4.3. The WHO Disability Assessment Schedule

A modified version of the World Health Organization Disability Assessment Schedule (WHODAS-II) (see Chwastiak & Von Korff, 2003, for information on psychometric properties of the original WHODAS-II) was used in the WMH Surveys to assess disability due to mental or physical disorders. It assessed six domains of functioning: "understanding and communicating," "self-care," "getting around," "getting along with others," "participation," and "life activities."

The rationale for modifying the WHODAS-II for the WMH Surveys was to reduce respondent burden, to substitute a validated method of assessing work disability for WHODAS-II items specifically assessing disability in occupational role, and to obtain estimates of activity limitation days. The key changes were as follows: (1) For the "understanding and communicating," "getting around," "self-care," and "getting along with others" domains, a filter question was used to determine whether additional disability questions had to be asked for each domain. Respondents who answered "no" to the filter questions for each of the first four domains were not asked subsequent questions about the corresponding domain. (2) For these four domains, a question about number of days with activity interference in the past month that referred to the activities mentioned in the filter question was asked. (3) A series of questions about activity limitations days was substituted for the WHODAS-II "life activities" domain questions. (4) Items from the "participation" domain concerning stigma, discrimination, and family burden were only asked of respondents with prior responses indicating significant functional disability. More information about this instrument can be found elsewhere (Von Korff et al. 2008).

The WHODAS-II is typically scored on a 0–100 scale, with higher scores indicating greater disability, although a standard scoring method has not been defined by the WHO. A score of 100 indicates the maximum possible score. The WMH Surveys followed this approach. For the "understanding and communicating," "getting around," "self-care," and "getting along with others" domains, the modified WHODAS-II was scored by estimating (on a 0–100 scale) the percent of the maximum possible score observed for the sum of the severity items and the percent of the maximum number of days of activity limitation in the prior month. These two scores were multiplied and then divided by 100 so that the resulting score ranged from 0 to 100. For these subscales, we compared multiplicative scoring, additive scoring, and scores based on item response methods. We found that the different scoring methods gave highly correlated results. Since they yielded nearly identical results, multiplicative scoring was employed because the European Survey Coordinating Group had previously decided to use this method.

For the "life activities" domain, a weighted sum of activity limitation days in the prior month was estimated. The following terms were added together: (1) the number of days totally unable to carry out normal activities in the prior month (item FD4); (2) one-half the number of days of reduced activities (item FD7); (3) one-half the number of days of reduced quality or care in work activities (item FD8); and (4) one-quarter the number of days requiring extreme effort to perform at one's usual level (item FD9). If this sum exceeded 30, it was recoded to equal 30 so that the sum had a range from 0 to 30. The sum was then divided by 30 and multiplied by 100 so that the resulting "life activities" score also ranged from 0 to 100. A Global Disability Scale score was estimated by averaging the scores of the "understanding and communicating," "getting around," "self-care," "getting along with others," and "life activities" domain scores.

4.4.4. Sheehan Disability Scale

Disability associated with specific mental disorders or physical conditions was assessed with the Sheehan Disability Scales (SDS) (Hambrick et al. 2004; Leon et al. 1997), a widely used self-report measure. The SDS consist of four questions, each asking the respondent to rate on a 0–10 scale the extent to which a particular disorder "interfered with" activities in one of four role domains during the month in the past year when the disorder was most severe. The four domains include (1) "your home management, like cleaning, shopping, and taking care of the (house/apartment)" (home); (2) "your ability to work" (work); (3) "your social life" (social); and (4) "your ability to form and maintain close relationships with other people" (close relationships).

The 0–10 response options were presented in a visual analog format with labels for the response options of none (0), mild (1–3), moderate (4–6), severe (7–9), and very severe (10). A global SDS score was also created by assigning each respondent the highest SDS domain score reported across the four domains. The SDS are "condition specific"; therefore, they were administered separately for each of the mental disorders. In the case of the physical disorders, the SDS were administered only for one physical disorder per respondent. This disorder was selected randomly from among all the physical disorders reported by the respondent as being in existence during the 12 months before interview. This method of selection underrepresents comorbid physical disorders, which may be more severe than pure disorders, as a function of number of such disorders. In order to correct this bias, a weight was applied to each case equal to the number of physical conditions reported by the respondent for some analyses reported in this volume.

4.4.5. Childhood Family Adversities

The following childhood adversities were assessed in many, but not all, of the WMH Surveys: physical abuse, sexual abuse, neglect, parental death, parental divorce, other parental loss, parental mental disorder, parental substance-use disorders, parental criminal behavior, family violence, and family economic adversity (see Table 4.3). Detailed information on how each of these adversities was assessed in the WMH Surveys is provided in the Appendix to this chapter. Analyses related to childhood adversities that are included in this book are limited to countries that assessed all or most of the aforementioned childhood adversities and age of onset for physical disorders. These countries are Mexico, Colombia, the United States, Belgium, France, Germany, Italy, the Netherlands, Spain, and Japan.

The aim in the assessment of childhood adversities was to focus on adversities occurring in a familial context, not all possible childhood adversities. Thus, natural disasters or exposures to war conflict were not assessed in this section. The rationale for focusing on adversities occurring in a familial context was that these are more likely to be sustained over long periods of time and, thereby, more likely to have chronic health effects.

In analyses of the association of childhood adversities with adult onset of physical disorders reported in this volume, respondents who reported that the experience occurred before the age of 18 and met the criteria specified for a given adversity (specified in Appendix) were coded as having experienced childhood family adversity. Information on how these analyses were carried out is provided in the following section.

While the validity of retrospective report of childhood adversities is an important methodological question, there is evidence supporting the validity of retrospective recall of major childhood adversities (Hardt & Rutter 2004). The meta-analysis reported by Hardt and Rutter (2004) concluded that

Retrospective reports in adulthood of major adverse experiences in childhood, even when these are of a kind that allow reasonable operationalisation, involve a substantial rate of false negatives, and substantial measurement error. On the other hand, although less easily quantified, false positive reports are probably rare. Several studies have shown some bias in retrospective reports. However, such bias is not sufficiently great to invalidate retrospective case-control studies of major adversities of an easily defined kind. Nevertheless, the findings suggest that little weight can be placed on the retrospective reports of details of early experiences or on reports of experiences that rely heavily on judgement or interpretation. Retrospective studies have a worthwhile place in research, but further research is needed to examine possible biases in reporting.

Table 4.3. Items for the assessment of childhood family adversities

Adversity	Number of items	Items
Physical abuse	3	"When you were growing up, how often did someone in your household do any of the things (on List B: slapped, hit, pushed, grabbed, shoved, or threw something at them) to you – often, sometimes, rarely, or never?" "Who did this to you (biological father, adoptive father, stepfather, biological mother, adoptive mother, or stepmother)?" "As a child, were you ever badly beaten up by your parents or the people who raised you?"
Sexual abuse	2	"The next two questions are about sexual assault. The first is about rape. We define this as someone either having sexual intercourse with you or penetrating your body with a finger or object when you did not want them to, either by threatening you or by using force. Did this ever happen to you?" "Other than rape, were you ever sexually assaulted or molested?"
Neglect	6	"How often were you made to do chores that were too difficult or dangerous for someone your age (often, sometimes, rarely, or never)?" "How often were you left alone or unsupervised when you were too young to be alone (often, sometimes, rarely, or never)?" "How often did you go without things you need like clothes, shoes, or school supplies because your parents or caregivers spent the money on themselves (often, sometimes, rarely, or never)?" "How often did your parents or caregivers make you go hungry or not prepare regular meals (often, sometimes, rarely, or never)?" "How often did your parents or caregivers ignore or fail to get you medical treatment when you were sick or hurt (often, sometimes, rarely, or never)?" "How much effort did [woman/man who raised the respondent] put into watching over you and making sure you had a good upbringing (a lot, some, a little, or not at all?)?"
Parental depression	2	"During the years you were growing up, did [woman/man who raised the respondent] ever have periods lasting 2 weeks or more where he/she was sad or depressed most of the time (yes, no)?" "During the time [his/her] depression was at its worst, did he/she also have other symptoms like low energy, changes in sleep or appetite, and problems with concentration?"

(continued)

Table 4.3 (continued)

Adversity	Number of items	Items
Parental generalized anxiety disorder	2	"During the time you were growing up, did [woman/man who raised the respondent] ever have periods of a month or more when she was constantly nervous, edgy, or anxious?" "During the time [his/her] nervousness was at its worst, did he/she also have other symptoms like being restless, irritable, easily tired, and difficulty falling asleep?"
Parental panic disorder	1	"Did [woman/man who raised the respondent] ever complain about anxiety attacks where all of a sudden she felt frightened, anxious, or panicky?"
Parental substance-use disorder	2	"Did [woman/man who raised the respondent] ever have a problem with alcohol or drugs?" "Did she have this problem during all, most, some, or only a little of your childhood?"
Parental criminal behavior	2	"Was she ever involved in criminal activities like burglary or selling stolen property?" "Was he/she ever arrested or sent to prison?"
Family violence	2	"How often did [your parents/the people who raised you] do any of these things (on List A) to each other while you were growing up – (often, sometimes, rarely, or never)?" "When you were a child, did you ever witness serious physical fights at home, like when your father beat up your mother?"
Family economic adversity	5	"During your childhood and adolescence, was there ever a period of six months or more when your family received money from government assistance program like welfare, aid to families with dependent children, general assistance, or temporary assistance for needy families?" "Who was the male head of your household for most of your childhood (biological father, adoptive father, stepfather, someone else, or no male head)?" "How much of your childhood did [your mother/she] either work for pay or work in a family business (all, most, some, a little, or not at all)?" Who was the female head of your household for most of your childhood (biological mother, adoptive mother, stepmother, someone else, or no female head)?" "How much of your childhood did [your father/male head of household] either work for pay or work in a family business (all of the time, most, some, a little, or not at all)?"

4.5. ANALYTIC METHODS

4.5.1. Weights

Sample weights were employed in most of the analyses reported in the volume so that reported data provide unbiased estimates for the populations surveyed. Part One data were weighted to adjust for differential probabilities of selection and to match population distributions on sociodemographic and geographic data. The Part Two sample was additionally weighted for the oversampling of Part One respondents with core disorders.

4.5.2. Odds Ratios

Logistic regression analysis (Hosmer & Lemeshow 2000) was used to estimate some associations presented in this book. The logistic regression coefficients were transformed to ORs for ease of interpretation. Significance of each logistic regression effect was determined using a Wald X^2-test statistic.

4.5.3. Accounting for the Complex Sample Design

All analyses were based on weighted data and implemented in SUDAAN (Research Triangle Institute 2002). Significance tests, standard errors, and 95% confidence intervals were estimated using the Taylor series method to adjust for the weighting and clustering of the data. All significance tests were made using two-sided tests evaluated at the 0.05 level of significance.

4.5.4. Pooled Odds Ratios

Some chapters present pooled estimates of ORs, a meta-analytic method used to summarize results across surveys. The pooled estimate of the OR is calculated by weighting by the inverse of the variance of the estimate for each survey, and the 95% confidence intervals of the estimate were similarly estimated.

4.5.5. Analyses of Childhood Psychosocial Stressors and Adult Onset of Chronic Physical Disorders

The association of childhood adversities and early-onset mental disorders with adult-onset physical disorders was studied with survival analyses, using retrospective self-report of age of onset of the physical condition. These analyses are reported in this volume for diabetes, heart disease, hypertension, asthma/chronic obstructive lung disease, back pain, headache, and arthritis. Persons who had not developed the physical condition by the time of the survey interview were censored at their current age. The start of the period at risk of adult onset for each physical condition was set at age 20. Persons who reported that physical condition developed before age 21 were excluded from these analyses.

First, Kaplan–Meier curves were developed for graphical comparison of the age-specific cumulative proportion of respondents reporting onset of each physical condition, comparing three categories of number of childhood adversities: none, one, and two or more adversities. Kaplan–Meier curves were also used to compare onset of the physical condition for persons with and without early-onset depression/anxiety disorder.

Then, Cox proportional hazards models were developed to estimate the relative risk of adult onset of each physical condition as a function of categories of number of childhood adversities and early-onset depression/anxiety disorder status. In these analyses, time to age of onset of the physical condition from age 20 was the dependent variable. The number of different childhood adversities in four categories none, one, two, and three or more and early-onset mental disorders were independent variables. The "no adversities" category and persons without early-onset depression/anxiety disorder served as the reference groups. All associations were expressed as hazard ratios (HRs), measuring the relative risk after adjustment for potential confounders including current age and sex. Since comparable information regarding educational attainment was not available for the French survey, educational status was treated as missing for France. We repeated the main analyses controlling for age, sex, and education, with education entered as a dichotomous variable split at the median level for each country, for all surveys except France. The results were consistently similar to those not controlling for education, so the analyses including the French survey (but not controlling for education) are reported in this volume.

To account for the possibility of differential recall of childhood adversities among those with a current mood or anxiety disorder, we performed an additional analysis on the association between adversities and each physical condition while adjusting for current (12-month) mood or anxiety disorder.

Childhood adversities and early-onset mental disorders were included in the Cox models both separately and simultaneously to investigate to what extent they were independently associated with the risk of adult onset of each physical condition.

We screened for interaction of childhood adversities and early-onset mental disorders in predicting adult onset of each physical condition. We also estimated the HRs for specific childhood adversities (adjusted for age and sex) and for specific mental disorders (adjusted for age and sex).

Country was included in all analyses as a stratifying variable, which allowed each country to have a unique hazard function. Confidence intervals (95%) were estimated for all HRs. Statistical significance was evaluated with $p = .05$ for a two-sided test. The analyses were performed using the SURVIVAL procedure in SUDAAN statistical software to account for the complex sample design (Research Triangle Institute 2002).

4.6. LIMITATIONS AND STRENGTHS

This chapter provides an overview of the methods employed in the WMH Surveys and detailed accounts of key measurement and analytic methods pertinent to the research results reported in this book. In considering the methods of the WMH Surveys, there are limitations that require careful consideration.

A significant limitation of the WMH Surveys in studying mental–physical comorbidity was that ascertainment of chronic physical conditions was necessarily limited to self-report. This chapter summarizes evidence from prior research regarding the validity of self-reported chronic physical diseases including diabetes, heart disease, asthma, and arthritis. The key question is whether survey research on mental–physical comorbidity yields results that contribute to improved understanding of the extent and nature of mental–physical comorbidity, of risk factors for mental–physical comorbidity, and regarding the health consequences of mental–physical comorbidity. The substantive chapters in this book place the WMH Survey results within the context of prior research that has ascertained chronic disease status by means other than self-report, when such research is available. In general, the results reported here are consonant with prior research. Where there are uncertainties and methodological questions, these are duly noted. While chronic pain status is typically ascertained via self-report, information reported here regarding pain severity and duration was less than is available in many population surveys of chronic pain conditions. We hope that the research reported here will provide a basis for future studies that are able to use more complete and rigorous methods to study mental–physical comorbidity, risk factors for co-occurrence of mental and physical disorders, and the consequences of mental–physical comorbidity.

These important limitations need to be balanced against the unique contributions and strengths of the WMH Surveys. Never before has mental–physical comorbidity been studied in large general population samples with standardized methods in such a diverse set of countries. The ascertainment of mental disorders employed the most rigorous methods available for use in large population surveys. The WMH Surveys also provided unique and innovative information on the relationships between childhood psychosocial adversities and risks of developing physical conditions, and downstream consequences of mental–physical comorbidity for social role disability. The large number of cases with specific mental and physical disorders developed through in-person interviews with tens of thousands of individuals worldwide provides unprecedented ability to study the co-occurrence of mental and physical disorders for conditions that have relatively low prevalence rates in general population samples.

While future researchers will undoubtedly be able to improve on the methods employed to study mental–physical comorbidity in diverse countries worldwide, the research methods implemented in the WMH Surveys represent a distinct advance over prior cross-national studies of the relationships between mental and physical disorders.

4.7. SUMMARY

This chapter has illustrated the opening point – namely, the attention to methodological details and the extraordinary "behind-the-scenes" work that made possible the results on mental–physical comorbidity reported in this volume. Throughout this effort, the need for country-specific adaptations was harmonized with the goal of obtaining standardized cross-national population-based data and estimates. This accomplishment is remarkable, considering the sensitive nature of many of the survey questions on mental health and childhood adversities. The sensitive nature of the survey questions highlights the need for carefully trained and closely supervised lay interviewers and the care that was taken in carrying out fieldwork. The data collected through tens of thousands of interviews then had to be coded and cleaned and complex computer algorithms developed and written to create the variables used in analyses. The research reported in this book represents the efforts not only of the authors of the chapters, but also of those persons interviewed, the interviewers, the field supervisors and survey staff, all the individuals who prepared the data for analysis, and the investigators and statisticians who have analyzed and reported the results in this book and in peer-reviewed journals. Although an effort of such scope inevitably suffers from methodological flaws and compromises, the results of these surveys on mental–physical comorbidity will provide a basis for more refined and ambitious research efforts in the coming decades.

REFERENCES

Aguilar-Salinas, C. A., Velazquez Monroy, O., Gomez-Perez, F. J., Gonzalez Chavez, A., Esqueda, A. L., Molina Cuevas, V., Rull-Rodrigo, J. A., & Tapia Conyer, R. (2003). Characteristics of patients with type 2 diabetes in Mexico: Results from a large population-based nationwide survey. *Diabetes Care*, **26**, 2021–6.

Alberts, M., Urdal, P., Steyn, K., Stensvold, I., Tverdal, A., Nel, J. H., & Steyn, N. P. (2005). Prevalence of cardiovascular diseases and associated risk factors in a rural black population of South Africa. *European Journal of Cardiovascular Prevention and Rehabilitation*, **12**, 347–54.

American Psychiatric Association. (1994). *Diagnostic and Statistical Manual of Mental Disorders*, 4th ed. Washington, DC: American Psychiatric Press.

Baker, M., Stabile, M., & Deri, C. (2001). What do self-reported, objective, measures of health measure? *Journal of Human Resources*, **39**, 1067–93.

Bautista, L. E., Orostegui, M., Vera, L. M., Prada, G. E., Orozco, L. C., & Herran, O. F. (2006). Prevalence and impact of cardiovascular risk factors in Bucaramanga, Colombia: Results from the Countrywide Integrated

Noncommunicable Disease Intervention Programme (CINDI/CARMEN) baseline survey. *European Journal of Cardiovascular Prevention and Rehabilitation,* **13**, 769–75.

Bergmann, M. M., Byers, T., Freedman, D., & Mokdad, A. (1998). Validity of self-reported diagnoses leading to hospitalization: A comparison of self-reports with hospital records in a prospective study of American adults. *American Journal of Epidemiology,* **147**, 969–77.

Burney, P. G. J., Chinn, S., Jarvis, D., Luczynska, C., & Lai, E. (1996). Variations in the prevalence of respiratory symptoms, self-reported asthma attacks, and use of asthma medication in the European Community Respiratory Health Survey (ECRHS). *European Respiratory Journal,* **9**, 687–95.

Chwastiak, L., & Von Korff, M. (2003). Disability in depression and back pain: Evaluation of the World Health Organization Disability Assessment Schedule (WHO DAS II) in a primary care setting. *Journal of Clinical Epidemiology,* **56**, 507–14.

Fan, V. S., Au, D., Heagerty, P., Deyo, R. A., McDonell, M. B., & Fihn, S. D. (2002). Validation of case-mix measures derived from self-reports of diagnoses and health. *Journal of Clinical Epidemiology,* **55**, 371–80.

Felson, D. T., Naimark, A., Anderson, J., Kazis, L., Castelli, W., & Meenan, R. F. (1987). The prevalence of knee osteoarthritis in the elderly. The Framingham Osteoarthritis Study. *Arthritis and Rheumatism,* **30**, 914–18.

First, M. B., Spitzer, R. L., Gibbon, M., & Williams, J. B. (2002). *Structured Clinical Interview for DSM-IV Axis I Disorders, Research Version, Nonpatient Edition* (SCID-I/NP). New York: New York State Psychiatric Institute.

Goldman, N., Lin, I. F., Weinstein, M., & Lin, Y. H. (2003). Evaluating the quality of self-reports of hypertension and diabetes. *Journal of Clinical Epidemiology,* **56**, 148–54.

Hambrick, J. P., Turk, C. L., Heimberg, R. G., Schneier, F. R., & Liebowitz, M. R. (2004). Psychometric properties of disability measures among patients with social anxiety disorder. *Journal of Anxiety Disorders,* **18**, 825–39.

Hardt, J., & Rutter, C. (2004). Validity of adult retrospective reports of adverse childhood experiences: Review of the evidence. *Journal of Child Psychology and Psychiatry,* **45**, 260–73.

Harkness, J., Pennell, B. E., Villar, A., Gebler, N., Aguilar-Gaxiola, S., & Bilgen, I. (2008). Translation procedures and translation assessment in the World Mental Health Survey Initiative. In *The WHO World Mental Health Surveys: Global Perspectives on the Epidemiology of Mental Disorders,* ed. R. C. Kessler & T. B. Ustun, pp. 91–103. Cambridge: Cambridge University Press.

Haro, J. M., Arbabzadeh-Bouchez, S., Brugha, T. S., de Girolamo, G., Guyer, M. E., Jin, R., Lepine, J. P., Mazzi, F., Reneses, B., Vilagut, G., Sampson, N. A., & Kessler, R. C. (2006). Concordance of the Composite International Diagnostic Interview Version 3.0 (CIDI 3.0) with standardized clinical assessments in the WHO World Mental Health Surveys. *International Journal of Methods in Psychiatric Research,* **15**, 167–80.

Heeringa, S., Wells, J. E., Hubbard, F., Mneimneh, Z., Chiu, W. T., Sampson, N., & Berglund, P. (2008). Sample designs and sampling procedures. In *The WHO World Mental Health Surveys: Global Perspectives on the Epidemiology of Mental Disorders,* ed. R. C. Kessler & T. B. Ustun, pp. 14–32. Cambridge: Cambridge University Press.

Hosmer, D. W., & Lemeshow, S. (2000). *Applied Logistic Regression.* New York: John Wiley & Sons.

Kehoe, R., Wu, S. Y., Leske, M. C., & Chylack, L. T., Jr. (1994). Comparing self-reported and physician-reported medical history. *American Journal of Epidemiology,* **139**, 813–18.

Kessler, R. C., Abelson, J., Demler, O., Escobar, J. I., Gibbon, M., Guyer, M. E., Howes, M. J., Jin, R., Vega, W. A., Walters, E. E., Wang, P., Zaslavsky, A., & Zheng, H. (2004). Clinical calibration of DSM-IV diagnoses in the World Mental Health (WMH) version of the World Health Organization (WHO) Composite International Diagnostic Interview (WMHCIDI). *International Journal of Methods in Psychiatric Research,* **13**, 122–39.

Kessler, R. C., & Ustun, T. B. (2004). The World Mental Health (WMH) Survey Initiative Version of the World Health Organization (WHO) Composite International Diagnostic Interview (CIDI). *International Journal of Methods in Psychiatric Research,* **13**, 93–121.

Kessler, R. C., & Ustun, T. B. (2008). *The WHO World Mental Health Surveys: Global Perspectives on the Epidemiology of Mental Disorders.* Cambridge: Cambridge University Press.

Kish, L. (1965). *Survey Sampling.* New York: John Wiley & Sons.

Knight, M., Stewart-Brown, S., & Fletcher, L. (2001). Estimating health needs: The impact of a checklist of conditions and quality of life measurement on health information derived from community surveys. *Journal of Public Health and Medicine*, 23, 179–86.

Kriegsman, D. M. W., Penninx, B. W. J. H., Eijk, J. Th. Mv., Boeke, A. J. P., & Deeg, D. J. H. (1996). Self-reports and general practitioner information on the presence of chronic diseases in community dwelling elderly. A study on the accuracy of patients' self-reports and on determinants of inaccuracy. *Journal of Clinical Epidemiology*, 49, 1407–17.

Leon, A. C., Olfson, M., Portera, L., Farber, L., & Sheehan, D. V. (1997). Assessing psychiatric impairment in primary care with the Sheehan Disability Scale. *International Journal of Psychiatry in Medicine*, 27, 93–105.

Lin, E. H. B., Katon, W., Von Korff, M., Tang, L., Williams, J. W., Kroenke, K., Hunkeler, E., Harpole, L., Hegel, M., Arean, P., Hoffing, M., Penna, R. D., Langston, C., & Unutzer, J. (2003). Effect of improving depression care on pain and functional outcomes among older adults with arthritis: A randomized controlled trial. *The Journal of the American Medical Association*, 290, 2428–34.

Molnar, B. E., Buka, S. L., & Kessler, R. C. (2001). Child sexual abuse and subsequent psychopathology: Results from the National Comorbidity Survey. *American Journal of Public Health*, 91, 753–60.

National Center for Health Statistics. (1994). Evaluation of National Health Interview Survey diagnostic reporting. *Vital and Health Statistics 2*, 120, 1–116.

Nyenwe, E. A., Odia, O. J., Ihekwaba, A. E., Ojule, A., & Babatunde, S. (2003). Type 2 diabetes in adult Nigerians: A study of its prevalence and risk factors in Port Harcourt, Nigeria. *Diabetes Research and Clinical Practice*, 62, 177–85.

Ormel, J., Kempen, G. I. J. M., Penninx, B. W. J. H., Brilman, E. I., Beekman, A. T. F., & Sonderen, Ev. (1997). Chronic medical conditions and mental health in older people: Disability and psychosocial resources mediate specific mental health effects. *Psychological Medicine*, 27, 1065–77.

Pearce, N., Douwes, J., & Beasley, R. (2000). The rise and rise of asthma: A new paradigm for the new millennium? *Journal of Epidemiology and Biostatistics*, 5, 5–16.

Pennell, B., Mneimneh, Z., Bowers, A., Chardoul, S., Wells, J. E., Carmen Viana, M., Dinkelmann, K., Gebler, N., Florescu, S., He, Y., Huang, Y., Tomov, T., & Vilagut, G. (2008). Implementation of the World Mental Health Surveys. In *The WHO World Mental Health Surveys: Global Perspectives on the Epidemiology of Mental Disorders*, ed. R. C. Kessler & T. B. Ustun, pp. 33–57. Cambridge: Cambridge University Press.

Penninx, B. W. J. H., Beekman, A. T. F., Ormel, J., Kriegsman, D. M. W., Boeke, A. J. P., Eijk, J. T., & Deeg, D. J. (1996). Psychological status among elderly people with chronic diseases: Does type of disease play a part? *Journal of Psychosomatic Research*, 40, 521–34.

Research Triangle Institute. (2002). *Sudaan 8.0.1*. North Carolina: Research Triangle Institute.

Schoenborn, C. A., Adams, P. F., & Schiller, J. S. (2003). Summary health statistics for the U.S. population: National Health Interview Survey, 2000. *Vital Health Statistics*, 10, 1–83.

Stansfeld, S. A., Fuhrer, R., Shipley, M. J., & Marmot, M. G. (2002). Psychological distress as a risk factor for coronary heart disease in the Whitehall II Study. *International Journal of Epidemiology*, 31, 248–55.

Statistics Netherlands. (1999) *Blaise Developer's Guide*. Herleen: Department of Statistical Informatics.

Tretli, S., Lund-Larsen, P. G., & Foss, O. P. (1982). Reliability of questionnaire information on cardiovascular disease and diabetes: Cardiovascular disease study in Finnmark county. *Journal of Epidemiology and Community Health*, 36, 269–73.

Von Korff, M., Crane, P., Alonso, J., Vilagut, G., Angermeyer, M., Bruffaerts, R., de Girolamo, G., Gureje, O., de Graaf, R., Huang, Y., Iwata, N., Karam, E., Kovess, V., Lara, C., Levinson, D., Posada-Villa, J., Scott, K., & Ormel, J. (2008). Modified WHODAS-II provides valid measure of global disability but filter items increased skewness. *Journal of Clinical Epidemiology*, 61, 1132–43.

World Health Organization. (1993). *ICD-10 Classification of Mental and Behavioural Disorders*. Geneva, Switzerland: World Health Organization.

Yates, W. R., Mitchell, J., Rush, A. J., Trivedi, M. H., Wisniewski, S. R., Warden, D., Hauger, R. B., Fava, M., Gaynes, B. N., Husain, M. M., & Bryan, C. (2004). Clinical features of depressed outpatients with and without co-occurring general medical conditions in STAR*D. *General Hospital Psychiatry*, 26, 421–9.

APPENDIX: ASSESSMENT OF CHILDHOOD FAMILY ADVERSITY (See Table 4.3 for Items)

Respondents were classified as having experienced "physical abuse" when they indicated that when they were growing up, their father or mother (including biological, step, or adoptive parent) slapped, hit, pushed, grabbed, shoved, or threw something at them or that they were beaten up as a child by the persons who raised them.

For "sexual abuse," the following questions were asked: "The next two questions are about sexual assault. The first is about rape. We define this as someone either having sexual intercourse with you or penetrating your body with a finger or object when you did not want them to, either by threatening you or using force, or when you were so young that you didn't know what was happening. Did this ever happen to you?" or "Other than rape, were you ever sexually assaulted or molested?" Sexual abuse was the only adversity where information was not collected that would distinguish whether the perpetrator was a family member or someone else. However, previous research using a similar measure but which did allow such a distinction showed that a good indirect way to distinguish family from nonfamily sexual abuse is to ask about number of instances of victimization, with cases involving one or two instances typically perpetrated by a stranger and those involving three or more instances typically perpetrated by a family member (Molnar, Buka, & Kessler 2001). In the WMH Surveys, therefore, respondents who reported that any of these experiences occurred to them three times or more were coded as having experienced sexual abuse (within the family context).

For the assessment of "neglect," two neglect scales were created. These were based on responses to the neglect items: "How often were you made to do chores that were too difficult or dangerous for someone your age?"; "How often were you left alone or unsupervised when you were too young to be alone?"; "How often did you go without things you need like clothes, shoes, or school supplies because your parents or caregivers spent the money on themselves?"; "How often did your parents or caregivers make you go hungry or not prepare regular meals?"; "How often did your parents or caregivers ignore or fail to get you medical treatment when you were sick or hurt?" The *serious* neglect scale was the sum of the number of neglect items where the respondent replied "often" or "sometimes," plus 1 if the respondent rated either of his or her parents as having spent little or no effort in watching over them to ensure they had a good upbringing. The *severe* neglect scale is the sum of the number of neglect items where respondents replied "often," plus 1 if the respondent rated either of his or her parents as having spent no effort in watching over them to ensure they had a good upbringing. Both the serious and severe neglect scales ranged from 0 to 6. For the final definition of "neglect," the respondent had to have a score of at least 1 on the *severe* neglect scale and at least 2 on the *serious* neglect scale.

(Note that the coding of the "neglect" domain was determined empirically on the basis of frequency distributions, to derive estimates in keeping with existing literature on the prevalence of these experiences in the general population.)

For "parental death," "parental divorce," or "other parental loss," respondents were first asked whether they lived with both of their parents when they were brought up. If respondents replied in the negative, they were asked: "Did your biological mother or father die, were they separated or divorced, or was there some other reason?" According to their answers to these questions, respondents were classified as having experienced parental death (i.e., when they indicated that one or both parents died), parental divorce (i.e., when they indicated that their parents divorced), and other parental loss (i.e., when respondents replied either that they were adopted, went to boarding school, or were in foster care or that they left home before the age of 16).

For "parental mental illness," the following questions were asked: *Parental depression* was assessed by the following diagnostic items: (1) "During the years you were growing up, did [woman/man who raised the respondent] ever have periods lasting 2 weeks or more where she was sad or depressed most of the time?"; and (2) "During the time when [his/her] depression was at its worst, did [he/she] also have other symptoms like low energy, changes in sleep or appetite, and problems with concentration?" A positive response to Depression item 1 was followed up with a frequency question: "Was this during all, most, some, or only a little of your childhood?" *Parental generalized anxiety disorder* (GAD) was assessed by the following diagnostic items: (1) "During the time you were growing up, did [woman/man who raised the respondent] ever have periods of a month or more when she was constantly nervous, edgy, or anxious?"; and (2) "During the time her nervousness was at its worst, did she also have other symptoms like being restless, irritable, easily tired, and difficulty falling asleep?" A positive response to GAD item 1 was followed up with a frequency question: "Was this during all, most, some, or only a little of your childhood?" *Parental panic disorder* was assessed by the following item: "Did [woman/man who raised the respondent] ever complain about anxiety attacks where all of a sudden she felt frightened, anxious, or panicky?" Respondents who replied positively to both diagnostic items for depression *and* who replied "all or most of the time" to the frequency item *and* who reported that their parents got professional help for depression *or* that depression interfered a lot with their parents' life or activities were coded as respondents with parental depression. Similar logic applied to characterizing respondents whose parents had GAD. Respondents who responded positively to the single-parental panic disorder item were coded as having parents with panic disorder.

Similarly, "parental substance-use disorder" was assessed with the following items: (criterion a) "Did [woman/man who raised the respondent] ever have a problem with alcohol or drugs" and (criterion b) "Did [he/she] have this problem during all, most, some, or only a little of your childhood?" Respondents who replied positively on the first and "all" and "most" on the second item were then asked (criterion c) whether the problem interfered a lot with life or activities of the man or woman who raised the respondent, or (criterion d) whether they had sought professional help for this problem. Those respondents who replied affirmatively on criteria (a) and (b) and on either (c) or (d) were coded as having had parents with a substance-use disorder.

"Parental criminal behavior" was assessed by the following questions: "Was [the woman/man who raised the respondent] ever involved in criminal activities like burglary or selling stolen property?" and "Was [the woman/man who raised the respondent] ever arrested or sent to prison?" Respondents who replied positively on either question were classified as having experienced criminal behavior in the family.

Respondents were coded as having experienced "family violence" when they indicated that they "were often hit, shoved, pushed, grabbed, or slapped while growing up" or "witnessed physical fights at home, like when your father beat up your mother."

"Family economic adversity" was coded positive if there was a positive response to either item (a) or item (b). Item (a) was "During your childhood and adolescence, was there ever a period of six months or more when your family received money from a government assistance program like Welfare, Aid to Families with Dependent Children, General Assistance, or Temporary Assistance for Needy Families?" (This item was modified to be relevant to the welfare programs in each country where the survey was administered). Item (b) was If there was no male head of the family and the female head did *not* work all or most of the time during respondent's childhood; or if there was no female head of the family and the male head did *not* work all or most of respondent's childhood; or if there was no female head and no male head of the family.

5 The Pattern and Nature of Mental–Physical Comorbidity: Specific or General?

OYE GUREJE

5.1. INTRODUCTION

Several studies have found an elevated prevalence of mental disorders, most commonly mood disorder, among persons with chronic pain conditions such as arthritis (Dickens et al. 2003; Lowe et al. 2004) and spinal pain (Currie & Wang 2004; Von Korff et al. 2005a). Prevalence studies conducted in both general populations and clinical settings have also found depression to be commonly associated with diabetes (Anderson et al. 2001; Eaton 2002), asthma (Brown, Khan, & Mahadi 2000; Goodwin & Eaton 2003; Goodwin, Jacobi, & Thefeld 2003), heart disease (Lett et al. 2004; Rudisch & Nemeroff 2003), and obesity (Friedman & Brownell 1995; Onyike et al. 2003; Stunkard, Faith, & Allison 2003). These comorbidities are of considerable clinical significance since research has also shown that the co-occurrence of mental disorders with these chronic physical conditions bodes ill for the outcomes of the latter. That is, persons with these physical conditions who also have a mental disorder, such as depression, are likely to experience worse functional disability, a poorer quality of life, and, in some instances, higher mortality, than those whose chronic physical conditions are not comorbid with mental disorders (de Groot et al. 2001; Lowe et al. 2004; Rudisch & Nemeroff 2003; Ten Thoren & Peterman 2000; Von Korff et al. 2005a).

Recent reports from the World Mental Health Surveys Initiative have focused on the relationship between mental disorders and several chronic physical conditions (Demyttenaere et al. 2007; Gureje et al. 2008; He et al. 2008; Ormel et al. 2007; Scott et al. 2007a, 2007b, 2008). These reports have broadened our understanding of the comorbidity between chronic physical conditions and common mental disorders. They have done this in two specific ways: First, they have been used to explore the relationship of not only depressive disorder but also of specific anxiety disorders, as well as substance-use disorders with chronic physical conditions. Second, the reports have examined the applicability of previous findings to developing countries, as prior research has largely been based on studies conducted in developed countries.

Understandably, these reports have focused on one physical disorder at a time. Thus, reports have been produced for spinal pain, arthritis, headache, diabetes, asthma, heart disease, as well as obesity. Examined individually, the association between mental disorders and a physical disorder, for example, a chronic pain condition, may lead to a relatively narrow explanation of the nature of the comorbidity. When a more diverse set of physical conditions is considered in the context of comorbidity with mental disorders, however, a clearer picture emerges. For example, the question of whether the relationship between mental disorders and physical conditions is specific or general is better addressed by looking at a broad spectrum of both mental disorders and physical conditions.

In this chapter, the profile and pattern of comorbidity between several chronic physical conditions and specific mood, anxiety, and substance-use disorders are explored. We used pooled data from the 18 participating surveys to assess the strength of association between specific chronic physical conditions and specific mental disorders. The aim is to determine whether the pattern of mental–physical comorbidity suggests specific relationships between mental disorders and physical health conditions or whether the pattern reflects a more general pattern of association.

5.2. APPROACH

5.2.1. Mental Disorder Status

Disorders considered in this chapter include anxiety disorders (generalized anxiety disorder, panic disorder and/or agoraphobia, post-traumatic stress disorder, and social phobia), mood disorders (dysthymia and major depressive disorder), and alcohol abuse/dependence. Disorders were assessed using the definitions and criteria of the *Diagnostic and Statistical Manual of Mental Disorders, Fourth Edition* (DSM-IV) (American Psychiatric Association 1994). The Composite International Diagnostic Interview (CIDI) organic exclusion rules were applied in making all diagnoses.

5.2.2. Chronic Pain and Medical Conditions

Each survey asked about the presence of chronic physical conditions using an adaptation of the questions in the U.S. Health Interview Survey (National Center for Health Statistics 1994). Questions about arthritis, chronic back/neck pains, headache, asthma, diabetes, and heart disease were included. Using self-reported information for height and weight, obesity was defined as a body mass index (BMI) of 30 kg/m^2 or greater. Persons with BMI less than 18.5 kg/m^2 were excluded from these analyses as other research shows a U-shaped relationship between BMI and the prevalence of mood disorder. Height and weight were self-reported by all respondents. Even though there is empirical evidence that self-reported height and weight correlate highly with objective measures, the data on obesity are likely to be affected by underreporting of weight.

This chapter reports 12-month prevalence rates for specific mental disorders among persons with the specified physical conditions during the prior year. Logistic regression was used to assess the association of the physical condition with mental disorder status after adjusting for age and sex. The regression models were estimated using the Taylor series method (Wolter 1985) with SUDAAN software (Research Triangle Institute 2002), taking into account the complex survey design.

We estimated adjusted odds ratios to assess the association of any mood disorder (major depressive disorder or dysthymia), any anxiety disorder (generalized anxiety disorders, panic disorder and/or agoraphobia, social phobia, or posttraumatic stress disorder), and alcohol abuse/dependence with the specified pain or medical condition. A pooled estimate of these odds ratios across surveys was also estimated. These odds ratios, the pooled estimate of the odds ratio, and the confidence intervals of the pooled estimate are displayed for each survey using a "funnel graph" (Bird et al. 2005). The line running through the middle of the funnel graph is the estimate of the odds ratio pooled across all the surveys. The 95% confidence interval of the pooled estimate is

The Pattern and Nature of Mental–Physical Comorbidity

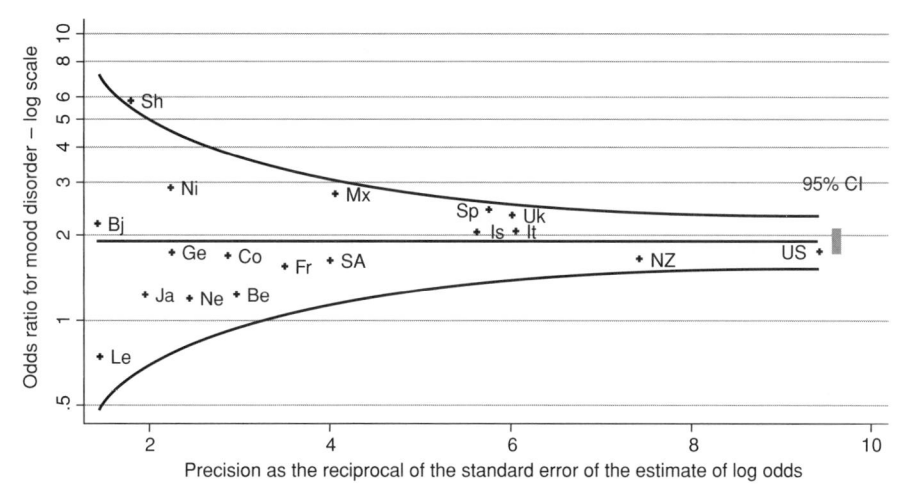

Figure 5.1. Estimates of the odds ratios (age and sex adjusted) for any mood disorder for persons with versus without arthritis. (Be, Belgium; Bj, Beijing; Co, Colombia; Fr, France; Ge, Germany; Is, Israel; It, Italy; Ja, Japan; Le, Lebanon; Mx, Mexico; Ne, the Netherlands; Ni, Nigeria; NZ, New Zealand; SA, South Africa; Sh, Shaghai; Sp, Spain; Uk, Ukraine; US, the United States.)

the bar immediately to the right of that line. The odds ratio estimates for each of the individual surveys are the points on the graph. The funnel lines above and below the pooled estimate show where a survey-specific odds ratio estimate would differ significantly from the pooled estimate (given the precision of the pooled estimate). That is, if a point falls within the funnel lines, then the survey-specific and pooled odds ratio estimates do not differ by more than would be expected by chance variation. If a survey-specific odds ratio estimate falls outside of the funnel lines, then its 95% confidence intervals do not include the pooled estimate. In other words, it differs from the pooled estimate by more than expected on the basis of chance variation. For example, in Figure 5.1, which shows the odds ratios for the association of arthritis and mood disorders, the pooled estimate of the odds ratio is about 2.0. All the survey-specific odds ratio estimates fall within the funnel, except for Shanghai, which means that the pooled estimate of the odds ratio consistently falls within the 95% confidence intervals of the survey-specific estimates. In contrast, Figure 5.2 shows the odds ratios for the association of arthritis and anxiety disorders. In Figure 5.2, the pooled estimate differs significantly from the survey-specific estimates for 3 surveys out of 18: for Lebanon (Le), for Germany (Ge), and for Shanghai (Sh). We did not estimate odds ratios or do funnel plots for alcohol abuse/dependence for arthritis and diabetes due to small cell sizes. Also, no plots were done for obesity for the same reason.

The funnel graph provides a quick way of seeing how closely the survey-specific estimates cluster around the pooled estimate of the odds ratio, and whether there is more variation in survey-specific odds ratio estimates than would be expected on the basis of chance. The funnel graph also shows which of the survey-specific estimates are most precise (i.e., have the smallest confidence intervals). The more precise estimates are to the right of the funnel graph, while the less precise estimates are to the left of the funnel graph. A

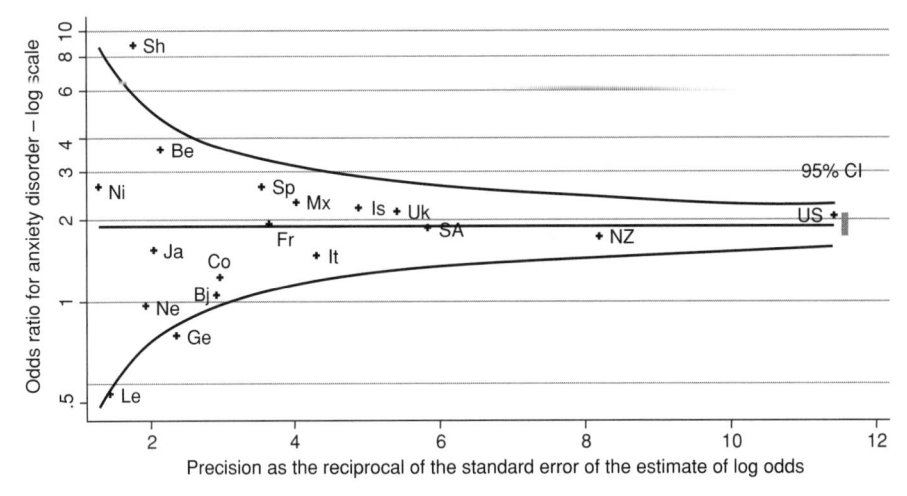

Figure 5.2. Estimates of the odds ratios (age and sex adjusted) for any anxiety disorder for persons with versus without arthritis. (Be, Belgium; Bj, Beijing; Co, Colombia; Fr, France; Ge, Germany; Is, Israel; It, Italy; Ja, Japan; Le, Lebanon; Mx, Mexico; Ne, the Netherlands; Ni, Nigeria; NZ, New Zealand; SA, South Africa; Sh, Shaghai; Sp, Spain; Uk, Ukraine; US, the United States.)

more technical explanation of these funnel graphs is provided in a technical note to this chapter.*

5.3. FINDINGS

Using estimates combining data from all 18 surveys, persons with arthritis, spinal pain, or headache in the prior year were more likely to also have major depression and dysthymia in the prior year (Table 5.1). After adjusting for age and sex, the pooled estimate of the odds ratios of major depression and dysthymia among persons with arthritis, back pain, or headache ranged between 1.9 (CI = 1.7–2.1) and 3.2 (CI = 2.8–3.8). The pattern of association of anxiety disorders with specific chronic pain conditions was broadly similar. Generalized anxiety disorder, panic disorder and/or agoraphobia, social phobia, as well as posttraumatic stress disorder were all likely to be comorbid with each of the chronic pain conditions. Here too, the pooled estimates of the odds ratios were all significantly greater than 1, ranging between 1.8 (CI = 1.6–2.1) and 3.3 (CI = 2.9–3.8). The pooled estimates of the odds ratios of substance-use disorders (alcohol abuse/dependence or drug abuse/dependence) among persons with the three pain conditions were somewhat smaller than those observed for mood or anxiety disorders. Nevertheless, none was less than 1. Surprisingly, the odds ratios of

---

* Technical note regarding the funnel graphs: The funnel graph plots the odds ratio for each survey on a log scale (y-axis) against the precision of the estimate of each odds ratio (x-axis). Precision is the reciprocal of the standard error of the odds ratio estimate. Precision increases as the standard error of the estimate becomes smaller. The "funnel" in these graphs shows the 95% confidence interval band for a survey estimate that would include the pooled estimate of the odds ratio at varying levels of precision. Each survey's estimate was plotted on the funnel graph, showing whether the 95% confidence interval of each estimate includes the pooled estimate of the odds ratio, given the estimated precision of that survey's estimate. On this graph, the less precise estimates are to the left (where the funnel is wider) and the more precise estimates are to the right (where the funnel is narrower).

The Pattern and Nature of Mental–Physical Comorbidity

Table 5.1. Age and sex adjusted odds ratio for mental disorders for persons with arthritis, spinal pain, and headache[a]

	Arthritis	Spinal pain	Headache
Mood disorder			
Major depressive disorder	1.9 (1.7–2.1)	2.3 (2.1–2.5)	2.8 (2.5–3.1)
Dysthymia	2.4 (2.0–2.7)	2.8 (2.5–3.2)	3.2 (2.8–3.8)
Anxiety disorder			
Generalized anxiety disorder	2.3 (1.9–2.6)	2.7 (2.4–3.1)	3.3 (2.9–3.8)
Agoraphobia or panic disorder	2.2 (1.9–2.5)	2.1 (1.9–2.4)	2.7 (2.8–3.1)
Social phobia	1.8 (1.6–2.1)	1.9 (1.7–2.2)	2.3 (2.0–2.6)
Posttraumatic stress disorder	1.9 (1.6–2.2)	2.6 (2.2–3.0)	3.1 (2.7–3.6)
Substance-use disorders			
Alcohol abuse/dependence	1.5 (1.2–1.9)	1.6 (1.4–1.9)	1.4 (1.1–1.6)
Drug abuse/dependence	1.8 (1.2–2.6)	1.8 (1.4–2.4)	2.3 (1.7–3.2)

[a] Both mental disorders and chronic pain conditions present in the prior 12 months.

drug abuse/dependence (ranging from 1.8 to 2.3) were generally higher than those of alcohol abuse/dependence (ranging from 1.4 to 1.6).

The elevated odds ratios indicate that persons with both depressive and anxiety disorders are more likely to have a wide range of chronic physical conditions and that persons with these chronic physical conditions are also more likely to have specific mood and anxiety disorders diagnosed according to DSM-IV criteria.

Estimates for each of the participating World Mental Health Surveys of the prevalence rates of depressive and anxiety disorders (as a group) by chronic physical conditions (chronic pain conditions and chronic physical diseases) are presented in Table A.5.1 (see Appendix tables). Survey-specific estimates of the prevalence rates of chronic pain conditions by mental disorder status are presented in Table A.5.2. Survey-specific estimates of the prevalence rates of chronic physical diseases by mental disorder status are presented in Table A.5.3.

Figures 5.1 and 5.2 show the funnel graph of the age and sex adjusted odds ratios for any mood and anxiety disorder, respectively, for the 18 countries for persons with arthritis. Both figures are strikingly similar in pattern. The pooled estimate of the odds ratio is 1.9 for any mood disorder as well as for any anxiety disorder. As can be seen from the two figures, with several exceptions for any anxiety disorder (Germany, Shanghai, and Lebanon), the 95% confidence intervals of the individual odds ratio estimates included the pooled estimate of the odds ratio (i.e., the survey-specific odds ratio estimates fell within the funnel lines). The few instances where this pattern did not apply were estimates with low precision (falling to the left side of the funnel graph). These figures suggest that the strength of association of mood disorder with arthritis is similar to that of anxiety disorder and that persons with arthritis are more likely than those without arthritis to experience mood and anxiety disorders. Figures A.5.1, A.5.2, and A.5.3 (see Appendix figures) present the funnel graphs of the age and sex adjusted odds ratios for any mood disorder, anxiety disorder, and substance-use disorder, respectively, for persons with spinal pain in the 18 surveys. The pooled estimate of odds

Table 5.2. Age and sex adjusted odds ratios for mental disorders among persons with asthma, diabetes, heart disease, and obesity[a]

	Asthma	Diabetes	Heart diseases	Obesity
Mood disorders				
Major depressive disorder	1.6 (1.4–1.8)	1.4 (1.2–1.6)	2.1 (1.8–2.4)	1.1 (1.1–1.2)
Dysthymia	1.7 (1.4–2.1)	1.3 (1.0–1.7)	2.4 (2.0–3.0)	1.1 (1.0–1.2)
Anxiety disorders				
Generalized anxiety disorder	1.7 (1.4–2.1)	1.6 (1.3–2.0)	2.1 (1.7–2.5)	1.1 (1.0–1.2)
Agoraphobia or panic disorder	1.7 (1.4–2.0)	1.5 (1.1–1.9)	2.7 (2.2–3.3)	1.3 (1.1–1.4)
Social phobia	1.3 (1.1–1.5)	1.3 (1.0–1.6)	1.9 (1.5–2.5)	1.0 (0.9–1.2)
Posttraumatic stress disorder	1.8 (1.4–2.3)	1.3 (1.0–1.8)	2.3 (1.8–2.9)	1.3 (1.2–1.5)
Substance-use disorders				
Alcohol abuse/dependence	1.7 (1.4–2.1)	1.1 (0.9–1.6)	1.4 (1.0–1.9)	1.1 (1.0–1.2)
Drug abuse/dependence	1.9 (1.4–2.6)	1.8 (0.9–3.6)	2.7 (1.5–4.9)	1.0 (0.9–1.2)

[a] The mental disorders present in the prior 12 months.

ratio for any mood disorder was 2.3 (CI = 2.1–2.5). Other than Mexico, Italy, and the United States, whose 95% confidence interval bands did not include the pooled estimate for mood disorder, all other surveys had 95% confidence intervals that included the pooled estimate for mood disorder. The same pattern was true for any anxiety disorder, for which the pooled estimate was 2.2 (Figure A.5.2). For alcohol-use disorder, the pooled estimate was 1.6 (Figure A.5.3). All these figures suggest that across most countries, persons with chronic spinal pain were more likely than those without to have mood disorders, anxiety disorders, and alcohol-use disorders. The strength of this association was similar for both mood and anxiety disorders, but alcohol-use disorder was less strongly associated with spinal pain.

The patterns of associations of mood, anxiety, and substance-use disorders with headache across the surveys were similar to those for arthritis and spinal pain. Figures A.5.4–A.5.6 show the graphs of the odds ratios, adjusted for age and sex in each instance. The pooled estimates of the odds ratios for mood (OR = 2.8) and anxiety (OR = 2.7) disorders were very similar, while both were significantly higher than that for alcohol-use disorders (OR = 1.4). In each instance, only a few countries had 95% of the confidence intervals of their odds ratios not included in the pooled estimate. Thus, for most countries, persons with chronic headache were almost three times more likely than those without to have mood and anxiety disorders, while their risk for alcohol-use disorders, while being greater than 1, was nevertheless considerably less.

Table 5.2 shows the associations of mood, anxiety, and substance-use disorders with asthma, diabetes, heart disease, and obesity. Elevated risks of all the mental disorders shown on the table were found among persons with asthma. Strikingly, the odds ratios clustered around 1.6–1.9 for all the mental disorders except social phobia with an odds ratio of 1.3. All were significant. The pattern for heart disease was similar. All the odds ratios fell within the range of 1.9–2.7, with exception of alcohol abuse/dependence with an odds ratio of 1.4. Again, all were significant. A weaker but still significant pattern of associations was found for mood and anxiety disorders with diabetes, with odds ratios ranging between 1.3 and 1.6. The associations of substance-use disorders with diabetes were not as strong, and did not quite reach statistical significance despite the large numbers of persons included in these analyses. The associations of the mental disorders with obesity were weaker still, but except in the case of drug abuse/dependence and social phobia, the 95% confidence intervals of the odds ratios were greater than 1. Thus, the results suggest that mental disorders had the strongest associations with heart diseases and asthma, and weaker but still generally significant associations with diabetes and obesity.

Figures A.5.7, A.5.8, and A.5.9 display the funnel graph of the age and sex adjusted odds ratios for any mood, anxiety, and alcohol-use/dependence disorder, respectively, for the 17 countries (Nigeria being excluded because of sparse numbers) for persons with asthma. The pooled odds ratios were 1.6, 1.5, and 1.7, respectively. As can be seen from the figures, other than Colombia and Spain for mood disorder, Ukraine for anxiety disorder, and Colombia for alcohol-use disorder, all the surveys had the 95% confidence intervals of the individual odds ratio that included the pooled estimate of the odds ratio. The few instances where this pattern did not apply were survey estimates with low precision. These figures support a view that persons with asthma are more likely than those without asthma to have mood, anxiety, and alcohol-use disorders and that the strengths of association with these disorders were remarkably similar.

The funnel graphs in Figures A.5.10 and A.5.11 are for 17 surveys (Nigeria being excluded here as well due to sparse numbers). These graphs display the age and sex adjusted odds ratios for any mood and anxiety disorder, respectively, for persons with diabetes. The pooled estimate of odds ratio for any mood disorder was 1.34, and for any anxiety disorder it was 1.26. Other than Mexico for mood disorder and Beijing for anxiety disorder, all other surveys had 95% confidence intervals that included the pooled estimate. Here again, the patterns of association suggest that, but for a few instances, persons with diabetes were more likely than those without to have mood and anxiety disorders, even though the strengths of both associations were considerably lower than that for asthma and heart disease.

The patterns of associations of mood, anxiety, and alcohol-use disorders with heart disease across the surveys are presented in Figures A.5.12–A.5.14. The pooled estimates of the odds ratios were 2.1 for mood disorders, 2.2 for anxiety disorders, and 1.4 for alcohol-use disorders. Only in the instance of anxiety disorder were there surveys whose 95% confidence intervals did not include the pooled estimate. Two of these surveys, Nigeria and Shanghai, had estimates with low precision, while two, Israel and New Zealand, surveys with high precision also had odds ratio estimates whose confidence intervals did not include the pooled estimate. Both Israel and New Zealand had odds ratio estimates that were lower than the pooled estimate. Thus, for most countries, persons with heart disease were considerably more likely to have mood, anxiety, and alcohol-use disorders, with the likelihood being double for the first two groups of disorders. However, there was potentially important heterogeneity in results across countries for anxiety disorders.

5.4. DISCUSSION

This chapter presents data from 18 surveys in countries that vary widely in culture and socioeconomic status, regarding the association between diverse physical disorders and selected common mental disorders. The physical conditions included chronic pain conditions (spinal pain, headache, and arthritis), a chronic respiratory condition (asthma), metabolic disorders (obesity and diabetes), and cardiovascular disorder (heart disease). The findings were broadly consistent; the presence of chronic physical conditions is associated with elevated likelihood of comorbid mental conditions. Mood and anxiety disorders showed similar patterns of association with each of the physical conditions. While alcohol-use disorders were more likely to occur at an increased level in persons with these physical conditions than those without, the strength of association tended to be weaker and less consistent than that for mood and anxiety disorders. These associations were broadly similar across diverse countries in both the developing and developed worlds.

The physical conditions that we examined are common. As reviewed in the earlier chapters of this book, as many as 25–50% of the adult population may suffer from some form of chronic pain, and worldwide the prevalence of asthma, diabetes, heart diseases, and obesity is on the rise. Previous studies have also suggested that the co-occurrence of mental disorders with these physical conditions negatively affects their management and outcomes. Several studies have suggested that chronic pain patients with coexisting psychiatric disorders have poorer treatment outcomes and increased disability. Unrecognized or untreated psychiatric disorders have the potential to compromise the successful rehabilitation of patients with chronic pain (Dersh, Polatin, & Gatchel 2002). Comorbid depression is associated with a twofold or greater increased risk for all-cause mortality in persons with heart disease (Evans et al. 2005; van Melle et al. 2004). Persons with diabetes experience increased functional disability and mortality, as well as increased health care costs when they are also depressed (Katon et al. 2005; Von Korff et al. 2005b). Overall, comorbidity of mental disorders with these chronic physical conditions portends a poorer outcome for the patients and higher health care costs for society.

The association of depression with chronic physical conditions has received considerable research attention, while anxiety disorders have received much less attention, and alcohol-use disorders have been rarely studied. This report has extended previous knowledge in this area not only by showing comparable association between mood and anxiety disorders with chronic physical disorders, but also by presenting data on individual anxiety and mood disorders with a range of physical disorders. By pooling data from several large survey samples, we were able to explore relationships that would have been difficult to study reliably in smaller single surveys. This chapter has also shown that the relationships between mental and physical disorders is not confined to just a few of physical disorders, or to "medically unexplained" chronic pain conditions, but extends to a broader range of physical disorders. This observation has implication for consideration of possible causes of comorbidity between mental and physical conditions.

The information presented here broadens the scope of understanding of mental–physical comorbidity by extending previous findings, largely made in industrialized and developed countries, to developing countries. These two groups of countries differ in important ways with respect to the occurrence and management of common chronic physical conditions. For example, access to health services differ between developed and developing countries.

The findings reported here suggest that the association between mental and physical disorders is not specific to a particular condition. That is, the association is not unique to chronic pain and depression or to anxiety and asthma. Rather, the evidence is that elevated risk of common mental disorders is common among persons with a broad range of chronic physical conditions. This observation has implications for consideration of the origin of the comorbidity between these two groups of disorders.

The link between mental disorders and chronic physical conditions is likely to be complex. Limitations in drawing causal inference have, in part, been due to the cross-sectional design of most studies. However, longitudinal studies suggest that simple causal relationships are unlikely. For example, studies of the association of chronic pain with depressive and anxiety disorders suggest a bidirectional relationship (Gureje, Simon, & Von Korff 2001). Also, even if diabetes might be intuitively expected to precede the onset of depression, prospective epidemiological studies provide evidence that depression increases the risk of developing diabetes (Eaton et al. 1996). Indeed, a recent report showed that comorbid depressive–anxiety disorder is more strongly associated with chronic physical conditions than is noncomorbid depressive or anxiety disorder alone (Scott et al. 2008). That pattern of association suggests a causal pathway that proceeds from mental disorder to chronic physical disorder rather than the reverse.

A shared origin or vulnerability is possible, however. The evidence produced in this report of a general rather than a specific association between mental and physical conditions is possibly indicative of a shared vulnerability. A population twin study has examined the extent to which genetic and environmental factors contribute to the covariance between symptoms of anxiety and depression on the one hand and spinal pain on the other hand (Reichborn-Kjennerud et al. 2002). The authors report that the correlation between spinal pain and symptoms of anxiety and depression was best explained by additive genetic and individual environmental factors. Genetic factors affecting both phenotypes were estimated to account for about 60% of the covariation. Evidence showing that early childhood adversities predict emergence of psychophysiological and pain disorders, as well as mental disorders, in adulthood supports the notion of a shared origin for comorbid mental and physical conditions (Sansone et al. 2006; Walker et al. 1999). A number of authors have offered important insights into the possible mechanisms through which these early experiences as well as later life trajectories may produce vulnerabilities for both mental and physical disorders (Chrousos & Kino 2007; Gluckman, Hanson, & Beedle 2007; McEwen 1998; McEwen & Stellar 1993).

In conclusion, depressive, anxiety, and, to a lesser extent, alcohol-use disorders are comorbid with a range of chronic pain and medical conditions. Comorbidity is common among persons with these chronic physical conditions irrespective of whether they reside in developed or developing countries. The pattern of comorbidity suggests general rather than specific relationships between mental disorders and chronic physical conditions. Even though the basis of comorbidity is not clearly understood, and cannot be explained by cross-sectional associations alone, the pattern of the relationship suggests that a shared origin or vulnerability, possibly with a distal rather than a proximal occurrence, may play a role in the co-occurrence of the two groups of disorders. Explanation of the general association of common mental disorders with diverse chronic physical disorders observed in the World Mental Health Surveys awaits further research.

REFERENCES

American Psychiatric Association. (1994). *Diagnostic and Statistical Manual of Mental Disorders*, 4th ed. Washington, DC: American Psychiatric Association.

Anderson, R. J., Freedland, K. E., Clouse, R. E., & Lustman, P. J. (2001). The prevalence of comorbid depression in adults with diabetes: A meta-analysis. *Diabetes Care*, **24**, 1069–78.

Bird, S. M., Coz, D., Farewell, V. T., Goldstein, H., Holt, T., & Smith, P. (2005). Performance indicators: Good, bad, and ugly. *Journal of the Royal Statistical Society, Series A*, **168**, 1–27.

Brown, E., Khan, D., & Mahadi, S. (2000). Psychiatric hospital in inner city outpatients with moderate or severe asthma. *International Journal of Psychiatry in Medicine*, **30**, 295–7.

Chrousos, G. P., & Kino, T. (2007). Glucocorticoid action networks and complex psychiatric and(or somatic disorders. *Stress*, **10**, 213–19.

Currie, S. R., & Wang, J. (2004). Chronic back pain and major depression in the general Canadian population. *Pain*, **107**, 60–4.

de Groot, M., Anderson, R., Freedland, K. E., Clouse, R. E., & Lustman, P. J. (2001). Association of depression and diabetes complications: A meta-analysis. *Psychosomatic Medicine*, **63**, 619–30.

Demyttenaere, K., Bruffaerts, R., Lee, S., Posada-Villa, J., Kovess, V., Angermeyer, M. C., Levinson, D., de Girolamo, G., Nakane, H., Mneimneh, Z., Lara, C., de Graaf, R., Scott, K. M., Gureje, O., Stein, D. J., Haro, J. M., Bromet, E. J., Kessler, R. C., Alonso, J., & Von Korff, M. (2007). Mental disorders among persons with chronic back or neck pain: Results from the World Mental Health Surveys. *Pain*, **129**, 332–42.

Dersh, J., Polatin, P. B., & Gatchel, R. J. (2002). Chronic pain and psychopathology: Research findings and theoretical considerations. *Psychosomatic Medicine*, **64**, 773–86.

Dickens, C., Jackson, J., Tomenson, B., Hay, E., & Creed, F. (2003). Association of depression and rheumatoid arthritis. *Psychosomatics*, **44**, 209–15.

Eaton, W. W. (2002). Epidemiologic evidence on the comorbidity of depression and diabetes. *Journal of Psychosomatic Research*, **53**, 903–6.

Eaton, W. W., Armenian, H., Gallo, J., Pratt, L., & Ford, D. E. (1996). Depression and risk for onset of type II diabetes. A prospective population-based study. *Diabetes Care*, **19**, 1097–102.

Evans, D. L., Charney, D. S., Lewis, L., Golden, R. N., Gorman, J. M., Krishnan, K. R., Nemeroff, C. B., Bremner, J. D., Carney, R. M., Coyne, J. C., Delong, M. R., Frasure-Smith, N., Glassman, A. H., Gold, P. W., Grant, I., Gwyther, L., Ironson, G., Johnson, R. L., Kanner, A. M., Katon, W. J., Kaufmann, P. G., Keefe, F. J., Ketter, T., Laughren, T. P., Leserman, J., Lyketsos, C. G., McDonald, W. M., McEwen, B. S., Miller, A. H., Musselman, D., O'Connor, C., Petitto, J. M., Pollock, B. G., Robinson, R. G., Roose, S. P., Rowland, J., Sheline, Y., Sheps, D. S., Simon, G., Spiegel, D., Stunkard, A., Sunderland, T., Tibbits, P., Jr., & Valvo, W. J. (2005). Mood disorders in the medically ill: Scientific review and recommendations. *Biological Psychiatry*, **58**, 175–89.

Friedman, M. A., & Brownell, K. D. (1995). Psychological correlates of obesity: Moving to the next research generation. *Psychological Bulletin*, **117**, 3–20.

Gluckman, P. D., Hanson, M. A., & Beedle, A. S. (2007). Early life events and their consequences for later disease: A life history and evolutionary perspective. *American Journal of Human Biology*, **19**, 1–19.

Goodwin, R. D., & Eaton, W. W. (2003). Asthma and the risk of panic attacks. *Psychological Medicine*, **33**, 879–85.

Goodwin, R. D., Jacobi, F., & Thefeld, W. (2003). Mental disorders and asthma in the community. *Archives of General Psychiatry*, **60**, 1125–30.

Gureje, O., Simon, G. E., & Von Korff, M. (2001). A cross-national study of the course of persistent pain in primary care. *Pain*, **92**, 195–200.

Gureje, O., Von Korff, M., Kola, L., Demyttenaere, K., He, Y., Posada-Villa, J., Lepine, J. P., Angermeyer, M. C., Levinson, D., de Girolamo, G., Iwata, N., Karam, A., Guimaraes Borges, G. L., de Graaf, R., Browne, M. O., Stein, D. J., Haro, J. M., Bromet, E. J., Kessler, R. C., & Alonso, J. (2008). The relation between multiple pains and mental disorders: Results from the World Mental Health Surveys. *Pain*, **135**, 82–91.

He, Y., Zhang, M., Lin, E. H., Bruffaerts, R., Posada-Villa, J., Angermeyer, M. C., Levinson, D., de Girolamo, G., Uda, H., Mneimneh, Z., Benjet, C., Graaf, R. D., Scott, K. M., Gureje, O., Seedat, S., Haro, J. M., Bromet, E. J., Alonso, J., von Korff, M., & Kessler, R. (2008). Mental disorders among persons with arthritis: Results from the World Mental Health Surveys. *Psychological Medicine*, **38**, 1–12.

Katon, W. J., Rutter, C., Simon, G., Lin, E. H., Ludman, E., Ciechanowski, P., Kinder, L., Young, B., & Von Korff, M. (2005). The association of comorbid depression with mortality in patients with type 2 diabetes. *Diabetes Care*, **28**, 2668–72.

Lett, H. S., Blumenthal, J. A., Babyak, M. A., Sherwood, A., Strauman, T., Robins, C., & Newman, M. F. (2004). Depression as a risk factor for coronary artery disease: Evidence, mechanisms and treatment. *Psychosomatic Medicine*, **66**, 305–15.

Lowe, B., Willand, L., Eich, W., Zipfel, S., Ho, A. D., Herzog, W., & Fiehn, C. (2004). Psychiatric comorbidity and work disability in patients with inflammatory rheumatic diseases. *Psychosomatic Medicine*, **66**, 395–402.

McEwen, B. S. (1998). Protective and damaging effects of stress mediators. *New England Journal of Medicine*, **338**, 171–9.

McEwen, B. S., & Stellar, E. (1993). Stress and the individual: Mechanisms leading to disease. *Archives of Internal Medicine*, **153**, 2093–3101.

National Center for Health Statistics. (1994). Evaluation of National Health Interview Survey – Diagnostic reporting. *Vital Health Statistics*, **2**, 1–116.

Onyike, C. U., Crum, R. M., Lee, H. B., Lyketsos, C. G., & Eaton, W. W. (2003). Is obesity associated with major depression? Results from the Third National Health and Nutrition Examination Survey. *American Journal of Epidemiology*, **158**, 1139–47.

Ormel, J., Von Korff, M., Burger, H., Scott, K., Demyttenaere, K., Huang, Y. Q., Posada-Villa, J., Pierre Lepine, J., Angermeyer, M. C., Levinson, D., de Girolamo, G., Kawakami, N., Karam, E., Medina-Mora, M. E., Gureje, O., Williams, D., Haro, J. M., Bromet, E. J., Alonso, J., & Kessler, R. (2007). Mental disorders among persons with heart disease – Results from World Mental Health Surveys. *General Hospital Psychiatry*, **29**, 325–34.

Reichborn-Kjennerud, T., Stoltenberg, C., Tambs, K., Roysamb, E., Kringlen, E., Torgersen, S., & Harris, J. R. (2002). Back-neck pain and symptoms of anxiety and depression: A population-based twin study. *Psychological Medicine*, **32**, 1009–20.

Research Triangle Institute. (2002). *SUDAAN: Professional Software for Survey Data Analysis Version 8.0.1*. North Carolina: Research Triangle Institute.

Rudisch, B., & Nemeroff, C. B. (2003). Epidemiology of comorbid coronary artery disease and depression. *Biological Psychiatry*, **54**, 227–40.

Sansone, R. A., Pole, M., Dakroub, H., & Butler, M. (2006). Childhood trauma, borderline personality symptomatology, and psychophysiological and pain disorders in adulthood. *Psychosomatics*, **47**, 158–62.

Scott, K. M., Bruffaerts, R., Simon, G. E., Alonso, J., Angermeyer, M., de Girolamo, G., Demyttenaere, K., Gasquet, I., Haro, J. M., Karam, E., Kessler, R. C., Levinson, D., Medina Mora, M. E., Oakley Browne, M. A., Ormel, J., Villa, J. P., Uda, H., & Von Korff, M. (2008). Obesity and mental disorders in the general population: Results from the World Mental Health Surveys. *International Journal of Obesity*, **32**, 192–200.

Scott, K. M., Bruffaerts, R., Tsang, A., Ormel, J., Alonso, J., Angermeyer, M. C., Benjet, C., Bromet, E., de Girolamo, G., de Graaf, R., Gasquet, I., Gureje, O., Haro, J. M., He, Y., Kessler, R. C., Levinson, D., Mneimneh, Z. N., Oakley Browne, M. A., Posada-Villa, J., Stein, D. J., Takeshima, T., & Von Korff, M. (2007a). Depression-anxiety relationships with chronic physical conditions: Results from the World Mental Health Surveys. *Journal of Affective Disorders*, **103**, 113–20.

Scott, K. M., Von Korff, M., Ormel, J., Zhang, M. Y., Bruffaerts, R., Alonso, J., Kessler, R. C., Tachimori, H., Karam, E., Levinson, D., Bromet, E. J., Posada-Villa, J., Gasquet, I., Angermeyer, M. C., Borges, G., de Girolamo, G., Herman, A., & Haro, J. M. (2007b). Mental disorders among adults with asthma: Results from the World Mental Health Survey. *General Hospital Psychiatry*, **29**, 123–33.

Stunkard, A., Faith, M. S., & Allison, K. C. (2003). Depression and obesity. *Biological Psychiatry*, **54**, 330–7.

Ten Thoren, C., & Peterman, F. (2000). Reviewing asthma and anxiety. *Respiratory Medicine*, **94**, 409–15.

van Melle, J. P., de Jonge, P., Spijkerman, T. A., Tijssen, J. G., Ormel, J., van Veldhuisen, D. J., van den Brink, R. H., & van den Berg, M. P. (2004). Prognostic association of depression following myocardial infarction with mortality and cardiovascular events: A meta-analysis. *Psychosomatic Medicine*, **66**, 814–22.

Von Korff, M., Crane, P., Lane, M., Miglioretti, D. L., Simon, G., Saunders, K., Stang, P., Brandenburg, N., & Kessler, R. (2005a). Chronic spinal pain and physical-mental comorbidity in the United States: Results from the national comorbidity survey replication. *Pain*, **115**, 331–9.

Von Korff, M., Katon, W., Lin, E. H., Simon, G., Ciechanowski, P., Ludman, E., Oliver, M., Rutter, C., & Young, B. (2005b). Work disability among individuals with diabetes. *Diabetes Care*, **28**, 1326–32.

Walker, E. A., Gelfand, A., Katon, W. J., Koss, M. P., Von Korff, M., Bernstein, D., & Russo, J. (1999). Adult health status of women with histories of childhood abuse and neglect. *The American Journal of Medicine*, **107**, 332–9.

Wolter, K. (1985). *Introduction to Variance Estimation*. New York: Springer-Verlag.

APPENDIX

Table A.5.1a. Prevalence (CI) of 12-month depressive, anxiety, and either depressive or anxiety disorder among persons with back/neck pain, and prevalence (CI) of 12-month depressive or anxiety disorder among persons without back/neck pain

	Mental disorder prevalence among persons with back/neck pain			Depressive or anxiety disorder prevalence among persons without back/neck pain
Country	Any depressive disorder	Any anxiety disorder	Either depressive or anxiety disorder	Either depressive or anxiety disorder
Beijing	4.1 (2.3, 7.0)	2.4 (1.2, 4.7)	5.0 (3.1, 8.0)	2.9 (1.9, 4.4)
Colombia	12.9 (9.3, 17.6)	10.4 (7.3, 14.7)	20.1 (15.6, 25.6)	9.4 (8.0, 11.0)
Lebanon	2.5 (1.0, 6.0)	3.6 (2.4, 5.6)	5.8 (3.5, 9.6)	3.7 (2.2, 6.1)
Mexico	11.1 (8.0, 15.2)	8.8 (6.3, 12.1)	15.8 (12.1, 20.3)	5.6 (4.7, 6.7)
Nigeria	2.6 (1.6, 4.1)	0.9 (0.3, 2.2)	2.9 (1.9, 4.6)	1.3 (0.8, 2.1)
South Africa	8.4 (6.7, 10.7)	12.9 (10.9, 15.3)	18.4 (15.8, 21.4)	9.5 (8.1, 11.1)
Shanghai	4.1 (1.2, 12.9)	3.5 (0.8, 13.6)	5.3 (2.0, 13.2)	1.3 (0.7, 2.4)
Ukraine	15.4 (12.6, 18.7)	11.5 (9.3, 14.0)	21.6 (18.3, 25.4)	9.1 (7.1, 11.8)
Belgium	9.7 (7.0, 13.3)	5.6 (3.4, 9.2)	13.3 (11.2, 15.8)	7.5 (5.4, 10.4)
France	10.9 (7.4, 15.8)	9.8 (7.1, 13.3)	17.2 (13.1, 22.4)	10.1 (7.9, 12.7)
Germany	5.1 (3.4, 7.7)	4.3 (2.8, 6.5)	8.5 (6.2, 11.6)	5.1 (3.9, 6.5)
Israel	11.1 (9.1, 13.5)	10.1 (8.2, 12.4)	17.0 (14.5, 19.8)	6.9 (6.1, 7.7)
Italy	4.9 (3.6, 6.6)	4.7 (3.3, 6.6)	7.8 (6.0, 10.0)	4.4 (3.6, 5.4)
Japan	4.0 (2.5, 6.4)	5.8 (3.7, 9.1)	7.6 (5.4, 10.7)	3.2 (2.4, 4.3)
The Netherlands	10.2 (7.0, 14.6)	11.2 (6.2, 19.3)	18.1 (12.5, 25.3)	7.5 (6.1, 9.3)
New Zealand	10.5 (8.9, 12.3)	16.4 (14.3, 18.8)	21.1 (18.7, 23.8)	12.2 (11.3, 13.2)
Spain	7.9 (5.7, 10.8)	4.6 (3.0, 7.1)	9.9 (7.2, 13.7)	4.9 (4.2, 5.8)
United States	16.2 (14.2, 18.5)	22.4 (20.2, 24.8)	28.7 (26.0, 31.6)	15.0 (13.8, 16.2)
Any developing country	9.0 (8.0, 10.2)	9.0 (8.1, 10.1)	15.0 (13.7, 16.5)	6.5 (6.0, 7.1)
Any developed country	10.6 (9.8, 11.4)	12.9 (12.0, 13.8)	18.4 (17.3, 19.5)	9.7 (9.2, 10.1)
All countries	10.0 (9.4, 10.7)	11.4 (10.7, 12.1)	17.1 (16.3, 18.0)	8.6 (8.2, 8.9)

Table A.5.1b. Prevalence (CI) of 12-month depressive, anxiety, and either depressive or anxiety disorders among persons with headache, and prevalence (CI) of 12-month depressive or anxiety disorder among persons without headache

Country	Mental disorder prevalence among persons with headache — Any depressive disorder	Any anxiety disorder	Either depressive or anxiety disorder	Depressive or anxiety disorder prevalence among persons without headache — Either depressive or anxiety disorder
Beijing	8.1 (4.3, 14.9)	5.6 (3.0, 10.3)	9.8 (5.7, 16.3)	3.0 (2.0, 4.5)
Colombia	14.1 (10.9, 18.1)	9.4 (6.9, 12.8)	20.8 (16.7, 25.5)	8.5 (7.4, 9.9)
Lebanon	6.4 (2.9, 13.6)	7.0 (1.6, 25.2)	12.1 (5.7, 23.8)	3.0 (1.8, 5.1)
Mexico	11.2 (8.2, 15.2)	13.6 (9.8, 18.7)	19.8 (15.1, 25.7)	5.6 (4.7, 6.7)
Nigeria	2.3 (1.3, 4.0)	1.8 (0.6, 5.2)	3.6 (2.0, 6.5)	1.3 (0.9, 2.1)
South Africa	7.3 (5.8, 9.0)	13.2 (11.2, 15.5)	17.6 (15.2, 20.2)	9.1 (7.6, 10.7)
Shanghai	11.3 (2.7, 36.5)	10.8 (2.3, 37.9)	14.3 (4.5, 37.5)	1.3 (0.8, 2.2)
Ukraine	17.6 (14.7, 21.0)	12.1 (9.9, 14.7)	23.4 (19.8, 27.4)	9.7 (7.6, 12.3)
Belgium	14.1 (8.7, 22.1)	9.1 (5.1, 15.7)	18.0 (12.2, 25.9)	7.4 (5.8, 9.4)
France	14.5 (10.6, 19.5)	10.9 (7.2, 16.1)	19.9 (15.5, 25.1)	10.4 (8.6, 12.4)
Germany	9.9 (6.1, 15.5)	10.8 (6.8, 16.7)	17.3 (11.7, 24.9)	4.7 (3.8, 5.9)
Israel	12.9 (10.5, 15.7)	10.5 (8.3, 13.2)	18.4 (15.5, 21.6)	7.1 (6.4, 8.0)
Italy	9.6 (6.8, 13.4)	9.3 (6.4, 13.3)	14.9 (11.0, 20.0)	4.4 (3.6, 5.4)
Japan	9.1 (4.8, 16.4)	12.0 (7.4, 18.9)	16.1 (10.2, 24.5)	3.2 (2.4, 4.1)
The Netherlands	13.2 (8.7, 19.5)	13.9 (8.6, 21.6)	21.8 (16.0, 28.9)	7.9 (6.2, 10.1)
New Zealand	14.8 (12.6, 17.3)	21.6 (18.6, 24.9)	28.4 (24.9, 32.1)	12.0 (11.1, 13.0)
Spain	13.4 (10.3, 17.3)	8.1 (5.8, 11.3)	16.7 (13.0, 21.1)	4.6 (4.0, 5.3)
United States	22.0 (18.9, 25.4)	30.4 (27.6, 33.3)	38.2 (35.0, 41.5)	14.6 (13.4, 15.8)
Any developing country	10.1 (9.0, 11.3)	11.3 (10.1, 12.6)	17.8 (16.3, 19.4)	6.0 (5.5, 6.6)
Any developed country	15.3 (14.1, 16.6)	17.9 (16.6, 19.3)	25.4 (23.9, 27.0)	9.5 (9.1, 9.9)
All countries	12.8 (11.9, 13.7)	14.7 (13.7, 15.7)	21.7 (20.6, 22.8)	8.3 (8.0, 8.7)

Table A.5.1c. Prevalence (CI) of 12-month depressive, anxiety, and either depressive or anxiety disorders among persons with arthritis, and prevalence (CI) of 12-month depressive or anxiety disorder among persons without arthritis

	Mental disorder prevalence among persons with arthritis			Depressive or anxiety disorder prevalence among persons without arthritis
Country	Any depressive disorder	Any anxiety disorder	Either depressive or anxiety disorder	Either depressive or anxiety disorder
Beijing	3.9 (1.5, 9.8)	2.3 (1.4, 4.0)	5.2 (2.6, 10.2)	3.4 (2.2, 5.2)
Colombia	9.3 (5.3, 15.7)	6.8 (3.8, 11.7)	14.1 (8.9, 21.6)	10.2 (8.9, 11.6)
Lebanon	1.4 (0.4, 4.9)	1.2 (0.4, 3.9)	2.3 (0.8, 6.1)	4.2 (2.8, 6.2)
Mexico	10.2 (7.0, 14.6)	7.7 (5.1, 11.4)	13.7 (10.1, 18.3)	6.3 (5.3, 7.5)
Nigeria	2.2 (1.4, 3.5)	1.3 (0.5, 3.4)	3.1 (1.8, 5.1)	1.3 (0.8, 2.1)
South Africa	7.6 (5.1, 11.2)	14.5 (11.3, 18.3)	19.0 (15.3, 23.3)	11.0 (9.7, 12.5)
Shanghai	5.7 (1.5, 19.8)	4.4 (1.0, 17.7)	6.5 (2.2, 17.6)	1.5 (0.9, 2.5)
Ukraine	19.9 (15.4, 25.3)	12.8 (10.2, 15.9)	25.6 (20.7, 31.2)	11.6 (9.7, 13.7)
Belgium	6.2 (3.4, 11.0)	6.2 (3.2, 11.6)	10.5 (6.4, 16.6)	8.2 (6.5, 10.4)
France	7.1 (4.6, 10.8)	7.8 (5.4, 11.1)	12.1 (8.5, 17.0)	11.4 (9.3, 13.9)
Germany	4.2 (2.2, 7.9)	1.6 (0.7, 3.3)	5.1 (2.9, 8.9)	5.8 (4.7, 7.1)
Israel	10.7 (8.1, 14.0)	9.3 (7.0, 12.4)	16.2 (13.0, 20.0)	7.9 (7.1, 8.7)
Italy	6.0 (4.7, 7.5)	4.3 (3.1, 6.1)	7.7 (6.2, 9.6)	4.5 (3.6, 5.7)
Japan	2.2 (0.9, 5.5)	3.3 (1.3, 8.1)	3.9 (1.7, 8.4)	3.9 (3.0, 5.1)
The Netherlands	5.2 (2.8, 9.4)	5.7 (2.9, 10.7)	7.9 (4.5, 13.6)	9.5 (7.6, 11.9)
New Zealand	6.4 (5.2, 7.9)	11.4 (9.7, 13.3)	13.8 (12.0, 15.9)	13.9 (12.9, 15.0)
Spain	7.7 (6.2, 9.7)	4.1 (3.2, 5.3)	9.2 (7.6, 11.1)	4.7 (3.9, 5.7)
United States	9.6 (8.3, 11.1)	16.5 (14.5, 18.8)	20.0 (18.0, 22.1)	16.7 (15.5, 17.9)
Any developing country	8.9 (7.6, 10.4)	8.4 (7.2, 9.7)	14.0 (12.4, 15.8)	7.6 (7.1, 8.2)
Any developed country	7.7 (7.0, 8.4)	10.4 (9.5, 11.4)	14.1 (13.1, 15.1)	10.7 (10.2, 11.1)
All countries	8.0 (7.4, 8.6)	9.9 (9.2, 10.7)	14.0 (13.2, 14.9)	9.5 (9.2, 9.9)

Table A.5.1d. Prevalence (CI) of 12-month depressive, anxiety, and either depressive or anxiety disorders among persons with any chronic pain condition, and prevalence (CI) of 12-month depressive or anxiety disorder among persons with no pain condition

Country	Mental disorder prevalence among persons with any pain[a] — Any depressive disorder	Any anxiety disorder	Either depressive or anxiety disorder	Depressive or anxiety disorder prevalence among persons with no pain — Either depressive or anxiety disorder
Beijing	4.3 (2.6, 6.9)	3.3 (2.2, 5.1)	5.9 (4.0, 8.7)	2.2 (1.3, 3.7)
Colombia	11.2 (9.3, 13.4)	9.0 (6.9, 11.5)	17.5 (14.9, 20.4)	7.8 (6.5, 9.3)
Lebanon	3.6 (1.9, 6.9)	5.3 (2.4, 11.4)	8.4 (5.2, 13.2)	2.5 (1.2, 5.0)
Mexico	9.6 (7.4, 12.4)	8.6 (6.7, 10.9)	14.8 (12.0, 18.1)	4.3 (3.6, 5.2)
Nigeria	2.0 (1.3, 2.9)	0.8 (0.3, 1.9)	2.4 (1.6, 3.7)	1.2 (0.7, 2.2)
South Africa	6.7 (5.6, 8.0)	11.5 (10.0, 13.2)	15.9 (14.0, 18.0)	8.0 (6.4, 10.1)
Shanghai	3.6 (1.4, 9.0)	2.7 (0.9, 8.1)	4.7 (2.3, 9.1)	0.9 (0.4, 2.0)
Ukraine	13.9 (11.8, 16.2)	10.3 (8.7, 12.3)	19.7 (17.0, 22.7)	6.4 (4.2, 9.6)
Belgium	9.1 (6.4, 12.7)	5.6 (3.6, 8.5)	12.2 (9.4, 15.7)	6.3 (4.7, 8.3)
France	8.7 (6.5, 11.4)	8.9 (7.2, 11.1)	14.5 (11.9, 17.6)	8.7 (6.3, 12.0)
Germany	5.3 (4.0, 6.8)	5.1 (3.5, 7.3)	9.1 (6.9, 11.8)	4.1 (3.2, 5.2)
Israel	10.2 (8.7, 11.9)	8.7 (7.4, 10.2)	15.1 (13.4, 17.1)	5.4 (4.7, 6.3)
Italy	5.1 (4.2, 6.2)	4.7 (3.5, 6.1)	7.6 (6.3, 9.1)	3.6 (2.7, 4.8)
Japan	3.1 (1.9, 5.0)	4.6 (3.0, 7.0)	6.0 (4.1, 8.7)	3.1 (2.3, 4.0)
The Netherlands	8.5 (6.1, 11.5)	10.2 (6.8, 14.9)	15.3 (11.8, 19.7)	6.4 (4.8, 8.6)
New Zealand	8.6 (7.6, 9.6)	13.9 (12.5, 15.4)	18.0 (16.4, 19.7)	11.2 (10.2, 12.4)
Spain	7.2 (5.8, 8.9)	3.9 (3.0, 5.1)	8.9 (7.2, 10.8)	4.0 (3.1, 5.0)
United States	12.2 (10.9, 13.5)	18.6 (17.1, 20.2)	23.5 (21.8, 25.4)	12.9 (11.5, 14.4)
Any developing country	7.8 (7.2, 8.6)	8.4 (7.7, 9.2)	13.8 (12.8, 14.8)	5.1 (4.5, 5.7)
Any developed country	9.1 (8.5, 9.6)	11.5 (10.8, 12.1)	16.3 (15.5, 17.0)	8.2 (7.7, 8.7)
All countries	8.6 (8.2, 9.1)	10.4 (9.9, 10.9)	15.4 (14.8, 16.0)	7.1 (6.7, 7.4)

[a] Any pain includes back/neck pain, headache, arthritis, and "other" chronic pain.

Table A.5.1e. Prevalence (CI) of 12-month depressive, anxiety, and either depressive or anxiety disorders among persons with diabetes, and prevalence (CI) of 12-month depressive or anxiety disorder among persons without diabetes

Country	Any depressive disorder	Any anxiety disorder	Either depressive or anxiety disorder	Either depressive or anxiety disorder (without diabetes)
Beijing	3.1 (0.6, 14.9)	0.3 (0.0, 2.1)	3.4 (0.7, 14.3)	3.6 (2.4, 5.2)
Colombia	8.1 (4.3, 14.8)	6.6 (3.4, 12.3)	12.3 (7.4, 20.0)	10.4 (9.1, 11.8)
Lebanon	3.1 (0.6, 14.1)	1.5 (0.4, 5.7)	3.8 (1.0, 13.9)	4.1 (2.7, 6.1)
Mexico	9.0 (5.8, 13.8)	4.5 (2.2, 8.7)	10.2 (6.7, 15.1)	6.7 (5.7, 7.9)
Nigeria	0.0 (–, –)	0.0 (–, –)	0.0 (–, –)	1.6 (1.1, 2.3)
South Africa	4.3 (2.1, 8.4)	13.5 (9.5, 18.8)	16.5 (11.8, 22.7)	11.6 (10.3, 13.0)
Shanghai	1.5 (0.2, 10.9)	3.0 (0.4, 20.5)	4.5 (0.9, 19.0)	2.1 (1.2, 3.9)
Ukraine	19.5 (10.7, 32.9)	11.9 (5.8, 22.7)	25.9 (14.2, 42.4)	14.1 (12.0, 16.5)
Belgium	3.7 (1.0, 12.6)	4.4 (1.8, 10.2)	8.1 (3.8, 16.5)	8.7 (6.8, 11.0)
France	6.4 (2.8, 14.0)	5.6 (1.3, 21.5)	10.8 (4.5, 24.1)	11.6 (9.7, 13.9)
Germany	5.7 (2.9, 11.0)	0.5 (0.1, 3.9)	5.7 (2.9, 11.0)	5.7 (4.7, 6.9)
Israel	7.5 (5.2, 10.8)	6.5 (4.4, 9.4)	12.3 (9.3, 16.0)	8.4 (7.5, 9.2)
Italy	6.0 (2.6, 13.2)	3.9 (0.9, 15.5)	8.7 (3.7, 19.0)	5.3 (4.5, 6.2)
Japan	3.2 (1.0, 9.4)	3.8 (1.2, 11.4)	4.1 (1.4, 11.4)	3.9 (3.0, 5.0)
The Netherlands	3.3 (1.3, 8.5)	3.2 (1.2, 8.3)	4.0 (1.7, 9.1)	9.8 (8.1, 11.7)
New Zealand	5.6 (3.7, 8.5)	10.4 (7.9, 13.7)	12.9 (9.8, 16.7)	13.9 (13.0, 15.0)
Spain	4.2 (2.6, 6.8)	1.8 (0.9, 3.6)	4.7 (2.9, 7.5)	5.7 (4.9, 6.6)
United States	8.5 (5.9, 12.2)	14.2 (11.6, 17.1)	17.7 (14.5, 21.5)	17.6 (16.5, 18.7)
Any developing country	6.4 (4.9, 8.4)	8.3 (6.3, 10.8)	12.8 (10.4, 15.8)	8.2 (7.6, 8.7)
Any developed country	6.5 (5.4, 7.8)	8.2 (7.1, 9.5)	12.0 (10.5, 13.6)	11.3 (10.9, 11.7)
All countries	6.5 (5.6, 7.6)	8.3 (7.3, 9.4)	12.2 (10.9, 13.6)	10.2 (9.8, 10.5)

The Pattern and Nature of Mental–Physical Comorbidity

Table A.5.1f. Prevalence (CI) of 12-month depressive, anxiety, and either depressive or anxiety disorders among persons with COPD or asthma, and prevalence (CI) of 12-month depressive or anxiety disorder among persons without COPD or asthma

	Mental disorder prevalence among persons with COPD or asthma			Depressive or anxiety disorder prevalence among persons without COPD or asthma
Country	Any depressive disorder	Any anxiety disorder	Either depressive or anxiety disorder	Either depressive or anxiety disorder
Beijing	3.7 (1.2, 10.9)	4.1 (0.9, 16.8)	6.6 (1.9, 20.1)	3.5 (2.4, 5.0)
Colombia	22.3 (12.8, 36.0)	6.4 (3.1, 12.4)	28.7 (18.5, 41.7)	9.8 (8.6, 11.2)
Lebanon	4.1 (0.4, 29.7)	1.7 (0.3, 10.8)	4.1 (0.4, 29.7)	4.1 (2.7, 6.0)
Mexico	5.4 (2.5, 11.4)	7.5 (3.9, 14.0)	9.0 (4.8, 16.2)	6.8 (5.7, 8.0)
Nigeria	5.1 (1.7, 14.8)	0.0 (–, –)	5.1 (1.7, 14.8)	1.5 (1.0, 2.2)
South Africa	8.9 (5.2, 14.7)	17.0 (11.9, 23.6)	22.4 (16.5, 29.7)	11.1 (9.8, 12.6)
Shanghai	2.0 (0.3, 11.3)	0.0 (–, –)	2.0 (0.3, 11.3)	2.2 (1.3, 3.9)
Ukraine	19.7 (13.4, 27.9)	14.3 (8.7, 22.8)	27.0 (19.0, 36.8)	13.8 (11.7, 16.3)
Belgium	9.7 (4.4, 20.0)	5.0 (2.1, 11.6)	13.1 (6.1, 25.8)	8.3 (6.3, 10.8)
France	10.3 (6.3, 16.6)	13.4 (8.6, 20.1)	18.3 (13.4, 24.5)	10.8 (9.2, 12.8)
Germany	6.3 (2.6, 14.3)	4.2 (2.0, 8.5)	9.5 (4.9, 17.6)	5.4 (4.4, 6.7)
Israel	8.5 (6.4, 11.2)	6.5 (4.7, 9.0)	12.7 (10.1, 15.8)	8.2 (7.3, 9.1)
Italy	7.5 (4.9, 11.4)	4.2 (1.5, 11.6)	10.3 (6.4, 16.0)	5.1 (4.2, 6.2)
Japan	3.2 (1.1, 8.9)	3.5 (1.3, 9.5)	3.9 (1.5, 9.8)	3.9 (3.0, 5.1)
The Netherlands	6.8 (3.6, 12.4)	14.0 (6.8, 26.7)	19.7 (11.4, 31.7)	8.2 (6.7, 10.1)
New Zealand	9.4 (8.0, 11.0)	13.4 (11.5, 15.6)	18.2 (15.9, 20.8)	12.9 (12.0, 13.9)
Spain	9.6 (6.5, 14.0)	7.5 (4.2, 12.8)	12.2 (8.6, 16.9)	5.2 (4.4, 6.1)
United States	11.6 (9.4, 14.2)	17.6 (14.8, 20.8)	22.7 (19.2, 26.6)	16.8 (15.5, 18.2)
Any developing country	10.6 (8.1, 13.8)	11.3 (8.7, 14.7)	19.0 (15.5, 23.1)	7.9 (7.4, 8.5)
Any developed country	9.4 (8.5, 10.4)	12.0 (10.9, 13.2)	17.2 (15.9, 18.6)	10.5 (10.1, 11.0)
All countries	9.6 (8.7, 10.6)	11.9 (10.9, 13.0)	17.5 (16.2, 18.8)	9.5 (9.2, 9.9)

COPD, chronic obstructive pulmonary disease.

Table A.5.1g. Prevalence (CI) of 12-month depressive, anxiety, and either depressive or anxiety disorders among persons with heart disease, and prevalence (CI) of 12-month depressive or anxiety disorder among persons without heart disease

Country	Mental disorder prevalence among persons with heart disease			Depressive or anxiety disorder prevalence among persons without heart disease
	Any depressive disorder	Any anxiety disorder	Either depressive or anxiety disorder	Either depressive or anxiety disorder
Beijing	3.1 (1.7, 5.5)	3.8 (2.1, 6.7)	5.5 (3.5, 8.6)	3.3 (2.3, 4.9)
Colombia	13.9 (8.5, 22.1)	10.5 (5.9, 18.1)	19.6 (12.6, 29.3)	10.1 (8.8, 11.6)
Lebanon	1.3 (0.2, 6.3)	1.3 (0.2, 6.3)	1.3 (0.2, 6.3)	4.2 (2.8, 6.2)
Mexico	9.2 (4.9, 16.5)	6.7 (2.9, 14.6)	12.4 (6.8, 21.4)	6.7 (5.7, 7.9)
Nigeria	2.4 (0.9, 6.3)	6.0 (1.0, 28.0)	8.0 (2.1, 26.5)	1.5 (1.0, 2.2)
South Africa	10.3 (7.2, 14.5)	20.2 (14.8, 26.9)	25.4 (19.4, 32.6)	11.0 (9.7, 12.4)
Shanghai	6.9 (1.8, 22.8)	6.0 (1.3, 23.7)	8.5 (2.8, 22.7)	1.3 (0.8, 2.3)
Ukraine	19.4 (15.9, 23.3)	14.1 (11.7, 16.8)	26.4 (22.0, 31.3)	10.4 (8.4, 12.9)
Belgium	7.4 (3.3, 15.4)	1.7 (0.7, 4.3)	8.4 (4.2, 16.2)	8.7 (6.6, 11.4)
France	6.4 (2.8, 13.9)	7.8 (2.4, 22.3)	11.9 (5.0, 25.6)	11.6 (9.9, 13.5)
Germany	5.0 (2.7, 8.8)	2.3 (1.1, 4.6)	5.5 (3.2, 9.4)	5.7 (4.7, 6.9)
Israel	8.4 (6.0, 11.6)	6.4 (4.5, 9.0)	12.4 (9.5, 15.9)	8.3 (7.5, 9.2)
Italy	7.8 (4.6, 12.7)	6.1 (2.6, 13.8)	11.8 (6.8, 19.7)	5.0 (4.2, 6.0)
Japan	5.0 (2.1, 11.4)	7.9 (3.6, 16.4)	9.4 (4.8, 17.6)	3.5 (2.6, 4.8)
The Netherlands	7.4 (3.3, 15.8)	8.5 (3.8, 17.9)	14.2 (7.5, 25.4)	9.0 (7.2, 11.0)
New Zealand	4.7 (3.2, 6.9)	7.8 (5.9, 10.2)	9.8 (7.5, 12.7)	14.2 (13.2, 15.3)
Spain	8.0 (4.6, 13.7)	4.5 (2.2, 8.8)	8.4 (4.9, 14.1)	5.5 (4.8, 6.4)
United States	9.2 (6.5, 12.8)	15.5 (11.5, 20.6)	18.7 (14.2, 24.1)	17.5 (16.4, 18.6)
Any developing country	12.7 (11.0, 14.7)	12.8 (10.9, 15.0)	20.4 (17.9, 23.2)	7.5 (6.9, 8.0)
Any developed country	7.1 (6.1, 8.3)	8.2 (7.0, 9.5)	12.2 (10.7, 13.8)	11.3 (10.8, 11.7)
All countries	9.1 (8.2, 10.1)	9.8 (8.8, 11.0)	15.1 (13.7, 16.5)	9.9 (9.6, 10.3)

The Pattern and Nature of Mental–Physical Comorbidity

Table A.5.1h. Prevalence (CI) of 12-month depressive, anxiety, and either depressive or anxiety disorders among persons with ulcers, and prevalence (CI) of 12-month depressive or anxiety disorder among persons without ulcers

	Mental disorder prevalence among persons with ulcers			Depressive or anxiety disorder prevalence among persons without ulcers
Country	Any depressive disorder	Any anxiety disorder	Either depressive or anxiety disorder	Either depressive or anxiety disorder
Beijing	4.9 (0.9, 21.8)	4.5 (0.8, 21.4)	5.9 (1.4, 21.7)	3.5 (2.4, 5.0)
Colombia	9.6 (6.4, 14.1)	10.0 (6.5, 15.0)	15.9 (11.2, 22.0)	9.8 (8.5, 11.2)
Lebanon	3.6 (0.9, 13.1)	7.1 (1.1, 35.1)	10.0 (2.4, 33.8)	3.9 (2.5, 5.9)
Mexico	10.1 (5.7, 17.2)	4.7 (2.5, 8.7)	12.8 (7.8, 20.2)	6.6 (5.6, 7.8)
Nigeria	5.0 (2.1, 11.5)	3.3 (0.6, 16.2)	7.8 (3.2, 17.8)	1.4 (0.9, 2.1)
South Africa	9.2 (5.5, 15.2)	18.0 (13.0, 24.4)	22.2 (17.1, 28.4)	11.2 (9.9, 12.7)
Shanghai	1.9 (0.6, 5.3)	2.0 (0.4, 8.9)	3.9 (1.5, 9.7)	2.1 (1.1, 3.8)
Ukraine	16.0 (11.1, 22.5)	11.6 (6.8, 19.2)	22.2 (15.3, 31.1)	13.7 (11.6, 16.2)
Belgium	13.2 (6.1, 26.4)	6.7 (2.9, 14.9)	15.9 (7.7, 29.9)	8.2 (6.1, 10.9)
France	3.8 (2.0, 7.1)	13.7 (5.8, 29.1)	15.3 (7.1, 29.8)	11.4 (9.3, 13.8)
Germany	4.9 (2.8, 8.6)	4.2 (2.2, 7.9)	7.4 (4.7, 11.4)	5.6 (4.6, 6.8)
Israel	7.9 (5.5, 11.1)	4.6 (2.9, 7.3)	10.8 (8.0, 14.4)	8.5 (7.7, 9.4)
Italy	10.3 (6.2, 16.7)	4.1 (1.8, 8.9)	11.9 (7.5, 18.4)	5.2 (4.3, 6.2)
Japan	2.6 (1.2, 5.7)	4.3 (2.1, 8.5)	5.1 (2.5, 10.3)	3.7 (2.9, 4.9)
The Netherlands	10.2 (5.5, 18.2)	17.2 (8.2, 32.3)	20.4 (10.5, 36.0)	8.9 (7.3, 10.8)
New Zealand	9.4 (7.0, 12.5)	14.3 (11.3, 18.0)	19.3 (15.6, 23.5)	13.6 (12.6, 14.6)
Spain	5.5 (3.3, 8.9)	3.5 (1.8, 6.7)	6.4 (3.9, 10.4)	5.6 (4.9, 6.5)
United States	15.1 (12.4, 18.2)	23.9 (20.6, 27.6)	29.4 (25.6, 33.4)	16.3 (15.3, 17.4)
Any developing country	9.3 (7.5, 11.4)	10.5 (8.5, 12.9)	16.2 (13.8, 19.0)	7.9 (7.3, 8.4)
Any developed country	9.9 (8.7, 11.2)	12.9 (11.5, 14.5)	17.9 (16.2, 19.7)	10.9 (10.4, 11.3)
All countries	9.7 (8.7, 10.8)	12.1 (10.9, 13.4)	17.3 (15.9, 18.8)	9.8 (9.4, 10.1)

Table A.5.1i. Prevalence (CI) of 12-month depressive, anxiety, and either depressive or anxiety disorders among persons with any chronic physical disorder, and prevalence (CI) of 12-month depressive or anxiety disorder among persons with no chronic physical disorder

Country	Mental disorder prevalence among persons with any chronic physical disorder[a]			Depressive or anxiety disorder prevalence among persons with no chronic physical disorder
	Any depressive disorder	Any anxiety disorder	Either depressive or anxiety disorder	Either depressive or anxiety disorder
Beijing	4.0 (2.2, 7.1)	2.9 (1.3, 6.7)	5.4 (3.1, 9.2)	3.2 (1.9, 5.1)
Colombia	10.9 (8.5, 14.0)	8.4 (6.1, 11.4)	16.0 (12.9, 19.8)	9.1 (7.8, 10.5)
Lebanon	2.9 (1.0, 7.8)	2.9 (0.7, 11.0)	5.1 (1.9, 12.9)	3.9 (2.5, 6.1)
Mexico	8.7 (6.5, 11.6)	5.9 (4.4, 7.9)	11.6 (9.0, 14.7)	6.2 (5.2, 7.5)
Nigeria	3.3 (1.8, 5.9)	1.6 (0.3, 6.8)	4.6 (2.3, 8.7)	1.3 (0.9, 2.0)
South Africa	7.3 (5.7, 9.2)	14.2 (11.9, 16.9)	18.5 (15.7, 21.6)	9.9 (8.5, 11.5)
Shanghai	3.3 (0.9, 11.4)	3.2 (0.7, 13.0)	4.4 (1.5, 12.4)	1.4 (0.8, 2.6)
Ukraine	17.2 (14.3, 20.6)	11.9 (10.0, 14.2)	23.1 (19.6, 27.0)	9.8 (7.7, 12.5)
Belgium	8.3 (5.9, 11.4)	4.2 (2.6, 6.8)	10.7 (8.1, 14.0)	8.0 (5.6, 11.3)
France	8.2 (5.7, 11.5)	10.7 (8.2, 14.0)	15.1 (12.3, 18.5)	10.5 (8.5, 12.8)
Germany	5.0 (3.4, 7.3)	2.9 (1.9, 4.5)	6.8 (5.0, 9.2)	5.4 (4.2, 6.8)
Israel	8.3 (6.9, 9.9)	6.2 (5.0, 7.6)	12.1 (10.4, 13.9)	7.3 (6.4, 8.2)
Italy	6.7 (5.1, 8.7)	5.5 (3.3, 8.9)	10.2 (7.6, 13.6)	4.4 (3.6, 5.4)
Japan	3.1 (1.8, 5.3)	3.6 (2.1, 6.0)	4.7 (2.9, 7.5)	3.6 (2.5, 5.0)
The Netherlands	6.7 (4.4, 10.0)	10.5 (6.6, 16.3)	15.0 (10.4, 21.0)	7.5 (5.9, 9.5)
New Zealand	7.9 (6.9, 9.0)	12.5 (11.1, 14.1)	16.4 (14.7, 18.2)	12.7 (11.7, 13.9)
Spain	6.3 (4.6, 8.5)	4.1 (2.8, 5.9)	7.5 (5.7, 9.8)	5.2 (4.3, 6.3)
United States	11.2 (9.7, 12.8)	17.2 (15.6, 18.9)	22.1 (20.1, 24.3)	15.4 (14.3, 16.6)
Any developing country	9.2 (8.2, 10.3)	9.6 (8.6, 10.7)	15.5 (14.2, 17.0)	6.7 (6.1, 7.3)
Any developed country	8.3 (7.7, 8.9)	10.6 (9.9, 11.3)	15.2 (14.3, 16.0)	9.8 (9.4, 10.3)
All countries	8.6 (8.1, 9.1)	10.3 (9.8, 10.9)	15.3 (14.5, 16.0)	8.6 (8.3, 9.0)

[a] Any chronic physical disorder includes diabetes, COPD or asthma, heart disease, ulcers, cancer, epilepsy, HIV/AIDS, stroke, and tuberculosis.

Table A.5.2a. Prevalence (CI) of back pain, headache, arthritis, and any chronic pain among persons with a 12-month depressive disorder

Country	Back pain	Headache	Arthritis	Any pain[a]
Beijing	49.4 (29.4, 69.7)	26.2 (15.6, 40.5)	14.0 (4.8, 34.6)	65.7 (44.6, 82.0)
Colombia	20.1 (14.6, 27.1)	35.1 (26.6, 44.8)	9.1 (5.4, 14.8)	49.0 (40.2, 57.9)
Lebanon	25.8 (10.6, 50.4)	40.2 (19.9, 64.4)	5.3 (1.6, 16.1)	52.9 (30.4, 74.2)
Mexico	32.0 (25.7, 39.1)	23.0 (17.8, 29.3)	18.1 (13.5, 23.9)	55.1 (48.1, 61.9)
Nigeria	37.5 (24.5, 52.6)	21.5 (12.9, 33.7)	33.5 (21.3, 48.3)	53.0 (36.9, 68.5)
South Africa	45.8 (36.3, 55.5)	48.8 (40.6, 57.1)	15.9 (10.8, 22.9)	66.8 (56.0, 76.0)
Shanghai	54.5 (21.8, 83.7)	45.7 (14.4, 80.8)	49.6 (17.6, 81.9)	69.5 (37.4, 89.6)
Ukraine	64.9 (58.1, 71.1)	60.4 (53.4, 67.0)	40.4 (34.8, 46.3)	83.7 (76.7, 88.8)
Belgium	31.5 (22.0, 42.8)	27.6 (17.5, 40.7)	20.5 (12.2, 32.2)	60.0 (45.5, 73.0)
France	34.3 (24.0, 46.5)	27.7 (19.5, 37.6)	30.8 (21.2, 42.6)	63.5 (52.8, 73.1)
Germany	27.8 (18.6, 39.3)	22.2 (14.3, 32.7)	14.7 (7.2, 27.9)	50.3 (39.9, 60.7)
Israel	32.4 (27.1, 38.2)	28.8 (23.7, 34.4)	17.0 (13.0, 21.8)	55.8 (49.9, 61.6)
Italy	40.1 (31.2, 49.6)	24.4 (18.0, 32.2)	44.7 (37.3, 52.3)	64.7 (56.4, 72.1)
Japan	27.8 (16.5, 42.9)	22.3 (11.7, 38.4)	9.8 (4.2, 21.1)	37.8 (25.3, 52.1)
The Netherlands	32.3 (21.3, 45.7)	25.0 (16.3, 36.4)	10.0 (4.9, 19.5)	51.1 (35.5, 66.4)
New Zealand	29.5 (25.5, 33.8)	25.2 (21.8, 28.9)	18.6 (15.7, 22.0)	49.7 (45.4, 54.0)
Spain	26.3 (21.2, 32.1)	27.2 (21.8, 33.3)	37.5 (31.8, 43.5)	57.0 (48.7, 65.0)
United States	36.3 (32.2, 40.6)	32.9 (27.4, 38.9)	30.8 (26.5, 35.3)	62.8 (57.3, 67.9)
Any developing country	42.6 (38.6, 46.7)	43.2 (39.5, 47.0)	21.7 (18.9, 24.8)	64.7 (60.6, 68.7)
Any developed country	32.5 (30.4, 34.7)	28.2 (25.9, 30.5)	24.0 (22.1, 26.0)	56.5 (54.0, 59.0)
All countries	35.5 (33.5, 37.4)	32.6 (30.6, 34.6)	23.3 (21.8, 25.0)	58.9 (56.8, 61.0)

[a] Any pain includes back/neck pain, headache, arthritis, and "other" chronic pain.

Table A.5.2b. Prevalence (CI) of back pain, headache, arthritis, and any chronic pain among persons with a 12-month anxiety disorder

Country	Back pain	Headache	Arthritis	Any pain[a]
Beijing	38.1 (23.4, 55.3)	23.5 (11.7, 41.8)	10.9 (5.8, 19.6)	66.8 (50.2, 80.1)
Colombia	16.9 (12.1, 23.2)	24.5 (18.6, 31.5)	6.9 (4.2, 11.0)	40.9 (33.6, 48.7)
Lebanon	25.7 (11.8, 47.3)	30.3 (7.9, 68.8)	3.2 (0.9, 10.9)	53.4 (23.0, 81.5)
Mexico	27.2 (21.1, 34.3)	30.0 (22.5, 38.8)	14.7 (10.2, 20.7)	52.6 (45.3, 59.8)
Nigeria	25.2 (6.8, 61.1)	33.6 (8.6, 73.3)	40.1 (12.0, 76.7)	40.9 (11.8, 78.2)
South Africa	40.1 (33.4, 47.3)	50.9 (43.7, 58.0)	17.3 (13.4, 22.1)	65.9 (58.0, 72.9)
Shanghai	79.3 (42.9, 95.1)	74.9 (34.7, 94.4)	65.5 (30.1, 89.3)	91.1 (86.1, 94.5)
Ukraine	66.3 (56.6, 74.8)	56.8 (48.6, 64.6)	35.5 (29.0, 42.6)	85.6 (75.3, 92.0)
Belgium	27.8 (16.5, 42.9)	27.0 (15.6, 42.6)	31.2 (20.5, 44.4)	55.9 (40.8, 69.9)
France	29.3 (20.0, 40.6)	19.8 (12.6, 29.7)	32.0 (21.8, 44.2)	62.3 (48.2, 74.6)
Germany	23.5 (15.5, 34.1)	24.7 (16.3, 35.4)	5.5 (2.7, 11.0)	49.2 (38.1, 60.3)
Israel	41.5 (34.7, 48.6)	33.1 (26.7, 40.1)	20.7 (15.7, 26.8)	66.9 (60.0, 73.2)
Italy	44.5 (34.1, 55.4)	27.3 (19.7, 36.5)	37.2 (28.1, 47.2)	67.9 (57.4, 76.8)
Japan	35.3 (23.6, 49.0)	26.0 (15.9, 39.6)	12.5 (5.5, 26.0)	48.7 (36.6, 60.9)
The Netherlands	34.9 (21.4, 51.3)	26.0 (15.5, 40.1)	10.8 (5.0, 21.9)	60.6 (47.0, 72.7)
New Zealand	30.0 (27.1, 33.1)	23.9 (21.2, 26.8)	21.5 (19.0, 24.2)	52.5 (49.4, 55.5)
Spain	26.2 (17.5, 37.4)	28.0 (19.5, 38.4)	34.0 (25.6, 43.5)	52.4 (42.0, 62.5)
United States	31.1 (28.1, 34.3)	28.3 (25.0, 31.9)	33.1 (29.6, 36.8)	59.8 (55.5, 63.9)
Any developing country	38.3 (34.3, 42.4)	43.4 (39.4, 47.4)	18.3 (15.8, 21.1)	62.4 (58.1, 66.6)
Any developed country	31.8 (30.0, 33.7)	26.6 (24.8, 28.5)	26.3 (24.4, 28.3)	57.6 (55.5, 59.8)
All countries	33.6 (31.8, 35.3)	31.1 (29.4, 32.8)	24.2 (22.6, 25.8)	58.9 (57.0, 60.9)

[a] Any pain includes back/neck pain, headache, arthritis, and "other" chronic pain.

Table A.5.2c. Prevalence (CI) of back pain, headache, arthritis, and any chronic pain among persons with either a 12-month depressive or anxiety disorder

Country	Back pain	Headache	Arthritis	Any pain[a]
Beijing	41.4 (28.7, 55.3)	21.4 (13.6, 32.0)	12.5 (5.7, 25.3)	61.5 (47.7, 73.8)
Colombia	18.7 (14.4, 23.9)	30.9 (24.9, 37.6)	8.3 (5.6, 12.1)	45.8 (39.4, 52.2)
Lebanon	26.5 (15.1, 42.2)	34.2 (17.4, 56.2)	3.9 (1.4, 10.1)	54.5 (33.5, 74.1)
Mexico	28.0 (23.4, 33.1)	25.0 (20.0, 30.8)	15.0 (11.9, 18.7)	52.1 (47.2, 56.9)
Nigeria	30.1 (17.9, 45.9)	23.8 (12.3, 41.1)	32.4 (19.0, 49.7)	46.6 (28.8, 65.2)
South Africa	40.9 (34.9, 47.2)	48.4 (42.7, 54.2)	16.2 (12.9, 20.3)	64.9 (57.9, 71.4)
Shanghai	54.9 (26.7, 80.3)	45.9 (18.5, 76.0)	44.7 (20.5, 71.8)	72.2 (50.1, 87.0)
Ukraine	63.3 (56.0, 70.0)	55.8 (49.7, 61.7)	36.1 (31.3, 41.1)	82.4 (75.4, 87.7)
Belgium	30.6 (24.1, 38.0)	24.8 (17.4, 34.2)	24.5 (17.5, 33.1)	56.9 (48.8, 64.6)
France	31.6 (23.5, 41.0)	22.2 (16.3, 29.4)	30.4 (21.6, 40.8)	62.1 (52.2, 71.0)
Germany	27.3 (19.8, 36.4)	23.1 (16.6, 31.2)	10.7 (5.8, 18.9)	51.5 (42.1, 60.8)
Israel	35.0 (30.5, 39.9)	28.9 (24.6, 33.6)	18.1 (14.7, 22.1)	58.3 (53.4, 63.1)
Italy	42.6 (35.3, 50.3)	25.3 (19.6, 32.1)	38.6 (32.1, 45.5)	63.7 (56.1, 70.6)
Japan	31.3 (22.1, 42.3)	23.6 (14.8, 35.4)	10.1 (4.9, 19.7)	43.4 (33.4, 54.0)
The Netherlands	33.5 (23.6, 45.2)	24.3 (16.6, 34.1)	9.0 (4.8, 16.3)	54.4 (44.3, 64.2)
New Zealand	28.8 (26.2, 31.6)	23.5 (21.0, 26.1)	19.5 (17.5, 21.7)	50.8 (48.0, 53.6)
Spain	25.8 (20.4, 32.0)	26.3 (21.1, 32.3)	34.6 (28.9, 40.8)	54.5 (46.0, 62.8)
United States	31.0 (28.3, 33.8)	27.7 (24.4, 31.1)	31.0 (28.0, 34.3)	58.8 (54.7, 62.8)
Any developing country	38.8 (35.6, 42.1)	41.8 (38.8, 44.7)	18.7 (16.7, 20.9)	62.2 (58.8, 65.5)
Any developed country	31.0 (29.5, 32.6)	25.7 (24.1, 27.3)	24.2 (22.7, 25.8)	55.7 (53.9, 57.6)
All countries	33.3 (31.8, 34.8)	30.4 (29.0, 31.8)	22.6 (21.4, 23.9)	57.6 (56.0, 59.3)

[a] Any pain includes back/neck pain, headache, arthritis, and "other" chronic pain.

Table A.5.3a. Prevalence (CI) of diabetes, lung disease, heart disease, ulcers, and any chronic physical disorder among persons with a 12-month depressive disorder

Country	Diabetes	Lung disease	Heart disease	Ulcers	Any physical disorder[a]
Beijing	6.1 (0.9, 32.1)	3.9 (1.3, 10.9)	13.1 (7.7, 21.5)	7.2 (1.4, 29.4)	29.0 (14.4, 49.8)
Colombia	4.3 (2.2, 8.2)	11.8 (6.6, 20.2)	6.7 (4.1, 10.9)	16.5 (10.9, 24.3)	34.5 (27.1, 42.6)
Lebanon	9.0 (1.9, 33.5)	3.0 (0.5, 15.1)	2.3 (0.4, 10.7)	6.7 (1.8, 22.3)	18.1 (6.6, 40.7)
Mexico	9.3 (6.0, 14.0)	3.2 (1.5, 6.6)	4.9 (2.6, 8.9)	8.4 (5.2, 13.2)	23.8 (18.3, 30.2)
Nigeria	0.0 (–, –)	9.9 (3.6, 24.5)	3.6 (1.5, 8.3)	14.2 (6.7, 27.5)	22.5 (14.0, 34.2)
South Africa	4.9 (2.5, 9.5)	12.2 (7.3, 19.8)	12.9 (8.8, 18.5)	10.5 (6.2, 17.1)	33.7 (27.9, 40.0)
Shanghai	3.4 (0.3, 26.2)	6.3 (1.0, 31.5)	48.8 (16.6, 82.1)	9.4 (2.9, 26.5)	49.7 (17.2, 82.4)
Ukraine	5.5 (3.3, 8.8)	8.6 (5.8, 12.6)	48.3 (42.8, 53.9)	12.8 (9.4, 17.1)	59.1 (51.9, 66.0)
Belgium	2.5 (0.7, 8.6)	13.1 (5.9, 26.8)	10.7 (4.1, 24.9)	13.1 (6.6, 24.4)	33.1 (21.6, 47.1)
France	4.0 (1.9, 8.4)	15.7 (10.8, 22.2)	5.3 (2.3, 11.9)	3.2 (1.8, 5.7)	28.7 (21.6, 37.1)
Germany	8.0 (4.5, 14.0)	13.3 (5.8, 27.8)	12.9 (7.4, 21.5)	9.1 (5.9, 13.7)	35.0 (24.6, 47.1)
Israel	10.0 (6.9, 14.3)	15.4 (11.7, 20.1)	12.9 (9.3, 17.7)	10.1 (7.1, 14.2)	39.5 (33.9, 45.4)
Italy	5.7 (2.4, 13.0)	12.3 (7.7, 19.1)	11.7 (7.2, 18.5)	10.1 (5.7, 17.1)	31.3 (23.9, 39.9)
Japan	9.0 (3.4, 22.1)	9.9 (3.7, 23.9)	13.2 (5.3, 29.0)	12.6 (6.2, 24.0)	39.0 (24.7, 55.5)
The Netherlands	4.2 (1.8, 9.8)	12.3 (5.9, 24.1)	10.5 (4.8, 21.3)	7.8 (4.3, 13.6)	30.5 (19.5, 44.3)
New Zealand	4.1 (2.7, 6.1)	25.1 (21.9, 28.6)	4.7 (3.2, 6.8)	7.5 (5.6, 10.0)	37.0 (33.0, 41.0)
Spain	5.5 (3.6, 8.4)	15.2 (10.7, 21.1)	8.1 (5.5, 11.8)	6.4 (4.0, 10.0)	28.9 (21.9, 37.1)
United States	7.2 (5.1, 10.2)	17.9 (14.8, 21.4)	7.6 (5.7, 9.9)	16.7 (14.1, 19.6)	42.6 (38.0, 47.4)
Any developing country	5.5 (4.1, 7.2)	9.3 (7.1, 12.1)	19.2 (16.8, 21.9)	11.9 (9.7, 14.5)	38.1 (34.9, 41.4)
Any developed country	6.2 (5.2, 7.4)	18.5 (16.8, 20.2)	8.1 (7.0, 9.5)	10.7 (9.5, 12.0)	37.5 (35.3, 39.7)
All countries	6.0 (5.2, 7.0)	15.8 (14.5, 17.2)	11.4 (10.3, 12.6)	11.0 (9.9, 12.2)	37.7 (35.8, 39.5)

[a] Any physical disorder includes diabetes, COPD or asthma, heart disease, ulcers, cancer, epilepsy, HIV/AIDS, stroke, and tuberculosis.

Table A.5.3b. Prevalence (CI) of diabetes, lung disease, heart disease, ulcers, and any chronic physical disorder among persons with a 12-month anxiety disorder

Country	Diabetes	Lung disease	Heart disease	Ulcers	Any physical disorder[a]
Beijing	0.7 (0.1, 5.3)	5.7 (1.5, 19.2)	20.4 (10.9, 35.2)	8.7 (1.6, 36.0)	27.8 (11.2, 54.1)
Colombia	3.6 (1.7, 7.3)	3.5 (1.8, 6.8)	5.3 (3.0, 9.3)	17.8 (11.2, 27.2)	27.5 (19.6, 37.2)
Lebanon	2.9 (0.7, 11.2)	0.9 (0.2, 4.2)	1.6 (0.3, 8.3)	9.0 (1.1, 45.6)	12.4 (2.4, 44.4)
Mexico	4.9 (2.4, 9.9)	4.7 (2.5, 8.9)	3.8 (1.7, 8.6)	4.2 (2.4, 7.2)	17.3 (13.0, 22.6)
Nigeria	0.0 (–, –)	0.0 (–, –)	18.2 (2.8, 62.8)	18.9 (3.1, 63.1)	21.3 (4.1, 63.3)
South Africa	8.9 (6.0, 12.8)	13.5 (9.0, 19.7)	14.5 (10.3, 20.1)	11.7 (8.7, 15.5)	37.8 (31.6, 44.4)
Shanghai	12.0 (1.2, 60.4)	0.0 (–, –)	72.6 (32.0, 93.7)	17.5 (2.7, 61.9)	83.4 (32.2, 98.2)
Ukraine	4.6 (2.5, 8.3)	8.7 (4.9, 14.9)	48.1 (40.0, 56.4)	12.7 (7.3, 21.3)	56.2 (47.5, 64.5)
Belgium	4.4 (1.9, 9.8)	10.3 (5.0, 20.2)	3.7 (1.6, 8.7)	10.1 (4.9, 19.6)	25.6 (17.8, 35.4)
France	3.4 (0.8, 13.6)	19.3 (12.9, 27.9)	6.2 (2.2, 15.9)	11.0 (4.4, 24.6)	35.9 (27.2, 45.5)
Germany	0.7 (0.1, 5.1)	9.0 (4.6, 16.7)	6.0 (2.8, 12.1)	7.8 (4.2, 14.2)	20.7 (13.3, 30.8)
Israel	12.0 (8.2, 17.2)	16.8 (12.2, 22.6)	13.8 (9.8, 19.1)	8.3 (5.2, 13.1)	41.6 (34.9, 48.6)
Italy	4.3 (1.0, 16.1)	8.0 (2.8, 20.6)	10.6 (4.3, 24.0)	4.6 (2.1, 9.9)	29.4 (19.4, 41.9)
Japan	9.4 (3.4, 23.5)	9.5 (3.3, 24.4)	18.2 (7.7, 37.2)	18.1 (9.5, 31.9)	40.2 (25.8, 56.5)
The Netherlands	4.0 (1.5, 10.3)	25.2 (13.1, 42.8)	11.9 (5.2, 24.6)	12.9 (6.8, 23.3)	47.4 (34.9, 60.3)
New Zealand	4.9 (3.8, 6.2)	23.3 (20.7, 26.2)	5.0 (3.9, 6.4)	7.5 (6.0, 9.3)	38.0 (35.0, 41.2)
Spain	4.0 (2.0, 8.1)	20.1 (12.6, 30.4)	7.6 (4.0, 14.1)	6.9 (3.8, 12.3)	31.8 (22.6, 42.7)
United States	7.5 (6.2, 8.9)	16.9 (14.6, 19.5)	8.0 (6.3, 10.0)	16.5 (14.4, 18.8)	40.9 (37.6, 44.3)
Any developing country	6.3 (4.8, 8.3)	9.0 (6.7, 11.9)	17.3 (14.6, 20.4)	12.1 (9.8, 14.8)	35.7 (31.9, 39.6)
Any developed country	6.4 (5.6, 7.3)	19.0 (17.5, 20.6)	7.6 (6.6, 8.7)	11.3 (10.1, 12.6)	38.6 (36.7, 40.6)
All countries	6.3 (5.6, 7.2)	16.3 (15.0, 17.7)	10.2 (9.2, 11.3)	11.5 (10.4, 12.7)	37.8 (36.1, 39.6)

[a] Any physical disorder includes diabetes, COPD or asthma, heart disease, ulcers, cancer, epilepsy, HIV/AIDS, stroke, and tuberculosis.

Table A.5.3c. Prevalence (CI) of diabetes, lung disease, heart disease, ulcers, and any chronic physical disorder among persons with either a 12-month depressive or anxiety disorder

Country	Diabetes	Lung disease	Heart disease	Ulcers	Any physical disorder[a]
Beijing	4.5 (0.8, 22.2)	4.7 (1.7, 12.6)	15.6 (10.1, 23.3)	5.9 (1.5, 20.9)	26.7 (14.1, 44.8)
Colombia	3.9 (2.2, 6.7)	9.1 (5.6, 14.3)	5.7 (3.7, 8.7)	16.3 (11.2, 23.1)	30.2 (24.3, 36.8)
Lebanon	4.9 (1.2, 17.6)	1.3 (0.2, 7.3)	1.0 (0.2, 5.1)	8.2 (1.9, 28.9)	14.2 (5.0, 34.3)
Mexico	6.4 (4.2, 9.6)	3.3 (1.8, 5.9)	4.1 (2.3, 7.2)	6.5 (4.3, 9.6)	19.4 (15.4, 24.1)
Nigeria	0.0 (–, –)	7.0 (2.4, 18.7)	8.6 (2.2, 27.9)	15.5 (6.4, 33.3)	21.9 (11.3, 38.2)
South Africa	7.8 (5.4, 11.1)	12.7 (9.0, 17.6)	13.1 (9.6, 17.5)	10.3 (8.0, 13.1)	35.1 (30.0, 40.5)
Shanghai	8.2 (1.6, 33.1)	5.0 (0.8, 25.3)	47.4 (19.5, 77.0)	15.5 (5.6, 36.1)	53.0 (21.6, 82.2)
Ukraine	5.0 (3.1, 8.2)	8.2 (5.7, 11.9)	45.7 (39.8, 51.8)	12.3 (8.6, 17.4)	55.2 (48.5, 61.6)
Belgium	3.8 (1.9, 7.3)	12.5 (6.0, 24.2)	8.6 (3.7, 18.7)	11.1 (5.7, 20.3)	30.3 (20.7, 41.9)
France	4.0 (1.6, 9.5)	16.2 (12.1, 21.4)	5.8 (2.9, 11.1)	7.5 (3.3, 16.2)	31.0 (24.8, 38.0)
Germany	4.8 (2.6, 8.6)	12.0 (6.7, 20.5)	8.5 (5.1, 13.9)	8.1 (5.6, 11.5)	28.1 (21.4, 36.1)
Israel	11.4 (8.6, 15.0)	16.3 (13.0, 20.2)	13.4 (10.3, 17.2)	9.8 (7.2, 13.1)	40.5 (35.8, 45.5)
Italy	5.6 (2.5, 11.9)	11.3 (6.9, 17.9)	11.9 (6.7, 20.3)	7.7 (4.4, 13.2)	31.9 (24.6, 40.3)
Japan	6.8 (2.6, 16.8)	7.2 (2.8, 17.1)	14.7 (7.2, 27.5)	14.7 (7.8, 25.8)	35.5 (23.8, 49.4)
The Netherlands	3.0 (1.3, 6.5)	21.1 (11.8, 34.8)	11.8 (6.2, 21.3)	9.2 (5.1, 15.9)	40.1 (29.0, 52.5)
New Zealand	4.5 (3.5, 5.7)	23.7 (21.4, 26.3)	4.7 (3.7, 6.0)	7.5 (6.1, 9.2)	37.2 (34.4, 40.1)
Spain	4.8 (3.2, 7.1)	15.0 (11.3, 19.5)	6.6 (4.4, 9.7)	5.8 (3.7, 9.0)	26.9 (21.3, 33.5)
United States	7.3 (6.1, 8.7)	16.9 (14.7, 19.3)	7.5 (6.1, 9.1)	15.7 (13.9, 17.8)	40.9 (37.7, 44.2)
Any developing country	6.0 (4.8, 7.5)	9.2 (7.4, 11.3)	16.8 (14.8, 19.1)	11.4 (9.7, 13.4)	35.1 (32.3, 38.0)
Any developed country	6.3 (5.6, 7.1)	18.5 (17.2, 19.9)	7.7 (6.8, 8.6)	10.6 (9.7, 11.7)	37.6 (35.9, 39.3)
All countries	6.2 (5.6, 6.9)	15.8 (14.7, 16.9)	10.3 (9.5, 11.3)	10.9 (10.0, 11.8)	36.9 (35.4, 38.3)

[a] Any physical disorder includes diabetes, COPD or asthma, heart disease, ulcers, cancer, epilepsy, HIV/AIDS, stroke, and tuberculosis.

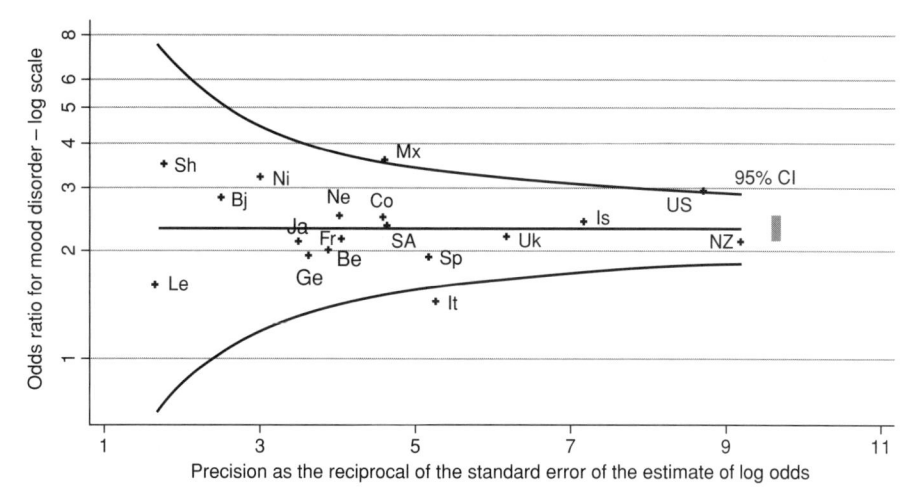

The Pattern and Nature of Mental–Physical Comorbidity

Figure A.5.1. Estimates of the odds ratios (age and sex adjusted) for any mood disorder for persons with versus without back/neck pain. (Be, Belgium; Bj, Beijing; Co, Colombia; Fr, France; Ge, Germany; Is, Israel; It, Italy; Ja, Japan; Le, Lebanon; Mx, Mexico; Ne, the Netherlands; Ni, Nigeria; NZ, New Zealand; SA, South Africa; Sh, Shaghai; Sp, Spain; Uk, Ukraine; US, the United States.)

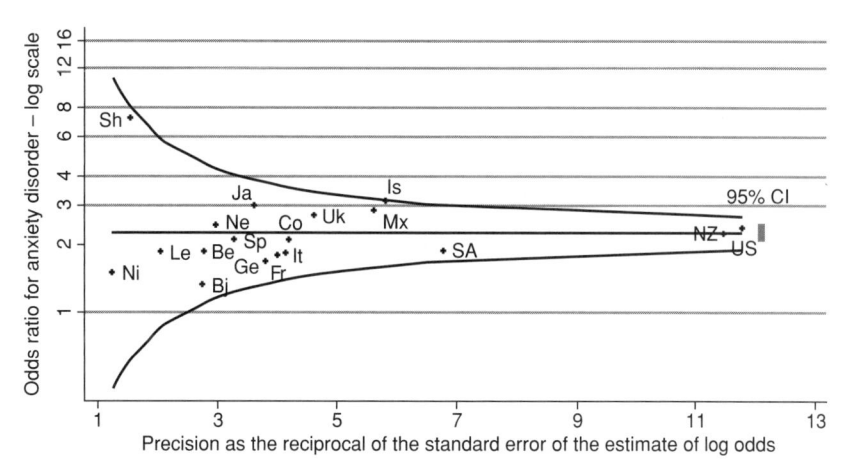

Figure A.5.2. Estimates of the odds ratios (age and sex adjusted) for any anxiety disorder for persons with versus without back/neck pain. (Be, Belgium; Bj, Beijing; Co, Colombia; Fr, France; Ge, Germany; Is, Israel; It, Italy; Ja, Japan; Le, Lebanon; Mx, Mexico; Ne, the Netherlands; Ni, Nigeria; NZ, New Zealand; SA, South Africa; Sh, Shaghai; Sp, Spain; Uk, Ukraine; US, the United States.)

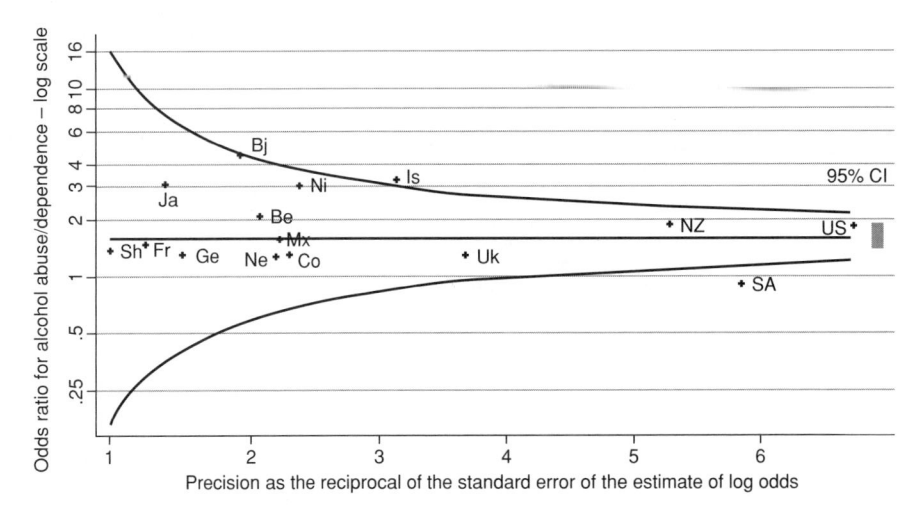

Figure A.5.3. Estimates of the odds ratios (age and sex adjusted) for alcohol-use/dependence disorders for persons with versus without back/neck pain. (Be, Belgium; Bj, Beijing; Co, Colombia; Fr, France; Ge, Germany; Is, Israel; Ja, Japan; Mx, Mexico; Ne, the Netherlands; Ni, Nigeria; NZ, New Zealand; SA, South Africa; Sh, Shaghai; Uk, Ukraine; US, the United States.)

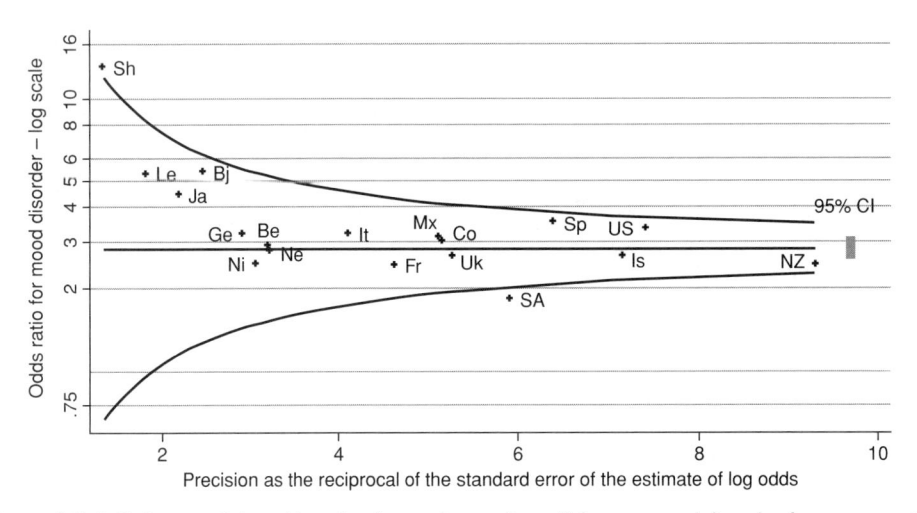

Figure A.5.4. Estimates of the odds ratios (age and sex adjusted) for any mood disorder for persons with versus without headache. (Be, Belgium; Bj, Beijing; Co, Colombia; Fr, France; Ge, Germany; Is, Israel; It, Italy; Ja, Japan; Le, Lebanon; Mx, Mexico; Ne, the Netherlands; Ni, Nigeria; NZ, New Zealand; SA, South Africa; Sh, Shaghai; Sp, Spain; Uk, Ukraine; US, the United States.)

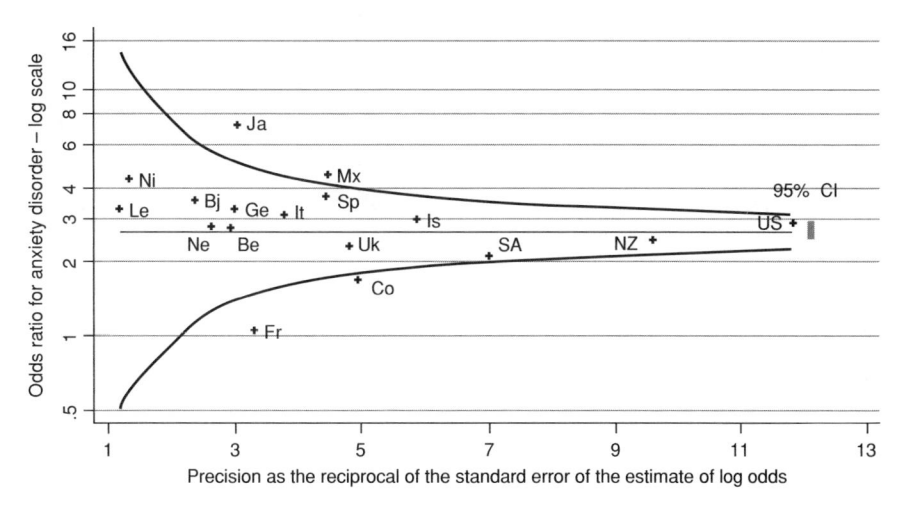

The Pattern and Nature of Mental–Physical Comorbidity

Figure A.5.5. Estimates of the odds ratios (age and sex adjusted) for any anxiety disorder for persons with versus without headache. (Be, Belgium; Bj, Beijing; Co, Colombia; Fr, France; Ge, Germany; Is, Israel; It, Italy; Ja, Japan; Le, Lebanon; Mx, Mexico; Ne, the Netherlands; Ni, Nigeria; NZ, New Zealand; SA, South Africa; Sp, Spain; Uk, Ukraine; US, the United States.)

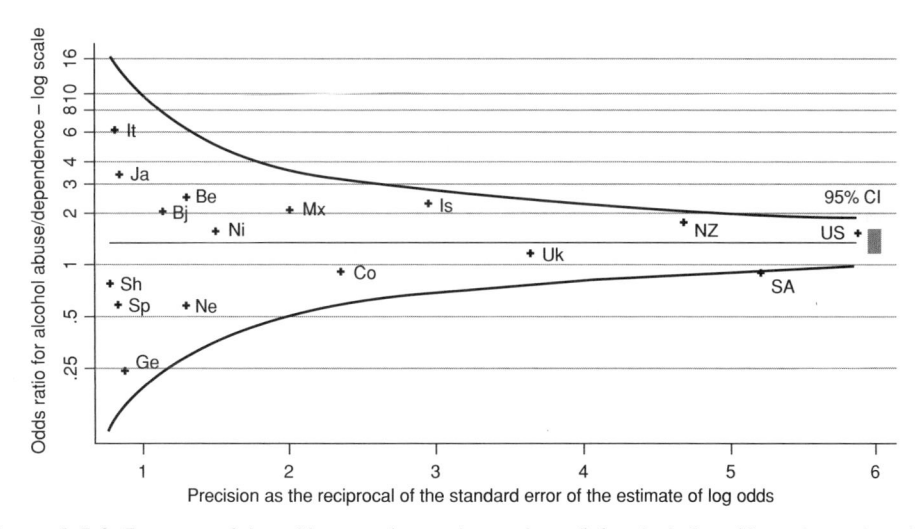

Figure A.5.6. Estimates of the odds ratios (age and sex adjusted) for alcohol-use/dependence disorders for persons with versus without headache. (Be, Belgium; Bj, Beijing; Co, Colombia; Ge, Germany; Is, Israel; It, Italy; Ja, Japan; Mx, Mexico; Ne, the Netherlands; Ni, Nigeria; NZ, New Zealand; SA, South Africa; Sh, Shaghai; Sp, Spain; Uk, Ukraine; US, the United States.)

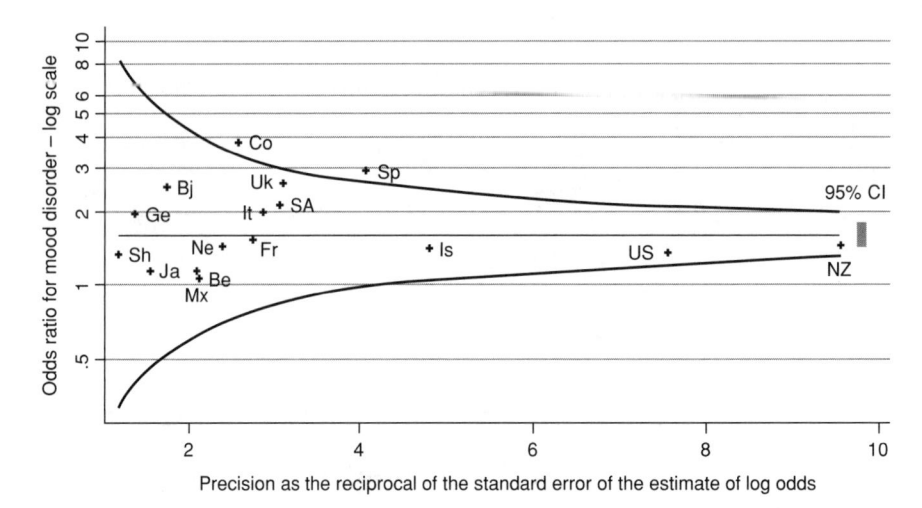

Figure A.5.7. Estimates of the odds ratios (age and sex adjusted) for any mood disorder for persons with versus without asthma. (Be, Belgium; Bj, Beijing; Co, Colombia; Fr, France; Ge, Germany; Is, Israel; It, Italy; Ja, Japan; Mx, Mexico; Ne, the Netherlands; NZ, New Zealand; SA, South Africa; Sh, Shaghai; Sp, Spain; Uk, Ukraine; US, the United States.)

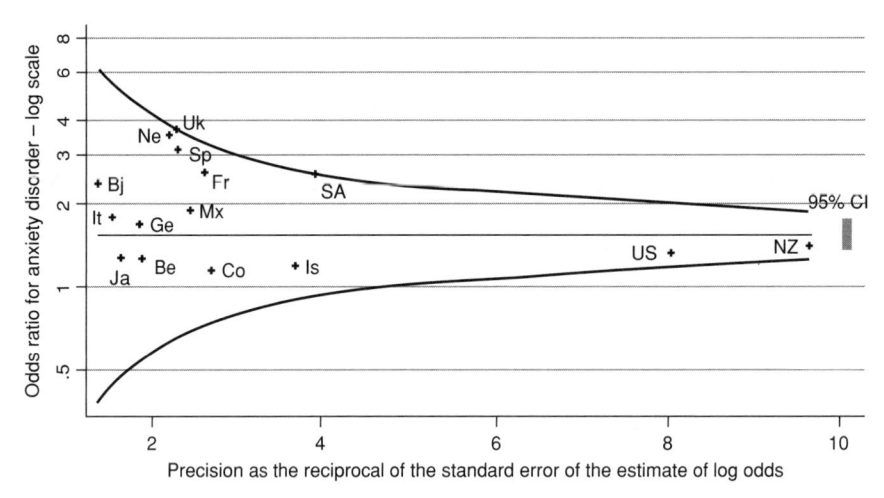

Figure A.5.8. Estimates of the odds ratios (age and sex adjusted) for any anxiety disorder for persons with versus without asthma. (Be, Belgium; Bj, Beijing; Co, Colombia; Fr, France; Ge, Germany; Is, Israel; It, Italy; Ja, Japan; Mx, Mexico; Ne, the Netherlands; Ni, Nigeria; NZ, New Zealand; SA, South Africa; Sp, Spain; Uk, Ukraine; US, the United States.)

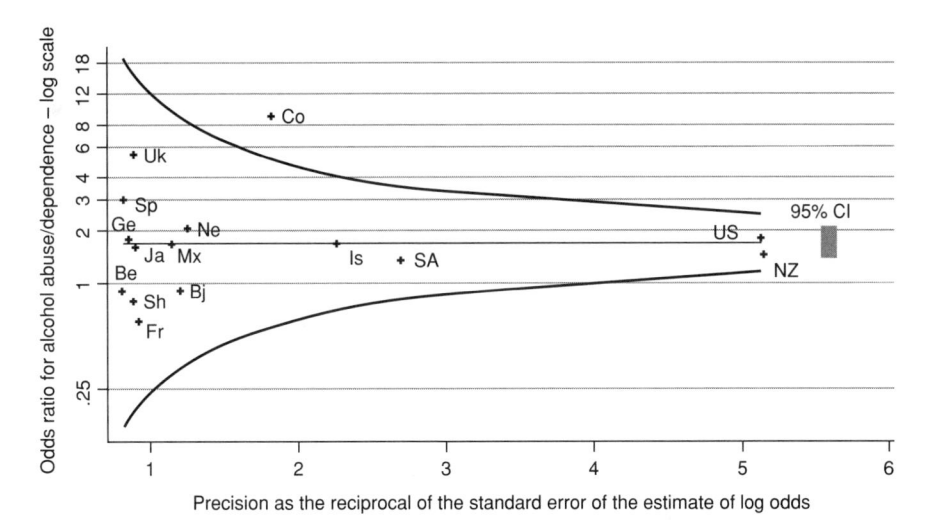

Figure A.5.9. Estimates of the odds ratios (age and sex adjusted) for alcohol-use/dependence disorders for persons with versus without asthma. (Be, Belgium; Bj, Beijing; Co, Colombia; Fr, France; Ge, Germany; Is, Israel; Ja, Japan; Mx, Mexico; Ne, the Netherlands; NZ, New Zealand; SA, South Africa; Sh, Shaghai; Sp, Spain; Uk, Ukraine; US, the United States.)

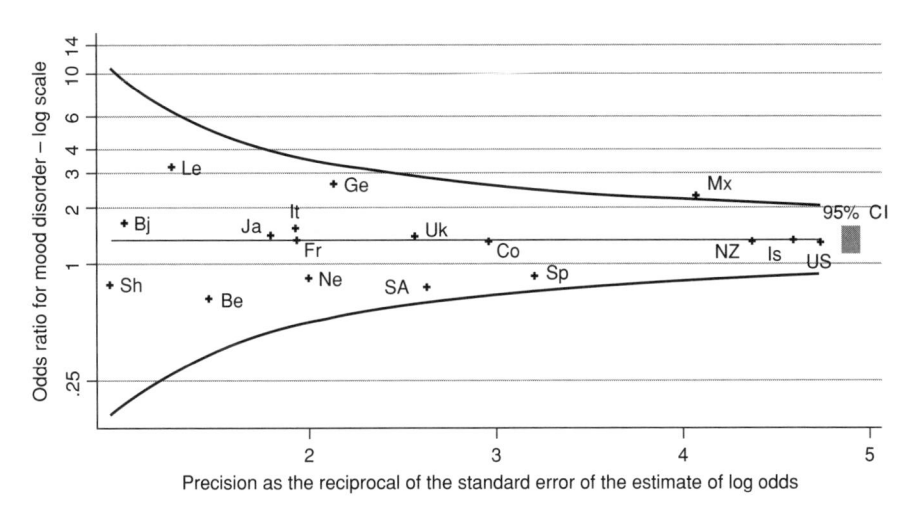

Figure A.5.10. Estimates of the odds ratios (age and sex adjusted) for any mood disorder for persons with versus without diabetes. (Be, Belgium; Bj, Beijing; Co, Colombia; Fr, France; Ge, Germany; Is, Israel; It, Italy; Ja, Japan; Le, Lebanon; Mx, Mexico; Ne, the Netherlands; NZ, New Zealand; SA, South Africa; Sh, Shaghai; Sp, Spain; Uk, Ukraine; US, the United States.)

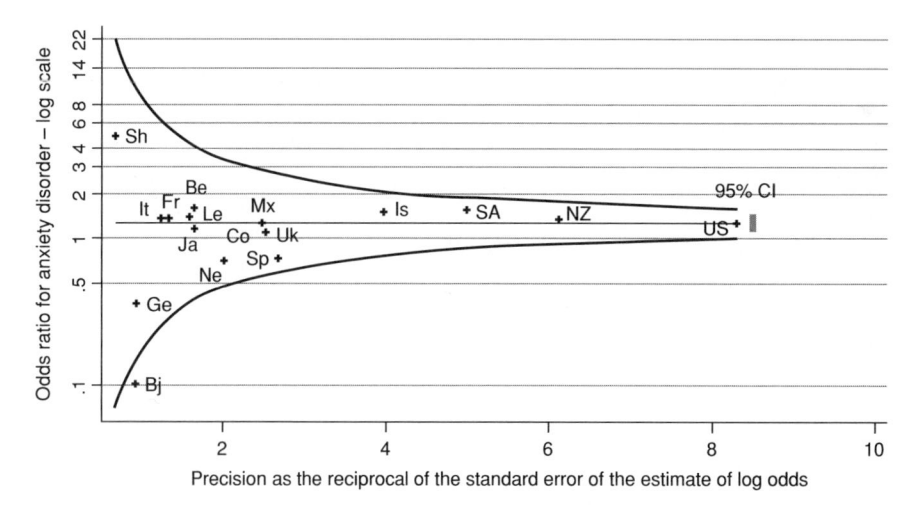

Figure A.5.11. Estimates of the odds ratios (age and sex adjusted) for any anxiety disorder for persons with versus without diabetes. (Be, Belgium; Bj, Beijing; Co, Colombia; Fr, France; Ge, Germany; Is, Israel; It, Italy; Ja, Japan; Le, Lebanon; Mx, Mexico; Ne, the Netherlands; NZ, New Zealand; SA, South Africa; Sh, Shaghai; Sp, Spain; Uk, Ukraine; US, the United States.)

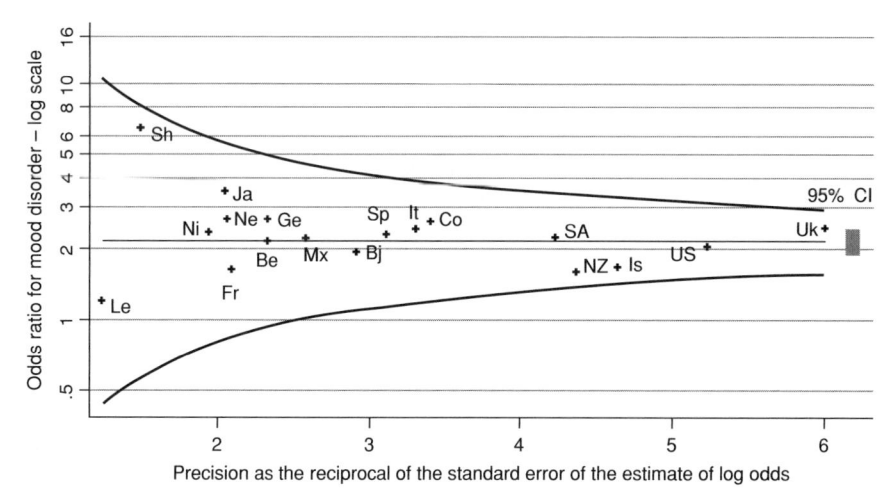

Figure A.5.12. Estimates of the odds ratios (age and sex adjusted) for any mood disorder for persons with versus without heart disease. (Be, Belgium; Bj, Beijing; Co, Colombia; Fr, France; Ge, Germany; Is, Israel; It, Italy; Ja, Japan; Le, Lebanon; Mx, Mexico; Ne, the Netherlands; Ni, Nigeria; NZ, New Zealand; SA, South Africa; Sh, Shaghai; Sp, Spain; Uk, Ukraine; US, the United States.)

The Pattern and Nature of Mental–Physical Comorbidity

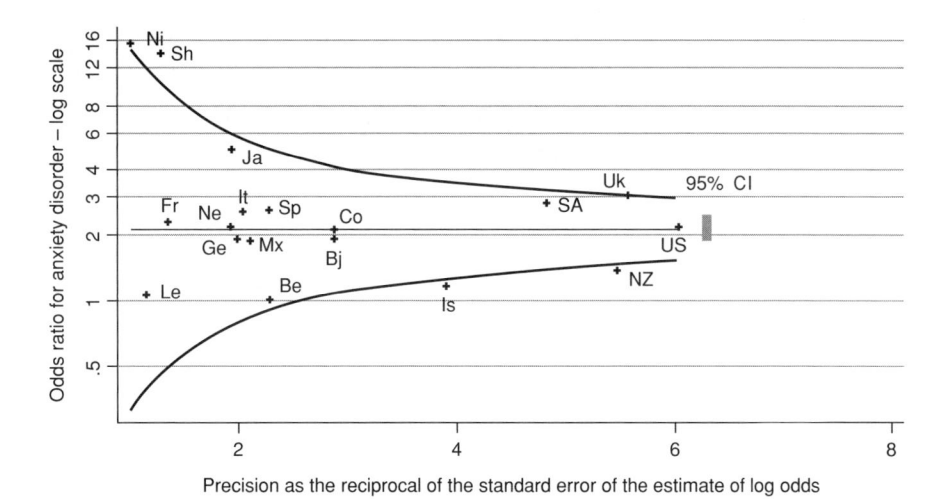

Figure A.5.13. Estimates of the odds ratios (age and sex adjusted) for any anxiety disorder for persons with versus without heart disease. (Be, Belgium; Bj, Beijing; Co, Colombia; Fr, France; Ge, Germany; Is, Israel; It, Italy; Ja, Japan; Le, Lebanon; Mx, Mexico; Ne, the Netherlands; Ni, Nigeria; NZ, New Zealand; SA, South Africa; Sh, Shaghai; Sp, Spain; Uk, Ukraine; US, the United States.)

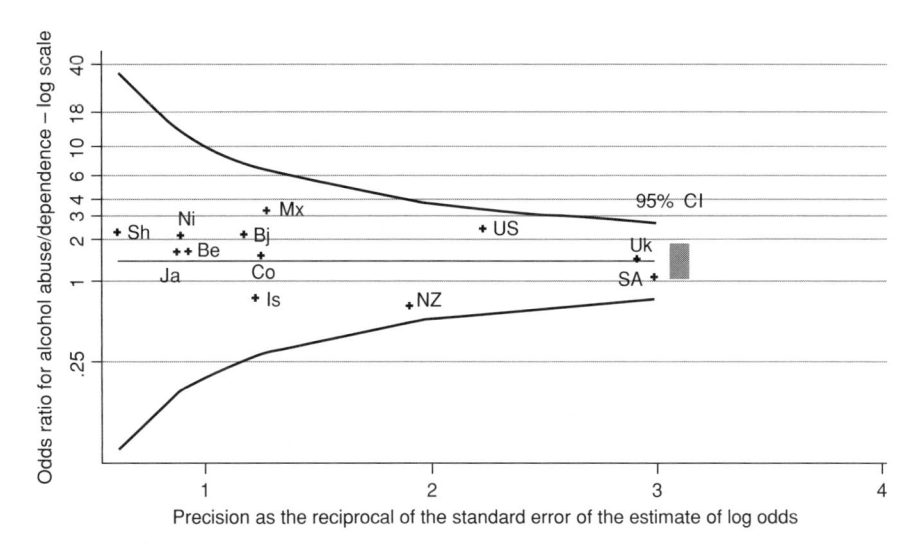

Figure A.5.14. Estimates of the odds ratios (age and sex adjusted) for alcohol-use/dependence disorders for persons with versus without heart disease. (Be, Belgium; Bj, Beijing; Co, Colombia; Is, Israel; Ja, Japan; Mx, Mexico; Ni, Nigeria; NZ, New Zealand; SA, South Africa; Sh, Shaghai; Uk, Ukraine; US, the United States.)

6 The Association of Age with Depressive and Anxiety Disorders, by Physical Comorbidity Status

KATE M. SCOTT

6.1. INTRODUCTION

One of the interesting questions in psychiatric epidemiology relates to what happens to the prevalence of mental disorders as we age – does it increase or decrease? From the perspective of the young, it often seems as if older age offers plenty to be despondent about, not least the increase in physical disease and disability. Interestingly though, many cross-sectional surveys of diagnosed mental disorders, including several of the World Mental Health (WMH) Surveys, have found a decrease in the prevalence of major depressive disorder (MDD) with increasing age (Alonso et al. 2004; Karel 1997; Kessler et al. 2003; Regier et al. 1988), and the picture for anxiety disorders is similar (Alonso et al. 2004; Jorm 2000).

Some researchers have been skeptical about these results, and methodological explanations have been sought. For example, the contribution of depression to premature mortality through suicide, and through its associated physical conditions such as cardiovascular disease, would reduce depression prevalence among older persons. There is also the fact that these surveys do not typically sample those living in institutions, which may bias the results (on the assumption that a greater proportion of older people live in institutions, and depression prevalence may be higher among the institutionalized). Another possibility is a cohort effect: the older groups in these surveys due to their different life experiences may have always had lower rates of mental disorder. That is, it might not be an age effect per se. With the exception of the cohort effects, however, most of these explanations are not thought to be sufficient to explain the age-related pattern (Hybels & Blazer 2002; Jorm 2000). As to whether the decrease in 12-month or 1-month depressive disorder with age is a cohort or age effect, there is probably insufficient evidence to draw conclusions about this (Jorm 2000), but it is notable that the same age-related decline in prevalence has now occurred in cross-national surveys conducted in the United States nearly a generation apart (Kessler et al. 2003; Regier et al. 1988). This is supportive of an age, rather than cohort explanation.

One methodological factor that does have a critical bearing on age patterns is whether researchers have used scale measures of depressive symptoms (e.g., the Centre for Epidemiologic Studies Depression Scale: CES-D) or structured/semistructured instruments that produce *Diagnostic and Statistical Manual of Mental Disorders, Fourth Edition* (DSM-IV), or International Classification of Mental and Behavioral Disorders (ICD-10), diagnoses of MDD. The WMH Surveys used the latter. Scale measures of depressive symptomatology often show an increase with age (Beekman et al. 1995; Hybels & Blazer 2002; Jorm 2000), though decreases (Henderson et al. 1998) and U-shaped patterns (Kessler et al. 1992; Newmann 1989) have also been observed. As illustration of the difference that the measurement of depression makes to estimates, the prevalence of "clinically significant depression" (measured by the CES-D and/or inclusive of subthreshold depression) among the >65 age group is generally in the range of 10–20% (Beekman et al. 1995; Snowdon 2001), compared with the prevalence of MDD, which is typically less than 3% (Alonso et al. 2004; Beekman et al. 1999; Troller et al. 2007; Wells, Golding, & Burnam 1989).

This contrast between the age patterning and prevalence estimates of CES-D depressive symptoms versus MDD has fueled suspicion about the validity of diagnostic criteria in older persons and their operationalization in standardized interviews such as the Composite International Diagnostic Interview (CIDI) (Beekman et al. 1995; Hybels & Blazer 2002; Mulsant & Ganguli 1999; O'Connor 2006; Snowdon 2001). It has been suggested that depression may manifest differently with age, with older people being more likely to report somatic symptoms and less likely to report required diagnostic symptoms of depressed mood and anhedonia (Christensen et al. 1999; Gallo, Anthony, & Muthén 1994; Hybels & Blazer 2002; Jorm 2000; Karel 1997). It has also been argued that the attribution of depressive symptoms to a comorbid physical condition increases with age independent of physical health status (Knäuper & Wittchen 1994), with the result that standardized diagnostic interviews may underdiagnose in older people because they exclude symptoms attributed to physical disease (Knäuper & Wittchen 1994; O'Connor 2006). Knäuper and Wittchen (1994) interpret their finding of increasing physical illness symptom attribution with age as a response to the complex stem questions and probing for physical causes for every depressive symptom in earlier versions of the CIDI. They suggest that changing the structure of the physical cause probe system so that it occurs after assessment of the complete depressive episode should address this problem. This change has been implemented in the version of the CIDI used in the surveys that form the basis of this report.

One of the few things that is not controversial about older age is that it is associated with an increase in the prevalence of chronic physical conditions. There is also substantial evidence that mental disorders are more common among persons with physical illness (Dew 1998; Evans et al. 2005; Harter, Conway, & Merikangas 2003; Scott et al. 2007; Wells et al. 1989). Moreover, longitudinal studies show that physical conditions are a potent risk factor for depression and anxiety onset (Brilman & Ormel 2001; Jordanova et al. 2007; Krishnan 2002; Schoevers et al. 2000). So, herein lies something of a paradox: an apparent decrease in diagnosed depression with increasing age, yet an undisputed increase in physical morbidity that is one of the key risk factors for mental disorders. To shed some light on this apparent anomaly we decided to disaggregate the age patterns in depressive and anxiety disorders into those with and without physical comorbidity. We hypothesized that we would see the usual decline in the prevalence of "noncomorbid" depression (without physical/pain condition comorbidity) with age. By contrast, we thought "comorbid" depression (with a comorbid chronic physical/pain condition) might in fact increase, or at least decrease less steeply, with age.

In this study based on 18 of the WMH Surveys we assessed whether there is an interaction of age with the presence of physical/pain condition comorbidity in the association with 12-month depressive or anxiety disorder, and we describe the association of age with 12-month mental disorders disaggregated into those with and without physical/pain condition comorbidity. The relative proportion of comorbid to noncomorbid depression in each age group was also determined. Relevant to the methodological issues raised earlier, we also show the percentage of depression cases excluded for organic (physical) causes in each age group. Our aims are thus both analytic and descriptive. Describing how mental–physical comorbidity varies across age groups in general population samples is important for guiding the work of both health care and mental health care professionals in appreciating the overall health problems of patients they treat.

6.2. APPROACH

6.2.1. Mental Disorder Status

This study included 12-month anxiety disorders (generalized anxiety disorder, panic disorder and/or agoraphobia, posttraumatic stress disorder, and social phobia) and depressive disorders (dysthymia and major depressive disorder). Anxiety and depressive disorders were aggregated into a single category on the basis of other findings from the WMH Surveys that anxiety and depressive disorders have equal and independent relationships with a wide range of chronic physical conditions (Scott et al. 2007).

CIDI organic exclusion rules were imposed for diagnoses of major depressive disorder and panic disorder. The probe for physical illness was applied at the episode level (i.e., after all individual symptom questions had been asked). Respondents were asked whether they considered that their episode of symptoms was *ever* "the result of physical causes such as physical illness or injury or the use of medication, drugs or alcohol." If they responded in the affirmative, they were then asked whether their episode was *always* the result of physical causes. If they responded in the affirmative again, they were asked to specify the causes that were recorded as open text. In all countries, a mental health clinician subsequently evaluated the open text responses and coded them as a legitimate organic exclusion. An episode of MDD was excluded on organic grounds only if the respondents indicated that their episodes were *always* due to physical causes and if the clinician coded them as legitimate organic exclusions. The percent of MDD episodes excluded as organic, by age group, for all countries combined was 4.4% (18–34 years), 6.6% (35–49 years), 8.0% (50–64 years), 8.9% (65–79 years), and 11.1% (>80 years).

6.2.2. Chronic Physical Conditions

For the analyses reported here, the "physical conditions" were aggregated and included stroke, heart attack, heart disease, asthma, chronic obstructive pulmonary disease (COPD), diabetes, ulcer, HIV/AIDS, epilepsy, tuberculosis, and cancer. The "pain conditions" were also aggregated and included arthritis, chronic back/neck problems, frequent or severe headaches, and other chronic pain.

Prevalence was estimated for four groups, those with (1) a 12-month depressive and/or anxiety disorder with a comorbid pain condition, (2) a 12-month depressive and/or anxiety disorder with a comorbid physical condition, (3) a 12-month depressive and/or anxiety disorder without a comorbid physical or pain condition, (4) a physical and/or pain condition without comorbid depressive and/or anxiety disorder. Groups (1) and (2) are not mutually exclusive. Group (4) is included to provide context for the mental disorder estimates.

Odds ratios for the association of age (reference level 18–34 years) with 12-month depressive and/or anxiety disorder were calculated for all countries combined, in logistic regression models controlling for gender. The interaction of age with physical/pain condition comorbidity (present vs. absent) in predicting 12-month depressive and/or anxiety disorder was assessed in a logistic

The Association of Age with Depressive and Anxiety Disorders

Table 6.1. Percent in the four mental and/or physical condition groups in each country

	% (95% CI)			
WMH country	Physical and/or pain condition (without depressive/anxiety disorders)	Depressive/anxiety disorders with pain condition	Depressive/anxiety disorders with physical condition	Depressive/anxiety disorders (without physical/pain condition)
Colombia	32.1 (29.3, 34.9)	4.8 (3.9, 5.8)	3.1 (2.4, 4.1)	4.4 (3.6, 5.4)
Mexico	27.7 (24.4, 31.3)	3.6 (2.9, 4.3)	1.3 (1.0, 1.7)	2.9 (2.4, 3.5)
United States	44.2 (42.4, 45.9)	10.3 (9.4, 11.3)	7.2 (6.5, 8.0)	5.1 (4.6, 5.8)
Japan	43.1 (37.7, 48.7)	1.7 (1.1, 2.5)	1.4 (0.9, 2.2)	1.7 (1.2, 2.3)
Beijing	41.7 (37.2, 46.3)	2.2 (1.5, 3.2)	1.0 (0.6, 1.6)	1.2 (0.7, 2.2)
Shanghai	46.0 (40.8, 51.3)	1.6 (0.8, 3.1)	1.2 (0.4, 3.4)	0.6 (0.2, 1.4)
New Zealand	45.4 (43.6, 47.3)	7.0 (6.4, 7.7)	5.2 (4.6, 5.7)	5.0 (4.5, 5.5)
Belgium	46.1 (42.5, 49.8)	4.9 (3.6, 6.7)	2.6 (1.8, 3.8)	2.9 (2.0, 4.3)
France	50.6 (46.1, 55.1)	7.2 (5.8, 8.8)	3.6 (2.8, 4.6)	3.3 (2.3, 4.7)
Germany	41.1 (37.9, 44.5)	2.9 (2.2, 3.9)	1.6 (1.2, 2.2)	2.2 (1.6, 2.9)
Italy	47.5 (44.3, 50.6)	3.4 (2.8, 4.2)	1.7 (1.3, 2.4)	1.6 (1.2, 2.2)
The Netherlands	39.4 (34.8, 44.2)	5.1 (3.9, 6.7)	3.8 (2.5, 5.5)	2.9 (1.9, 4.5)
Spain	41.3 (38.6, 44.1)	3.1 (2.5, 3.8)	1.5 (1.2, 1.9)	2.3 (1.8, 2.9)
Ukraine	54.0 (50.8, 57.2)	11.9 (10.1, 13.9)	7.9 (6.6, 9.5)	1.9 (1.2, 3.1)
Lebanon	30.3 (26.0, 35.1)	2.2 (1.4, 3.6)	0.6 (0.2, 1.6)	1.8 (0.9, 3.7)
Nigeria	33.0 (30.3, 35.9)	0.7 (0.5, 1.1)	0.3 (0.2, 0.7)	0.8 (0.4, 1.5)
Israel	41.7 (40.3, 43.1)	5.1 (4.4, 5.8)	3.5 (3.0, 4.1)	2.6 (2.2, 3.1)
South Africa	45.9 (43.2, 48.5)	7.7 (6.8, 8.7)	4.2 (3.5, 4.9)	3.4 (2.6, 4.5)

regression model on the pooled data set, controlling for gender.

A separate set of analyses using those with a 12-month depressive and/or anxiety disorder (i.e., cases) as denominator calculated the percent with a comorbid physical and/or pain condition, by age group, for all countries combined. All analyses were run with SUDAAN software (Research Triangle Institute 2002) to adjust for clustering and weighting.

6.3. FINDINGS

6.3.1. Prevalence of Mental and/or Physical Condition Groups

The percent with each of the four combinations of mental and/or physical conditions for each country is given in Table 6.1. Quite a lot of variability is apparent across individual surveys, but despite this variability, there is a pattern of mental disorder being more prevalent with pain/physical condition comorbidity than without it. Physical/pain conditions unaccompanied by mental comorbidity are a good deal more prevalent than when accompanied by mental comorbidity, in all countries.

6.3.2. Mental and/or Physical Condition Groups by Age

6.3.2.1. Prevalence by Age

The age patterns in the prevalence of the four mental and/or physical condition combinations are depicted in Figure 6.1. The prevalence of depressive and/or anxiety disorders in the absence of physical/pain condition comorbidity decreases with age. By contrast,

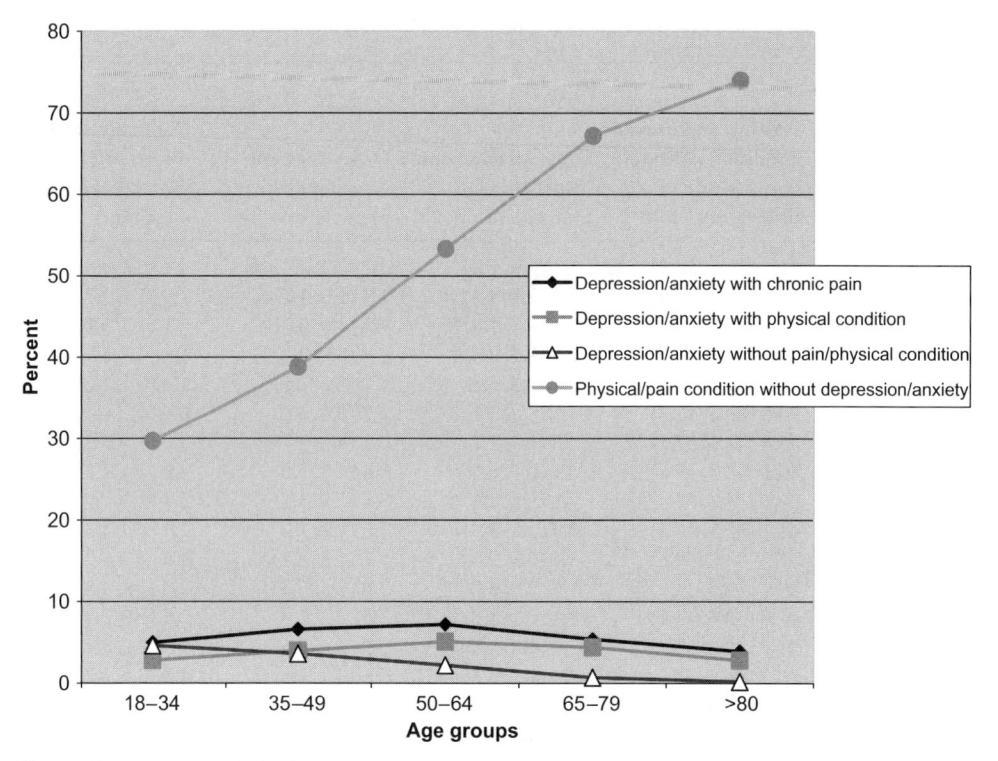

Figure 6.1. Percent with the four mental and/or physical condition combinations, by age group, all countries combined ($n = 42{,}697$).

the prevalence of physical/pain conditions in the absence of depressive and anxiety disorder increases sharply with age. The two mental–physical comorbidity groups display a similar age-related pattern of prevalence climbing slightly from younger to middle age and then reducing somewhat in the older groups.

6.3.2.2. Association of Age with Mental Disorders by Physical Comorbidity Status

The association of age with depression/anxiety (with and without physical/pain condition comorbidity), and with physical or pain condition without depression/anxiety comorbidity, is shown in Table 6.2. These data clarify the age curves shown in Figure 6.1, without the distraction of the differing prevalences across the four groups. The greatest change across the life span occurs in the decreasing odds ratio of depressive or anxiety disorder without physical/pain condition comorbidity. The two mental–physical comorbid groups show slightly different patterns in which the odds ratio of mental disorder comorbid with pain are the same in the 65–79 age group as the youngest group, but the odds ratios of mental disorder comorbid with physical condition are higher in the 65–79 age group compared to the youngest group. But all types of mental disorders (with or without comorbidity) decline in the oldest age group. The lack of substantive difference between the mental disorder groups in age patterns is confirmed in finding that the interaction of age and physical disorder comorbidity (present vs. absent) in the association with 12-month depressive or anxiety disorder was not significant ($p = .40$).

Table 6.2. Association of age (reference level 18–34 years) with 12-month mental disorders by physical/pain comorbidity status, and with physical/pain conditions in the absence of mental disorder, controlling for gender, all countries combined (n = 42,697)

Age groups in years (N)	Depressive/anxiety disorder with pain condition[a]	Depressive/anxiety disorder with physical condition[a]	Depressive/anxiety disorder without physical/pain condition[a]	Physical and/or pain condition without depressive/anxiety disorder[a]
18–34 (14,818)	1.0	1.0	1.0	1.0
35–49 (13,236)	1.3 (1.2, 1.5)*	1.4 (1.3, 1.6)*	0.8 (0.7, 0.9)*	1.5 (1.4, 1.6)*
50–64 (9,006)	1.5 (1.3, 1.6)*	1.9 (1.6, 2.2)*	0.5 (0.4, 0.5)*	2.7 (2.7, 2.9)*
65–79 (4,631)	1.0 (0.9, 1.2)	1.6 (1.3, 1.8)*	0.2 (0.1, 0.2)*	4.8 (4.4, 5.3)*
>80 (959)	0.7 (0.5, 1.0)*	0.9 (0.6, 1.3)	0.0 (0.0, 0.1)*	6.6 (5.5, 8.0)*

[a] Twelve-month DSM-IV depressive and/or anxiety disorders; *physical conditions* included stroke, heart attack, heart disease, asthma, COPD, diabetes, ulcer, HIV/AIDS, epilepsy, tuberculosis, and cancer; *pain conditions* included arthritis, 12-month chronic back/neck problems, 12-month frequent or severe headaches, and/or other 12-month chronic pain.
OR, odds ratio; CI, confidence interval.
* $p < .05$.

6.3.2.3. Proportion of Mental Disorder Cases with Physical/Pain Condition Comorbidity, by Age

The first column of Table 6.3 shows that mental disorders in the aggregate – that is, both with and without physical/pain condition comorbidity – decline in prevalence with age (Table 6.3). The second column shows the proportion of mental disorder cases with physical/pain condition comorbidity. This is greater than 50% at all ages, increases in a monotonic fashion with age, and comprises the vast majority of the oldest age group with mental disorders (Table 6.3).

6.4. DISCUSSION

When mental disorders were decomposed into those with versus without physical/pain condition comorbidity we found that those without comorbidity decreased monotonically with age, while those with comorbidity peaked in the middle years and then decreased in older age. Despite these apparent differences in age patterning, however, there was no significant difference in the relationship between mental disorders and age as a function of physical/pain condition comorbidity. In the aggregate, depressive and anxiety disorders decreased with age. It was also found that the overlap of mental and physical conditions was asymmetrical: among those with mental disorders, physical/pain condition comorbidity was more common than not, at all ages, and rises with age. By contrast, physical/pain conditions were more likely to occur without mental comorbidity than with it, at all ages.

These results are consistent with other general population surveys using standardized diagnostic measures in showing lower prevalences of depressive and anxiety disorders in older age groups relative to younger age groups. One issue that needs to be considered is whether the fact that we have sampled from the noninstitutionalized population, and effectively, given the demands of the CIDI, from a cognitively intact population, has been influential in producing this

Table 6.3. Percent with any 12-month depressive/anxiety disorder (cases), and proportion of cases with physical/pain condition comorbidity, by age group, all countries combined ($n = 42,697$)

Age groups in years (N)	Percent with any 12-month depressive/anxiety disorder[a] (%) (95% CI)	Proportion of cases (those with any 12-month depressive/anxiety disorder) with physical/pain condition comorbidity[a] (%)
18–34 (14,818)	10.7 (10.2, 11.3)	56.9
35–49 (13,236)	11.4 (10.8, 12.0)	68.6
50–64 (9,006)	10.4 (9.7, 11.1)	78.9
65–79 (4,631)	6.8 (6.1, 7.5)	89.2
>80 (959)	4.5 (3.5, 5.9)	95.3

[a] Twelve-month DSM-IV depressive and/or anxiety disorders; *physical conditions* included stroke, heart attack, heart disease, asthma, COPD, diabetes, ulcer, HIV/AIDS, epilepsy, tuberculosis, and cancer; *pain conditions* included arthritis, 12-month chronic back/neck problems, 12-month frequent or severe headaches, and/or other 12-month chronic pain.
CI, confidence interval.

age pattern. We think not. U.S. data indicate that rates of institutionalization are fairly low among those 65–79 years who form the majority of the older population (3% in those 65–69; 5% in those 70–74; 7% in those 75–79) (Siegler et al. 2002), and similar figures have been quoted for Australia (Troller et al. 2007). Troller et al. (2007) have calculated that inclusion of those living in aged-care facilities would have minimal impact on mental disorder prevalence among those 65 years and older. They also show that prevalence estimates of depression among older persons are unaffected whether those with mild cognitive impairment are included or excluded from analysis.

The next important methodological issue to consider is whether the application of organic exclusion criteria can explain the decline in mental disorder prevalence with age. Again, this seems unlikely. First, because the probes for organic causes were applied at the episode, not symptom, level, thus obviating the possibility that older persons would use organic attribution to deal with symptom-related probes (Knäuper & Wittchen 1994). Granted, it is still possible that older persons may be more likely to attribute entire episodes to organic causes (independent of actual health status), but at present we are not aware of evidence that this occurs, and in each of the WMH Surveys mental health clinicians judged the legitimacy of all such attributions. Second, although the data we present on the rates of organic exclusions show a clear increase with age, the proportion of cases excluded for organic causes is not high enough to explain the decline in mental disorder prevalence with age. For example, if the excluded cases were all reincluded, estimates of mental disorder in the youngest and oldest age groups would rise to 11.2 and 5.0%, respectively, compared with estimates of 10.7 and 4.5% with organic exclusions applied (and in fact this would be an overestimate of the impact of organic exclusions since the mental disorder estimates in this chapter combine depressive and anxiety disorders). Heithoff (1995) showed a similar result with Epidemiologic Catchment Area (ECA) data.

What we cannot rule out is the possibility that depression may manifest differently with age, which might mean that the declining prevalence we observe is an artifact of the fact that DSM-IV criteria become less valid with increasing age. The research on this is not consistent. Gallo et al. (1994), for example, find a negative association between age and reports of anhedonia, while Christensen et al. (1999) find the opposite (see also Karel 1997). A further consideration is the fact that these criticisms of diagnostic validity on the grounds of age differences in symptom manifestation and symptom attribution apply largely to depression diagnoses, yet anxiety disorders show the same decline with age (Alsonso et al. 2004; Troller et al. 2007; Wells et al. 1989). Nevertheless, it is also clear that fully structured lay-conducted interviews such as the CIDI produce considerably lower estimates of DSM-based depressive disorders among older populations than do semistructured interviews conducted by clinicians (Skoog 2004). The source of this discrepancy in prevalence, and its implications for conclusions about the validity of either the fully structured or semistructured interviews, remains to be clarified.

In sum, we find that despite the extremely prevalent reports of chronic pain/physical conditions among older age groups, the vast majority in the older general population do not have CIDI-diagnosed mental disorders. Methodological explanations notwithstanding, there are possible substantive explanations for this also, including age-related changes in expectations of declining health status (Karel 1997; Siegler et al. 2002). Another possibility is that if, as some researchers have speculated, older persons have greater psychological resources that reduce their vulnerability to depression (Blazer & Hybels 2005; Henderson et al. 1998; Karel 1997), these resources may also increase their ability to cope with the increased prevalence of physical illness. British researchers observing a sharp decrease in the prevalence of depressive and anxiety disorders at retirement age (Villamil, Huppert, & Melzer 2006) have suggested that it may be explained by reducing societal demands and expectations associated with the statutory retirement age. This cannot explain all of the decrease in mental disorder prevalence observed in the current report, as it continues to reduce in the >80 years age group relative to the 65–79 year age group (see also Troller et al. 2007), but different factors may be responsible for decreasing mental disorder prevalence at different ages, and retirement may well be an important factor in the younger old, which helps offset the psychological impact of increasing physical morbidity.

A less optimistic picture emerges when we consider the population with mental disorders though: physical condition comorbidity is the rule, not the exception, regardless of age. Past research has emphasized the need for improved detection and treatment of mental disorders in primary care (Coyne et al. 2002; Katon et al. 1992; Ormel et al. 1991). The present study highlights the need for health professionals, including mental health professionals, to address barriers to adequately manage physical comorbidity among those with mental disorders. Research among mental health professionals has identified barriers such as a lack of explicit allocation of responsibility for medical treatment, lack of service delivery integration, and pessimistic attitudes among treatment providers as to whether improved physical health is possible, or a priority, among those with mental illness (Brown, Inskip, & Barraclough 2000; Friedli & Dardis 2002; Hyland et al. 2003). Further research among primary care providers and hospital physicians may be warranted to identify whether there are barriers (e.g., attitudinal or time pressure) to a treatment focus on physical morbidity once a mental disorder has been diagnosed.

Several limitations of this study must be noted in addition to the sampling limitations already discussed. First, physical/pain conditions were ascertained by a standard checklist, rather than physician's examination, which contrasts with the detailed assessment of mental disorders. While acknowledging the limitation of self-report, methods research indicates that self-report of diagnosis (which was the measure for most of the physical conditions) generally shows good agreement with medical records data (Kehoe et al. 1994; Kriegsman et al. 1996; National Center for Health Statistics 1994). A second related issue is that the relative prevalence of mental and physical conditions observed here and their degree of overlap are influenced by which disorders we have chosen to include or exclude. Not all mental disorders were included, though we included most of the common disorders and those most closely associated with physical comorbidity. We also grouped together a larger number of physical/pain conditions. While this needs to be borne in mind when interpreting the results, it seems likely that the kind of asymmetry we observe here (a lower proportion of the population with physical conditions having mental disorder comorbidity relative to the proportion of the population with mental disorders who have physical comorbidity) is characteristic of general populations. Third, we have not included any data on disability, so although on a pure frequency basis it appears as if physical morbidity outweighs mental morbidity in older populations, this does not take into account the complicating and disabling contribution that depression makes to the morbidity of medical conditions (Buist-Bouwman et al. 2005; Kessler et al. 2003; Scott et al. 2009; Chapter 19).

In conclusion, this study provides a global population perspective on the age patterning of CIDI-diagnosed depressive and anxiety disorders, for the first time disaggregated into those with and without physical/pain condition comorbidity. No significant difference was found in the relationship between mental disorders and age as a function of physical/pain condition comorbidity. In the aggregate, depressive and anxiety disorders decreased with age, a result that cannot be explained by organic exclusion criteria. Physical/pain condition comorbidity among those with mental disorders is normative and increases with age.

ACKNOWLEDGMENT

Some material in this chapter appeared in Scott et al. (2008). This material is reprinted with the permission of *Psychological Medicine*.

REFERENCES

Alonso, J., Angermeyer, M. C., Bernert, S., Bruffaerts, R., Brugha, T. S., Bryson, H., de Girolamo, G., Graaf, R., Demyttenaere, K., Gasquet, I., Haro, J. M., Katz, S. J., Kessler, R. C., Kovess, V., Lépine J. P., Ormel, J., Polidori, G., Russo, L. J., Vilagut, G., Almansa, J., Arbabzadeh-Bouchez, S., Autonell, J., Bernal, M., Buist-Bouwman, M. A., Codony, M., Domingo-Salvany, A., Ferrer, M., Joo, S. S., Martínez-Alonso, M., Matschinger, H., Mazzi, F., Morgan, Z., Morosini, P., Palacín, C., Romera, B., Taub, N., & Vollebergh, W. A. (2004). Prevalence of mental disorders in Europe: Results from the European Study of the Epidemiology of Mental Disorders (ESEMeD) project. *Acta Psychiatrica Scandinavica Supplementum*, **420**, 21–7.

Beekman, A. T. F., Copeland, J. R. M., & Prince, M. J. (1999). Review of community prevalence of depression in later life. *British Journal of Psychiatry*, **174**, 307–11.

Beekman, A. T. F., Deeg, D. J. H., Van Tilburg, T., Smit, J. H., Hooijer, C., & Van Tilburg, W. (1995). Major and minor depression in later life: A study of prevalence and risk factors. *Journal of Affective Disorders*, **36**, 65–75.

Blazer, D. G., & Hybels, C. F. (2005). Origins of depression in later life. *Psychological Medicine*, **35**, 1241–52.

Brilman, E., & Ormel, J. (2001). Life events, difficulties and onset of depressive episodes in later life. *Psychological Medicine*, **31**, 859–69.

Brown, S., Inskip, H., & Barraclough, B. (2000). Causes of the excess mortality of schizophrenia. *British Journal of Psychiatry*, **177**, 212–17.

Buist-Bouwman, M. A., de Graaf, R., Vollebergh, W. A. M., & Ormel, J. (2005). Comorbidity of physical and mental disorders and the effect on work-loss days. *Acta Psychiatrica Scandinavica*, **111**, 436–43.

Christensen, H., Jorm, A. F., Mackinnon, A. J., Korten, A. E., Jacomb, P. A., Henderson, A. S., & Rodgers, B. (1999). Age differences in depression and anxiety symptoms: A structural equation modeling analysis of data from a general population sample. *Psychological Medicine*, **29**, 325–39.

Coyne, J. C., Thompson, R., Klinkman, M. S., & Nease, D. E., Jr. (2002). Emotional disorders in primary care. *Journal of Consulting & Clinical Psychology*, **70**, 798–809.

Dew, M. A. (1998). Psychiatric disorder in the context of physical illness. In *Adversity, Stress and Psychopathology*, ed. B. P. Dohrenwend, pp. 177–218. New York: Oxford University Press.

Evans, D. L., Charney, D. S., Lewis, L., Golden, R. N., Gorman, J. M., Krishnan, K. R., Nemeroff, C. B., Bremner, J. D., Carney, R. M., Coyne, J. C., Delong, M. R., Frasure-Smith, N., Glassman, A. H., Gold, P. W., Grant, I., Gwyther, L., Ironson, G., Johnson, R. L., Kanner, A. M., Katon, W. J., Kaufmann, P. G., Keefe, F. J., Ketter, T., Laughren, T. P., Leserman, J., Lyketsos, C. G., McDonald, W. M., McEwen, B. S., Miller, A. H., Musselman, D., O'Connor, C., Petitto, J. M., Pollock, B. G., Robinson, R. G., Roose, S. P., Rowland, J., Sheline, Y., Sheps, D. S., Simon, G., Spiegel, D., Stunkard, A., Sunderland, T., Tibbits, P., Jr., & Valvo, W. J. (2005). Mood disorders in the medically ill: Scientific review and recommendations. *Biological Psychiatry*, **58**, 175–89.

Friedli, L., & Dardis, C. (2002). Not all in the mind: Mental health service user perspectives on physical health. *Journal of Mental Health Promotion*, **1**, 36–46.

Gallo, J. J., Anthony, J. C., & Muthén, B. O. (1994). Age differences in the symptoms of depression: A latent trait analysis. *Journal of Gerontology*, **49**, 251–64.

Harter, M. C., Conway, K. P., & Merikangas, K. R. (2003). Associations between anxiety disorders and physical illness. *European Archives of Psychiatry & Clinical Neuroscience*, **253**, 313–20.

Heitoff, K. (1995). Does the ECA underestimate the prevalence of late-life depression? *Journal of the American Geriatric Society*, **43**, 2–6.

Henderson, A. S., Jorm, A. F., Korten, A., Jacomb, P., Christensen, H., & Rodgers, B. (1998). Symptoms of depression and anxiety during adult life: Evidence of a decline in prevalence with age. *Psychological Medicine*, **28**, 1321–8.

Hybels, C. F., & Blazer, D. (2002). Epidemiology and geriatric psychiatry. In *Textbook in Psychiatric Epidemiology*, ed. M. T. Tsuang & M. Tohen, pp. 603–28. New York: Wiley-Liss Inc.

Hyland, B., Judd, F., Davidson, S., Jolley, D., & Hocking, B. (2003). Case managers' attitudes to the physical health of their patients. *Australian and New Zealand Journal of Psychiatry*, **37**, 710–14.

Jordanova, V., Stewart, R., Goldberg, D., Bebbington, P., Brugha, T., Singleton, N., Lindesay, J. E., Jenkins, R., Prince, M., & Meltzer, H. (2007). Age variation in life events and their relationship with common mental disorders in a national survey population. *Social Psychiatry & Psychiatric Epidemiology*, **42**, 611–16.

Jorm, A. F. (2000). Does old age reduce the risk of anxiety and depression? A review of epidemiological studies across the adult life span. *Psychological Medicine*, **30**, 11–22.

Karel, M. J. (1997). Aging and depression: Vulnerability and stress across adulthood. *Clinical Psychology Review*, **17**, 847–79.

Katon, W., Von Korff, M., Lin, E., Bush, T., & Ormel, J. (1992). Adequacy and duration of antidepressant treatment in primary care. *Medical Care*, **30**, 67–76.

Kehoe, R., Wu, S. Y., Leske, M. C., & Chylack, L. T. (1994). Comparing self-reported and physician reported medical history. *American Journal of Epidemiology*, **139**, 813–18.

Kessler, R. C., Berglund, P., Demler, O., Jin, R., Koretz, D., Merikangas, K. R., Rush, A. J., Walters, E. E., & Wang, P. S. (2003). The epidemiology of major depressive disorder: Results from the National Comorbidity Survey Replication (NCS-R). *The Journal of the American Medical Association*, **289**, 3095–4105.

Kessler, R. C., Foster, C., Webster, P. S., & House, J. S. (1992). The relationship between age and depressive symptoms in two national surveys. *Psychology and Aging*, **7**, 119–26.

Knäuper, B., & Wittchen, H.-U. (1994). Diagnosing major depression in the elderly: evidence for response bias in standardized diagnostic interviews? *Journal of Psychiatry Research*, **28**, 147–64.

Kriegsman, D. M., Penninx, B. W., Van Eijk, J. T., Boeke, A. J., & Deeg, D. J. (1996). Self-reports and general practitioner information on the presence of chronic diseases in community dwelling elderly. *Journal of Clinical Epidemiology*, **49**, 1407–17.

Krishnan, K. R. R. (2002). Biological risk factors in late life depression. *Biological Psychiatry*, **52**, 185–92.

Mulsant, B.H., & Ganguli, M. (1999). Epidemiology and diagnosis of depression in late life. *Journal of Clinical Psychiatry*, **60**(suppl 20), 9–15.

National Center for Health Statistics. (1994). Evaluation of National Health Interview Survey diagnostic reporting. *Vital and Health Statistics 2*, **120**, 1–116.

Newman, J. P. (1989). Aging and depression. *Psychology and Aging*, **4**, 150–65.

O'Connor, D. W. (2006). Do older Australians truly have low rates of anxiety and depression? A critique of the 1997 National Survey of Mental Health and Wellbeing. *Australian and New Zealand Journal of Psychiatry*, **40**, 623–31.

Ormel, J., Koeter, M., Van Den Brink, W., & van de Willige, G. (1991). Recognition, management and course of anxiety and depression in general practice. *Archives of General Psychiatry*, **48**, 700–6.

Regier, D. A., Boyd, J. H., Burke, J. D. J., Rae, D. S., Myers, J. K., Kramer, M., Robins, L. N., George, L. K., Karno, M., & Locke, B. Z. (1988). One-month prevalence of mental disorders in the United States. *Archives of General Psychiatry*, **45**, 977–86.

Research Triangle Institute. (2002). *SUDAAN: Professional Software for Survey Data Analysis Version 8.0.1*. North Carolina: Research Triangle Institute.

Schoevers, R. A., Beekman, A. T. F., Deeg, D. J., Geerlings, M. I., Jonker, C., & Van Tilburg, W. (2000). Risk factors for depression in later life: Results of a prospective community based study (AMSTEL). *Journal of Affective Disorders*, **59**, 127–37.

Scott, K. M., Bruffaerts, R., Tsang, A., Ormel, J., Alonso, J., Angermeyer, M. C., Benjet, C., Bromet, E., de Girolamo, G., de Graaf, R., Gasquet, I., Gureje, O., Haro, J. M., He, Y., Kessler, R. C., Levinson, D., Mneimneh, Z. N., Oakley Browne, M. A., Posada-Villa, J., Stein, D. J., Takeshima, T., & Von Korff M. (2007). Depression-anxiety relationships with chronic physical conditions: Results from the World Mental Health surveys. *Journal of Affective Disorders*, **103**, 113–20.

Scott, K. M., Von Korff, M., Alonso, J., Angermeyer, M., Bromet, E. J., Bruffaerts, R., de Girolamo, G., de Graaf, R., Fernandez, A., Gureje, O., He, Y., Kessler, R. C., Kovess, V., Levinson, D., Medina-Mora, M. E., Mneimneh, Z., Oakley Browne, M. A., Posada-Villa, J., Tachimori, H., & Williams, D. (2008). Age patterns in the prevalence of DSM-IV depressive/anxiety disorders with and without physical co-morbidity. *Psychological Medicine*, **38**, 1659–69.

Scott, K. M., Von Korff, M., Alonso, J., Angermeyer, M. C., Bromet, E., Fayyad, J., de Girolamo, G., Demyttenaere, K., Gasquet, I., Gureje, O., Haro, J. M., He, Y., Kessler, R. C., Levinson, D., Medina Mora, M. E., Oakley Browne, M., Ormel, J., Posada-Villa, J., & Watanabe, M. (2009). Mental–physical comorbidity and its relationship with disability: Results from the World Mental Health Surveys. *Psychological Medicine*, **39**, 33–43.

Siegler, I. C., Bastian, L. A., Steffens, D. C., Bosworth, H. B., & Costa, P. T. (2002). Behavioural medicine and aging. *Journal of Consulting & Clinical Psychology*, **70**, 843–51.

Skoog, I. (2004). Psychiatric epidemiology of old age: The H70 study – the NAPE lecture 2003. *Acta Psychiatrica Scandinavica*, **109**, 4–18.

Snowdon, J. (2001). Is depression more prevalent in old age? *Australian and New Zealand Journal of Psychiatry*, **35**, 782–7.

Troller, J. N., Anderson, T. M., Sachdev, P. S., Brodaty, H., & Andrews, G. (2007). Age shall not weary them: Mental health in the middle-aged and the elderly. *Australian and New Zealand Journal of Psychiatry*, **41**, 581–9.

Villamil, E., Huppert, F. A., & Melzer, D. (2006). Low prevalence of depression and anxiety is linked to statutory retirement ages rather than personal work exit: A national survey. *Psychological Medicine*, **36**, 999–1009.

Wells, K. B., Golding, J. M., & Burnam, M. A. (1989). Affective, substance use, and anxiety disorders in persons with arthritis, diabetes, heart disease, high blood pressure, or chronic lung conditions. *General Hospital Psychiatry*, **11**, 320–7.

PART TWO

Risk Factors for Mental–Physical Comorbidity

7 The Development of Mental–Physical Comorbidity

KATE M. SCOTT

7.1 INTRODUCTION

How do mental and physical conditions come to be comorbid? In explanations of this, researchers have frequently hypothesized that one condition operates as a risk factor for the other, focusing on mechanisms that might lead from mental to physical disorder or from physical to mental disorder. These are variously referred to as direct, causal, or morbidity-mediated mechanisms (Carney et al. 2002; Neeleman, Sytema, & Wadsworth 2002; Rudisch & Nemeroff 2003), operating within antecedent and consequence models (Steptoe 2007b). An alternative approach is to consider risk factors common to mental and physical disorders, frequently referred to as indirect or underlying mechanisms (Neeleman et al. 2002; Stansfeld et al. 2002), operating within a shared determinants model (Steptoe 2007b). This chapter considers both direct and underlying factors, but special emphasis is given to the potential significance of underlying mechanisms acting as broad-spectrum risk factors for diverse physical and mental disorders over their developmental course. The review of research presented in this chapter provides a context for the following chapters regarding the possible role of childhood adversities and early-onset mental disorders in affecting risks of a range of chronic physical conditions.

7.2 MORBIDITY-MEDIATED (DIRECT) MECHANISMS

7.2.1. From Mental Disorder to Physical Condition: The Antecedent Model

While patients, clinicians, and scientists alike readily perceive that a serious physical disease might cause depression, it is less intuitively obvious that a mental disorder such as depression might lead to physical disease. Nonetheless, there is now a growing body of prospective research showing that depressive disorders, and possibly anxiety disorders, predict development of coronary heart disease (Goldston & Baillie 2008; Hemingway & Marmot 1999; Steptoe 2007a; Wulsin & Singla 2003) and non-insulin-dependent (type 2) diabetes (Engum 2007; Knol et al. 2006; Van den Akker et al. 2004). Prospective relationships have also been found between depression and cerebrovascular disease (Everson et al. 1998; Jonas & Mussolino 2000), between depressive disorders and chronic pain (Van Puymbroeck, Zautra, & Harakas 2007), and between anxiety and depressive disorders and subsequent asthma (Chida, Hamer, & Steptoe 2008; Hasler et al. 2005).

Among the diverse biological mechanisms postulated, several relate to the functioning of systems for managing stress and threat: the autonomic nervous system (through the sympathetic–adrenal–medullary (SAM) axis) and the neuroendocrine system (through the hypothalamic–pituitary–adrenocortical (HPA) axis). Disturbances in both these systems have been associated with depression and anxiety disorders (Goodyer 2007; Heim & Nemeroff 1999), though the neurobiology of these disorders is complex and likely extends beyond dysregulation of stress systems. Dysregulation of the hormonal products of the SAM and HPA axes, the catecholamines (e.g., adrenaline and noradrenaline) and the glucocorticoids (e.g., cortisol), has been associated with a range of adverse metabolic, cardiovascular, and immune system effects. These include elevated blood glucose levels, insulin resistance and obesity, enhanced blood clotting, increased blood pressure and reduced heart rate variability, both immunosuppression and increased inflammatory response, and a cascade of effects that contribute to atherosclerosis (Miller, Cohen, & Ritchey 2002; Musselman et al. 2007; Steptoe 2007a).

The findings of the World Mental Health Surveys regarding mental–physical comorbidity among persons with both anxiety and depression are interesting in this context. Comorbid depressive–anxiety disorder was more strongly associated with several physical conditions relative to noncomorbid depression or anxiety (Scott et al. 2007). Although this research was cross-sectional, this result makes more sense when viewed within an antecedent framework of mental disorder leading to physical disease (whereby comorbid mental disorders are more likely than noncomorbid disorders to lead to physical conditions) than in the reverse direction (which would imply that physical conditions are more likely to lead to comorbid mental disorders than to noncomorbid mental disorders). Other researchers have reported similar results using measures of depressive and anxiety symptoms (Stordal et al. 2003). These epidemiological findings are consistent with recent neurobiological research that offers a potential explanatory mechanism. Young, Abelson, and Cameron (2006) found that patients with comorbid depressive–anxiety disorder showed a greater release of the pituitary hormone ACTH (adrenocorticotropic hormone) in response to a social stress induction, relative to the two groups with noncomorbid depression and anxiety, even after controlling for depression severity. The authors suggested that the interacting neurobiology of anxiety and depressive disorders may operate to increase HPA axis activity further still in the comorbid group. Consistent with this, in a study of women with a history of childhood physical and sexual abuse, women with both current major depressive disorder and posttraumatic stress disorder exhibited a greater ACTH response to stress induction than women with either depression or an abuse history alone (Heim et al. 2000). One speculation is, therefore, that if people with both depression and anxiety show a more exaggerated HPA axis response to stress than those with single mental disorders, over time this could have biological consequences that might explain the stronger associations found in the World Mental Health Surveys between comorbid depression–anxiety disorder and physical conditions.

Mental disorders can also affect physical disease risks through behavioral pathways. Mental disorders have a well-established relationship with behavioral risk factors for chronic disease, such as smoking, poor diet, sedentary behavior, and excessive alcohol consumption (Davidson et al. 2001; Scott et al. 2006). Depression may also increase the risk of later-onset physical disease by affecting adherence to treatment of risk factors for specific diseases, whether that treatment involves behavior modification (e.g., smoking cessation, weight reduction, exercise, and dietary change) or adherence to medication (e.g., cholesterol-lowering medication) (Carney et al. 2002).

7.2.2. From Physical Condition to Mental Disorder: The Consequence Model

In considering the reverse causal pathway, from physical condition to mental disorder, it has been observed that this seems so reasonable as to even be expected (Evans et al. 2005). In fact, most people with chronic physical disease do not have mental disorders (Scott et al. 2008; Chapter 6). Nonetheless, it is possible that mental disorder consequent to physical disease explains a significant part of the epidemiological association of mental and physical morbidity. Facets of physical disease that may instigate depressive or anxiety disorders include disability, pain, disfigurement, stressful medical procedures, and fear of death. For example, disability or functional limitations have been found to prospectively increase the risk of subsequent depression onset (Penninx 2007; Prince et al. 1998), probably through mechanisms such as loss of perceived control and self-efficacy, restriction of social and leisure activities, restriction of ability to work, and increased dependence (Ormel et al. 1997). Chronic pain has also been found to lead to depression, particularly when severe and enduring (Campbell, Clauw, & Keefe 2003).

An important question is why some individuals with significant physical disease do not develop mood or anxiety disorders, while others do. Psychological processes play a critical role in mediating the emotional consequences of physical conditions. Leventhal, Diefenbach, and Leventhal (1992) have suggested that people actively seek to develop an understanding of their illness, an "illness representation," which incorporates information about five aspects of the illness: identity, cause, consequences, whether it can be cured or controlled, and its timeline. Illness representations are influenced by a range of psychosocial factors and, depending on the conclusions that people draw about their illness and its personal significance, are proposed to influence coping, mood, and adjustment (Weinman et al. 1996). While most research has been cross-sectional, some prospective research has found illness representations to be predictive of mood outcomes (Sharpe & Curran 2006).

Biological pathways from physical disease to mental disorder are also implicated, both directly, as physical disease frequently causes endocrine, neurochemical, metabolic, immunologic, and other disturbances that can themselves result in symptoms of anxiety and depression, and indirectly, via a range of medications (Cohen & Rodriguez 1995). The kind of behavioral changes required by the presence of disease can also be depression or anxiety provoking, such as major changes in diet or lifestyle, giving up smoking, the requirement for self-monitoring of disease parameters, and having to follow complex medication regimes (Cohen & Rodriguez 1995). Social factors are also important. Chronic physical disease may result in changes in social networks and key relationships, with significant consequences for emotional well-being (Cohen & Rodriguez 1995). On the positive side, social support has been found to buffer the effects of chronic illness (Sherbourne et al. 1992).

7.2.3. Bidirectionality

One thing that should be borne in mind is that although the preceding section teases out mental–physical comorbidity into separate directional pathways, there is much literature suggesting that the relationships between mental disorders on the one hand and cardiovascular disease, diabetes, respiratory disease, chronic pain, and risk factors such as obesity and smoking on the other are bidirectional

(Cohen & Rodriguez 1995; Dew 1998; Kiecolt-Glaser et al. 2002). Depression can facilitate the development of diabetes along the pathways just described, but then the resulting disability and lifestyle changes precipitated by the onset of diabetes can initiate or exacerbate depression. Bidirectionality is therefore likely to be an important factor maintaining mental–physical comorbidity. Moreover, this feedback loop between mental and physical disorders may be one mechanism by which mental–physical comorbidity has been found to have synergistic effects on disability (Scott et al. 2009; Chapters 17 and 19).

The antecedent and consequence models of morbidity-mediated causality can be contrasted with an alternative model of shared determinants. In this latter model, the comorbidity of mental and physical conditions is not a function of each condition increasing the risk of the other, but rather of the fact that they share common risk factors, and their co-occurrence is therefore a function of this shared etiology, rather than a causal connection (Anda et al. 2006). The research considered in the remainder of this chapter provides a framework for understanding how the integral action of early biological, psychological, behavioral, and social processes might increase risk for onset of both mental and physical conditions.

7.3. SHARED DETERMINANTS: A LIFE-SPAN PERSPECTIVE

In recent years there has been increasing recognition that attempting to determine the immediate antecedent causes of disease may be focusing the searchlight too narrowly and too late (in the natural history of the disease) (Anda et al. 2006). Research on the early-life origins of disease has, for the most part, addressed physical and mental outcomes separately, though a few studies have looked at common early-life risk factors for both mental and physical outcomes (Felitti 1998; Neeleman et al. 2002; Walker et al. 1999).

7.3.1. Latency Effects

Although it has long been understood that mental disorders may be influenced by childhood adversities, a life-span perspective on physical disease development is more recent. A major impetus for this has been research linking indices of poor fetal growth (such as low birth weight for gestational age) with adult-onset cardiovascular disease, insulin resistance and metabolic syndrome, non-insulin-dependent (type 2) diabetes, obesity, hypertension, and osteoporosis (Barker 1997; Barker et al. 2002; Gluckman, Hanson, & Beedle 2007; Hales 1997). Poor fetal growth can result from factors such as poor nutrition, maternal smoking, and/or stress during gestation; suboptimal nutrition can occur in both developed and developing countries due to nutrient imbalance and maternal constraint (Barker et al. 2002). Imbalanced nutrition and/or stress in utero are hypothesized to lead to changes in the infant's biology and metabolism via the mechanism of developmental plasticity. This is a phenomenon whereby, during particular critical or sensitive periods, the developing organism is "plastic" and is able to make biological adaptations in response to the environment (Barker 2007; Gluckman & Hanson 2007). Developmental plasticity may frequently be underpinned by epigenetic changes, in which the environment alters gene regulation or expression (Gluckman et al. 2007). This will facilitate adaptation to a postnatal environment that matches the environment that triggered the epigenetic changes. Under conditions of a constrained fetal environment, developmental plasticity is thought to lead to metabolic and other biological adaptations that, when "mismatched" to a postnatal environment of nutritional plenty, increase risk of the chronic physical diseases mentioned earlier (Gluckman & Hanson 2006; Godfrey et al. 2007).

This concept of critical or sensitive periods of development in which physiological responses may be "programmed" is an example of a *latency* model (Marmot 1997; Power & Hertzman 1997). Latency models are also likely to be relevant to the development of mental disorders, and possibly to the development of mental–physical comorbidity. There is now epidemiological research linking low birth weight to risk of adolescent and adult-onset depression (Gale & Martyn 2004; Thompson et al. 2001) and, when low birth weight occurs in conjunction with subsequent childhood abuse, with greater risk of mental disorders beyond the contribution of either factor alone (Nomura & Chemtob 2007). Low birth weight has also been linked to the co-occurrence of mental and physical problems in adulthood (Nomura et al. 2007). The main hypothesized mechanism for these connections has been the influence of gestational stress on HPA axis settings.

The critical periods for the setting of stress responsiveness are not necessarily just pre-birth. A substantial and compelling body of research with animals (primate and nonprimate) indicates that persistent changes in neurobiological and behavioral reactivity to stress can be instigated in early life by poor maternal care, maternal stress, or separation from the mother (Meaney 2001; Sanchez 2006). This is supported by evidence from clinical research with humans showing that individuals with a history of early-life adversity or abuse have heightened HPA axis activity compared to those without such a history (Heim et al. 2000; Heim, Plotsky, & Nemeroff 2004; Weiss, Longhurst, & Mazure 1999) and that individuals with a history of early-life adversity are at increased risk of both physical and mental health outcomes (Arnow 2004; Edwards et al. 2003; Felitti 1998; Walker et al. 1999).

What this all might suggest is that overexposure to glucocorticoids (or other forms of HPA axis dysregulation) at particular developmental junctures, or over extended periods of time, may be part of a common biological vulnerability to both mental and physical disorders. As noted earlier, HPA axis dysfunction is implicated in the long-term development of a range of physical disorders mediated by metabolic, cardiovascular, and immune systems (Chrousos & Kino 2007; Cohen, Janicki-Deverts, & Miller 2007; McEwen 1998). It is also implicated in depressive and anxiety disorders, through the effects of both the glucocorticoids and corticotrophin-releasing hormone – the activator of the HPA axis released by the hypothalamus (Bradley et al. 2008; Heim & Nemeroff 1999). Moreover, HPA axis dysregulation has been linked to cognitive and emotional dysfunction more broadly, through deleterious effects on several brain regions, in particular the hippocampus and amygdala, which have a high density of glucocorticoid receptors (Andersen & Teicher 2004; McEwen 2003; Teicher et al. 2003). To be sure, mental–physical comorbidity cannot be explained solely in terms of HPA axis dysregulation. But there is good evidence that early-life adversity, through its impact on the neuroendocrine and autonomic stress response, with its flow-on effects on the developing brain during a window of vulnerability, may initiate a particular pathway of neurobiological development such that risk is increased for a range of physical, emotional, and cognitive outcomes later in life (Teicher et al. 2002).

But the story does not end there.

7.3.2. Pathways and Cumulative Effects

Latency effects are not the only way that early life may influence later disease risk. *Pathways* and *cumulative* models focus on the influence that early-life adverse environments have on increasing exposure to later-life adverse environments or events. A pathways approach suggests that early environments shape subsequent life trajectories; cumulative models emphasize the cumulative effect of disadvantage at different points in the life course (Hertzman 1999; Maughan & McCarthy 1997; Power & Hertzman 1997). For example, a number of researchers documenting the social gradient in both physical and mental health outcomes have suggested that this comes about not simply through current socioeconomic circumstance, but through the influence of pathways and cumulative effects, through the effect of childhood socioeconomic status on subsequent educational attainment (Power & Hertzman 1997), and through the cumulative effect of poor socioeconomic status at different points in the life course (Singh-Manoux et al. 2004). Within pathways and cumulative models, the connection between childhood (economic, physical, and psychosocial) adversity and adult health outcomes has been proposed to be mediated by a complex range of psychological, biological, behavioral, and environmental factors (Felitti 1998; Maughan & McCarthy 1997; Pudrovska et al. 2005; Singh-Manoux et al. 2004).

7.3.3. A Synthesis?

The development of mental and physical conditions probably involves both latency and pathways/cumulative effects. The concept of *allostatic load* may encapsulate the operation of both. Allostatic load refers to the cumulative biological wear and tear that occurs through a chronic imbalance in the hormonal and neurotransmitter mediators of allostasis (the "maintenance of stability through change"), especially the glucocorticoids and catecholamines (McEwen 1998, 2007). It can come about through a variety of means: exposure to frequent or chronic stressors (relevant to the pathways/cumulative models of accumulating adversity); lack of desensitization to repeated stressors of the same type; inability to "turn off" stress responses after a stressor has terminated; inadequate stress response by some allostatic systems resulting in compensatory overactivity by others. (These last three mechanisms may result from a combination of latency and cumulative effects.)

Although the mechanisms by which allostatic load occurs are biological, the influencing factors are genetic, environmental, psychological, and behavioral (McEwen 1998). Gestational influences or early-life adversity may set the level of responsiveness of the HPA and SAM axes as discussed earlier. Early-life adversity may initiate a rolling sequence of difficult circumstances that facilitate the translation of individual biological reactivity into allostatic load. Psychological factors are instrumental in this process in influencing whether an experience is perceived as stressful (Lazarus & Folkman 1984). The influence of individual psychology is in part captured by personality constructs such as neuroticism, which has been linked prospectively to both mental and physical health outcomes (Neeleman, Bijl, & Ormel 2004; Neeleman et al. 2002). There is evidence that some of what characterizes personality, such as how one appraises the environment, and one's cognitive and emotional response to it, is itself shaped by childhood adversity and parental psychopathology (Alloy et al. 2004; Silk et al. 2006).

Individuals are not merely the passive recipients of the processes of development, but active agents in it. Behaviors such as smoking, drinking alcohol, overeating, and sexual activity can be part of the individual's stress-coping repertoire, but then have important physiological consequences that add to allostatic load and risk of disease, both physical and mental (Felitti 1998; McEwen 1998).

Mental disorders, in particular depression and anxiety disorders, can be viewed as the outcome of allostatic load, especially when recurrent, but they may also be viewed as contributors to it. The experience of depression and posttraumatic stress disorder, for example, involves ruminating on or reliving adverse experience, thus contributing to stress exposure (McEwen 2003). Moreover, mental disorders are associated with the negative health behaviors mentioned earlier.

In sum, the concept of allostatic load may offer a useful framework for understanding the longitudinal development of at least some mental–physical comorbidity, although of course no one theory can explain everything. To the extent that allostatic load may be applicable, the multiple physiological systems involved, together with the manifold environmental, psychological, and behavioral factors that mediate and moderate its development over time, help explain variation in the manifestation of mental–physical comorbidity across individuals.

7.4. CONCLUSION

The focus on direct, morbidity-mediated mechanisms that has dominated research on mental–physical comorbidity runs the risk of illuminating only part of a series of links that may extend much further, over the life span and across multiple aspects of human functioning. While there are plausible causal links between mental and physical conditions, some of the explanation of mental–physical comorbidity may lie in the developmental history of the individuals themselves, when considered from an ecological perspective. That developmental history considers whether there might be a continuity of adverse nutritional and psychosocial factors that has shaped the expression of genes, and subsequently the biological, psychological, and behavioral responses of the individual, responses that in turn help shape and select life trajectories and health outcomes – mental and physical. From a public health standpoint, a focus on early-life risk factors that have broad-spectrum effects on human development may be the most effective means of addressing the burden of physical and mental morbidity now increasingly prevalent on a worldwide basis.

This chapter has highlighted how a shared determinant such as childhood adversity could increase the risk of comorbid mental and physical conditions. Whether it does and the extent to which it does remain empirical questions. The research attempting to distinguish between shared determinant and morbidity-mediated models of mental–physical comorbidity is in its early days, and in addition to the fact that no one study will be able to provide definitive answers, there is unlikely to be only one answer. Direct, morbidity mechanisms may explain some instances of mental–physical comorbidity, and shared determinants may explain others.

The studies that follow in this section are concerned with the sequential comorbidity of early-onset mental disorders with chronic physical conditions that occur later in life, sometimes decades later. These studies find that childhood adversities and early-onset mental disorders independently predict a range of adult-onset physical conditions. The respective associations of childhood adversities and early-onset mental disorders with the physical outcomes are somewhat, but not greatly, reduced by adjustment for other predictors. These results suggest that the sequential comorbidity between early-onset mental disorders and subsequent physical conditions observed in the World Mental Health Surveys can be partly, but not substantially, explained by their shared risk factor of childhood adversity.

REFERENCES

Alloy, L. B., Abramson, L. Y., Gibb, B. E., Crossfield, A. G., Pieracci, A. M., Spasojevic, J., & Steinberg, J. A. (2004). Developmental antecedents of cognitive vulnerability to depression: Review of findings from the cognitive vulnerability to depression project. *Journal of Cognitive Psychotherapy: An International Quarterly*, 18, 115–33.

Anda, R. F., Felitti, V., Bremner, J. D., Walker, J. D., Whitfield, C., Perry, B. D., Dube, S. R., & Giles, W. H. (2006). The enduring effects of abuse and related adverse experiences in childhood. *European Archives of Psychiatry and Clinical Neuroscience*, 256, 174–86.

Andersen, S. L., & Teicher, M. H. (2004). Delayed effects of early stress on hippocampal development. *Neuropsychopharmacology*, 29, 1988–93.

Arnow, B. (2004). Relationships between childhood maltreatment, adult health and psychiatric outcomes, and medical utilisation. *Journal of Clinical Psychiatry*, 65, 10–15.

Barker, D. J. P. (1997). Fetal nutrition and cardiovascular disease in later life. *British Medical Bulletin*, 53, 96–108.

Barker, D. J. P. (2007). The origins of the developmental origins theory. *Journal of Internal Medicine*, 261, 412–17.

Barker, D. J. P., Eriksson, J. G., Forsen, T., & Osmond, C. (2002). Fetal origins of adult disease: Strength of effects and biological basis. *International Journal of Epidemiology*, 31, 1235–9.

Bradley, R. G., Binder, E. B., Epstein, M. P., Tang, Y., Nair, H. P., Liu, W., Gillespie, C. F., Berg, T., Evces, M., Newport, D. J., Stowe, Z. N., Heim, C. M., Nemeroff, C. B., Schwartz, A., Cubells, J. F., & Ressler, K. J. (2008). Influence of child abuse on adult depression: Moderation by the corticotropin-releasing hormone receptor gene. *Archives of General Psychiatry*, 65, 190–200.

Campbell, L. C., Clauw, D. J., & Keefe, F. J. (2003). Persistent pain and depression: A biopsychosocial perspective. *Biological Psychiatry*, 54, 399–409.

Carney, R. M., Freedland, K. E., Miller, G. E., & Jaffe, A. S. (2002). Depression as a risk factor for cardiac mortality and morbidity: A review of potential mechanisms. *Journal of Psychosomatic Research*, 53, 897–902.

Chida, Y., Hamer, M., & Steptoe, A. (2008). A bidirectional relationship between psychosocial factors and atopic disorders: A systematic review and meta-analysis. *Psychosomatic Medicine*, 70, 102–16.

Chrousos, G. P., & Kino, T. (2007). Glucocorticoid action networks and complex psychiatric and/or somatic disorders. *Stress*, 10, 213–19.

Cohen, S., Janicki-Deverts, D., & Miller, G. E. (2007). Psychological stress and disease. *The Journal of the American Medical Association*, 298, 1685–7.

Cohen, S., & Rodriguez, M. S. (1995). Pathways linking affective disturbances and physical disorders. *Health Psychology*, 14, 374–80.

Davidson, S., Judd, F., Jolley, D., Hocking, B., Thompson, S., & Hyland, B. (2001). Cardiovascular risk factors for people with mental illness. *Australian and New Zealand Journal of Psychiatry*, 35, 196–202.

Dew, M. A. (1998). Psychiatric disorder in the context of physical illness. In *Adversity, Stress and Psychopathology*, ed. B. P. Dohrenwend, pp. 177–218. New York: Oxford University Press.

Edwards, V. J., Holden, G. W., Felitti, V. J., & Anda, R. F. (2003). Relationship between multiple forms of childhood maltreatment and adult mental health in community respondents: Results from the adverse childhood experiences study. *The American Journal of Psychiatry*, 160, 1453–60.

Engum, A. (2007). The role of depression and anxiety in onset of diabetes in a large population-based study. *Journal of Psychosomatic Research*, 62, 31–8.

Evans, D. L., Charney, D. S., Lewis, L., Golden, J. M., Ranga Rama Krishnan, K., Nemeroff, C. B., Bremner, J. D., Carney, R. M., Coyne, J. C., Delong, M. R., Frasure-Smith, N., Glassman, A. H., Gold, P. W., Grant, I., Gwyther, L., Ironson, G., Johnson, R. L., Kanner, A. M., Katon, W. J., Kaufmann, P. G., Keefe, F. J., Ketter, T., Laughren, T. P., Leserman, J., Lyketsos, C. G., McDonald, W. M., McEwan, B. S., Miller, A. H., Musselman, D., O'Connor, C., Petitto, J. M., Pollock, B. G., Robinson, R. G., Roose, S. P., Rowland, J., Sheline, Y., Sheps, D. S., Simon, G., Spiegel, D., Stunkard, A., Sunderland, T., Tibbits, P., & Valvo, W. J. (2005). Mood disorders in the medically ill: Scientific review and recommendations. *Biological Psychiatry*, 58, 175–89.

Everson, S. A., Roberts, R. E., Goldberg, D. E., & Kaplan, G. A. (1998). Depressive symptoms and increased risk of stroke mortality over a 25-year

period. *Archives of Internal Medicine*, **158**, 1133–8.
Felitti, V. J. (1998). Relationship of childhood abuse and household dysfunction to many of the leading causes of death in adults. *American Journal of Preventive Medicine*, **14**, 245–58.
Gale, C. R., & Martyn, C. N. (2004). Birth weight and later risk of depression. *British Journal of Psychiatry*, **184**, 28–33.
Gluckman, P. D., & Hanson, M. A. (2006). *Mismatch: How Our World No Longer Fits Our Bodies*. Oxford: Oxford University Press.
Gluckman, P. D., & Hanson, M. A. (2007). Developmental plasticity and human disease: research directions. *Journal of Internal Medicine*, **261**, 461–71.
Gluckman, P. D., Hanson, M. A., & Beedle, A. S. (2007). Early life events and their consequences for later disease: A life history and evolutionary perspective. *American Journal of Human Biology*, **19**, 1–19.
Godfrey, K. M., Lillycrop, K. A., Burdge, G. C., Gluckman, P. D., & Hanson, M. A. (2007). Epigenetic mechanisms and the mismatch concept of the developmental origins of health and disease. *Pediatric Research*, **61**, 5R–10.
Goldston, K., & Baillie, A. J. (2008). Depression and coronary heart disease: A review of the epidemiological evidence, explanatory mechanisms and management approaches. *Clinical Psychology Review*, **28**, 289–307.
Goodyer, I. M. (2007). The hypothalamic-pituitary-adrenal axis: Cortisol, DHEA and mental and behavioral function. In *Depression and Physical Illness*, ed. A. Steptoe, pp. 280–98. London: Cambridge University Press.
Hales, C. N. (1997). Non-insulin-dependent diabetes mellitus. *British Medical Bulletin*, **53**, 109–22.
Hasler, G., Gergen, P. J., Kleinbaum, D. G., Ajdacic, V., Gamma, A., Eich, D., Rossler, W., & Angst, J. (2005). Asthma and panic in young adults. *American Journal of Respiratory and Critical Care Medicine*, **171**, 1224–30.
Heim, C., & Nemeroff, C. B. (1999). The impact of early adverse experiences on brain systems involved in the pathophysiology of anxiety and affective disorders. *Biological Psychiatry*, **46**, 1509–22.
Heim, C., Newport, D. J., Heit, S., Graham, Y. P., Wilcox, M., Bonsall, R., Miller, A. H., & Nemeroff, C. B. (2000). Pituitary-adrenal and autonomic responses to stress in women after sexual and physical abuse in childhood. *The Journal of the American Medical Association*, **284**, 592–7.
Heim, C., Plotsky, P. M., & Nemeroff, C. B. (2004). Importance of studying the contributions of early adverse experience to neurobiological findings in depression. *Neuropsychopharmacology*, **29**, 641–8.
Hemingway, H., & Marmot, M. (1999). Psychosocial factors in the aetiology and prognosis of coronary heart disease: Systematic review of prospective cohort studies. *British Medical Journal*, **318**, 1460–7.
Hertzman, C. (1999). The biological embedding of early experience and its effects on health in adulthood. *Annals of the New York Academy of Science*, **896**, 85–95.
Jonas, B. S., & Mussolino, M. E. (2000). Symptoms of depression as a prospective risk factor for stroke. *Psychosomatic Medicine*, **62**, 463–71.
Kiecolt-Glaser, J. K., McGuire, L., Robles, T. F., & Glaser, R. (2002). Emotions, morbidity, and mortality: New perspectives from psychoneuroimmunology. *Annual Review of Psychology*, **53**, 83–107.
Knol, M. J., Twisk, J. W., Beekman, A. T., Heine, R. J., Snoek, F. J., & Pouwer, F. (2006). Depression as a risk factor for the onset of type 2 diabetes mellitus: A meta-analysis. *Diabetologia*, **49**, 837–45.
Lazarus, R. S., & Folkman, S. (1984). *Stress, Appraisal and Coping*. New York: Springer.
Leventhal, H., Diefenbach, M., & Leventhal, E. A. (1992). Illness cognition: Using common sense to understand adherence and affect cognition interactions. *Cognitive Therapy and Research*, **16**, 143–63.
Marmot, M. G. (1997). Early life and adult disorder: Research themes. *British Medical Bulletin*, **53**, 3–9.
Maughan, B., & McCarthy, G. (1997). Childhood adversities and psychosocial disorders. *British Medical Bulletin*, **53**, 156–69.
McEwen, B. S. (1998). Protective and damaging effects of stress mediators. *New England Journal of Medicine*, **338**, 171–9.
McEwen, B. S. (2003). Mood disorders and allostatic load. *Biological Psychiatry*, **54**, 200–7.
McEwen, B. S. (2007). Physiology and neurobiology of stress and adaptation: Central role of the brain. *Physiological Reviews*, **87**, 873–904.
Meaney, M. J. (2001). Maternal care, gene expression, and the transmission of individual

differences in stress reactivity across generations. *Annual Review of Neuroscience*, 24, 1161–92.

Miller, G. E., Cohen, S., & Ritchey, A. K. (2002). Chronic psychological stress and the regulation of pro-inflammatory cytokines: A glucocorticoid resistance model. *Health Psychology*, 21, 536–41.

Musselman, D., Bowling, A., Gilles, N., Larsen, H., Betan, E., & Phillips, L. (2007). The interrelationship of depression and diabetes. In *Depression and Physical Illness*, ed. A. Steptoe, pp. 165–94. London: Cambridge University Press.

Neeleman, J., Bijl, R. V., & Ormel, J. (2004). Neuroticism, a central link between somatic and psychiatric morbidity: Path analysis of prospective data. *Psychological Medicine*, 34, 521–31.

Neeleman, J., Sytema, S., & Wadsworth, M. (2002). Propensity to psychiatric and somatic ill-health: Evidence from a birth cohort. *Psychological Medicine*, 32, 793–803.

Nomura, Y., Brooks-Gunn, J., Davey, C., Ham, J., & Fifer, W. P. (2007). The role of perinatal problems in risk of co-morbid psychiatric and medical disorders in adulthood. *Psychological Medicine*, 37, 1323–34.

Nomura, Y., & Chemtob, C. M. (2007). Conjoined effects of low birth weight and childhood abuse on adaptation and well-being in adolescence and adulthood. *Archives of Pediatrics and Adolescent Medicine*, 161, 186–92.

Ormel, J., Kempen, G. I., Penninx, B. W., Brilman, E. I., Beekman, A. T., & Van Sonderen, E. (1997). Chronic medical conditions and mental health in older people: Disability and psychosocial resources mediate specific mental health effects. *Psychological Medicine*, 27, 1065–77.

Penninx, B. W. (2007). Depression and physical disability. In *Depression and physical Illness*, ed. A. Steptoe, pp. 125–44. London: Cambridge University Press.

Power, C., & Hertzman, C. (1997). Social and biological pathways linking early life and adult disease. *British Medical Bulletin*, 53, 210–21.

Prince, M. J., Harwood, R. H., Thomas, A., & Mann, A. H. (1998). A prospective population-based cohort study of the effects of disablement and social milieu on the onset and maintenance of late-life depression: The Gospel Oak Project VII. *Psychological Medicine*, 28, 337–50.

Pudrovska, T., Schieman, S., Pearlin, L. I., & Nguyen, K. (2005). The sense of mastery as a mediator and moderator in the association between economic hardship and health in late life. *Journal of Aging and Health*, 17, 634–60.

Rudisch, B., & Nemeroff, C. B. (2003). Epidemiology of comorbid coronary artery disease and depression. *Biological Psychiatry*, 54, 227–40.

Sanchez, M. M. (2006). The impact of early adverse care on HPA axis development: Nonhuman primate models. *Hormones and Behaviour*, 50, 623–31.

Scott, K. M., Bruffaerts, R., Tsang, A., Ormel, J., Alonso, J., Angermeyer, M. C., Benjet, C., Bromet, E., de Girolamo, G., de Graaf, R., Gasquet, I., Gureye, O., Haro, J. M., He, Y., Kessler, R. C., Levinson, D., Mneimneh, Z. N., Oakley Browne, M. A., Posada-Villa, J., Stein, D. J., Takeshima, T., & Von Korff, M. (2007). Depression-anxiety relationships with chronic physical conditions: Results from the World Mental Health surveys. *Journal of Affective Disorders*, 103, 113–20.

Scott, K. M., Oakley Browne, M. A., McGee, M. A., & Wells, J. E. (2006). Mental-physical comorbidity in Te Rau Hinengaro: The New Zealand Mental Health Survey (NZMHS). *Australian and New Zealand Journal of Psychiatry*, 40, 882–8.

Scott, K. M., Von Korff, M., Angermeyer, M. C., Bromet, E., Bruffaerts, R., de Girolamo, G., de Graaf, R., Fernandez, A., Gureje, O., He, Y., Kessler, R., Kovess, V., Levinson, D., Medina Mora, M., Mneimneh, Z. N., Oakley Browne, M. A., Posada-Villa, J., Tachimori, H., & Williams, D. (2008). Age patterns in the prevalence of depressive/anxiety disorders with and without physical comorbidity. *Psychological Medicine*, 38, 1659–69.

Scott, K. M., Von Korff, M., Alonso, J., Angermeyer, M. C., Bromet, E., Fayyad, J., de Girolamo, G., Demyttenaere, K., Gasquet, I., Gureye, O., Haro, J. M., He, Y., Kessler, R. C., Levinson, D., Medina Mora, M., Oakley Browne, M. A., Ormel, J., Posada-Villa, J., Watanabe, M., & Williams, D. (2009). Mental-physical comorbidity and its relationship with disability: Results from the World Mental Health surveys. *Psychological Medicine*, 39, 33–43.

Sharpe, L., & Curran, L. (2006). Understanding the process of adjustment to illness. *Social Science & Medicine*, 62, 1153–66.

Sherbourne, C. D., Meredith, L. S., Rogers, W., & Ware, J. E. (1992). Social support and stressful life events: Age differences in their effects on health-related quality of life among the chronically ill. *Quality of Life Research*, 1, 235–46.

Silk, J. S., Shaw, D. S., Skuban, D. S., Oland, A. A., & Kovacs, M. (2006). Emotion regulation strategies in offspring of childhood-onset depressed mothers. *Journal of Child Psychology and Psychiatry*, 47, 69–78.

Singh-Manoux, A., Ferrie, J. E., Chandola, T., & Marmot, M. (2004). Socioeconomic trajectories across the life course and health outcomes in midlife: Evidence for the accumulation hypothesis? *International Journal of Epidemiology*, 33, 1072–9.

Stansfeld, S. A., Fuhrer, R., Shipley, M. J., & Marmot, M. G. (2002). Psychological distress as a risk factor for coronary heart disease in the Whitehall II study. *International Journal of Epidemiology*, 31, 248–55.

Steptoe, A. (2007a). Depression and the development of coronary heart disease. In *Depression and Physical Illness*, ed. A. Steptoe, pp. 53–86. London: Cambridge University Press.

Steptoe, A. (2007b). Integrating clinical with biobehavioural studies of depression and physical illness. In *Depression and Physical Illness*, ed. A. Steptoe, pp. 397–408. London: Cambridge University Press.

Stordal, E., Bjelland, I., Dahl, A. A., & Mykletun, A. (2003). Anxiety and depression in individuals with somatic health problems. The Nord-Trondelag Health Study (HUNT). *Scandinavian Journal of Primary Health Care*, 21, 136–41.

Teicher, M. H., Andersen, S. L., Polcari, A., Anderson, C. M., & Navalta, C. P. (2002). Developmental neurobiology of childhood stress and trauma. *Psychiatric Clinics of North America*, 25, 397–426.

Teicher, M. H., Andersen, S. L., Polcari, A., Anderson, C. M., Navalta, C. P., & Kim, D. M. (2003). The neurobiological consequences of early stress and childhood maltreatment. *Neuroscience and Biobehavioral Reviews*, 27, 33–44.

Thompson, C., Syddall, H., Rodin, I., Osmond, C., & Barker, D. J. P. (2001). Birthweight and the risk of depressive disorder in late life. *British Journal of Psychiatry*, 179, 450–5.

Van Den Akker, M., Schuurman, A., Metsemakers, J., & Buntinx, F. (2004). Is depression related to subsequent diabetes mellitus? *Acta Psychiatrica Scandinavica*, 110, 178–83.

Van Puymbroeck, C. M., Zautra, A. J., & Harakas, P. P. (2007). Chronic pain and depression: Twin burdens of adaptation. In *Depression and Physical Illness*, ed. A. Steptoe, pp. 145–64. London: Cambridge University Press.

Walker, E. A., Gelfand, A., Katon, W., Koss, M. P., Von Korff, M., & Russo, J. (1999). Adult health status of women with histories of childhood abuse and neglect. *American Journal of Medicine*, 107, 332–9.

Weinman, J., Petrie, K. J., Moss-Morris, R. E., & Horne, R. (1996). The illness perception questionnaire: A new method for assessing the cognitive representation of disease. *Psychology and Health*, 11, 431–45.

Weiss, E. L., Longhurst, J. G., & Mazure, C. M. (1999). Childhood sexual abuse as a risk factor for depression in women: Psychosocial and neurobiological correlates. *American Journal of Psychiatry*, 156, 816–28.

Wulsin, L. R., & Singla, B. M. (2003). Do depressive symptoms increase the risk for the onset of coronary disease: A systematic quantitative review. *Psychosomatic Medicine*, 65, 201–10.

Young, E. A., Abelson, J. L., & Cameron, O. G. (2006). Effect of comorbid anxiety disorders on the hypothalamic-pituitary-adrenal axis response to a social stressor in major depression. *Biological Psychiatry*, 56, 113–20.

8 Psychosocial Predictors of Adult-Onset Asthma

KATE M. SCOTT

8.1. INTRODUCTION

Asthma was once regarded as a quintessential psychosomatic condition, but views on its etiology have changed substantially to its current conceptualization as an atopic disease underpinned by inflammatory mechanisms triggered by gene–environment interactions (Chida, Hamer, & Steptoe 2008; Jenkins et al. 1994; Pearce, Douwes, & Beasley 2000). This is not to deny that asthma is often comorbid with mental disorders. A good deal of research among clinical and general practice samples (Afari et al. 2001; Brown, Khan, & Mahadi 2000; Goodwin et al. 2003; Kolbe et al. 2002; Nascimento et al. 2002; Perna et al. 1997; Shavitt, Gentil, & Mandetta 1992; Yellowlees et al. 1987, 1988) and general population samples (Goldney et al. 2003; Goodwin & Eaton 2003; Goodwin, Fergusson, & Horwood 2004; Goodwin, Jacobi, & Thefeld 2003; Janson et al. 1994; von Behren, Kreutzer, & Hernandez 2002) has established that asthma, particularly severe asthma, is related to both depressive and anxiety disorders. The World Mental Health (WMH) Surveys have confirmed this finding cross-nationally (Scott et al. 2007).

Despite the changing views on the nature of asthma, there is still interest in the role that psychosocial factors, including mental disorders, might play as contributing environmental factors in asthma onset and exacerbation. Much of the research in this area has recently been summarized in a meta-analysis and review of prospective studies investigating the relationship between psychosocial factors (stressful events, anxiety or depression symptoms, and poor social support) and atopic disorders among children and adults (Chida et al. 2008). This review found robust evidence for a bidirectional relationship between psychosocial factors and asthma, though the relationship is stronger in children, among whom most of this research has been conducted (Chida et al. 2008).

The current study, however, focuses on asthma beginning in adulthood (age 21 years and older). A small number of studies have found a relationship between earlier development of anxiety or depression and subsequent development of asthma during late adolescence or adulthood (Chida et al. 2008; Hasler et al. 2005; Wainwright et al. 2007). Considering psychosocial factors other than mental disorders, childhood adversity has been linked with incident asthma hospital admissions among adults aged 40–80 years (Wainwright et al. 2007), and associations have been observed between childhood sexual abuse and adult asthma activity (Romans et al. 2002). Clear evidence on the relationship between childhood adversity and adult-onset asthma is lacking, however, in part due to the variety of experience classified under "adversity." Chida et al. (2008), for example, did not find an association between some childhood adversities (stressful life event exposure) and asthma outcomes in adults, but other childhood adversities (dysfunctional relationships in childhood and parental mental disorder) did predict asthma.

A possible relationship between childhood adversity and adult asthma outcomes is of interest for a number of reasons. It may have implications for psychobiological pathways between early-life experience and adult disease. It may also explain the frequently observed comorbidity between mental disorders and asthma: this comorbidity may not come about through bidirectional causal mechanisms, but may in fact be a function of shared risk factors such as childhood adversity or other shared genetic or environmental factors (Hasler et al. 2005). Some research has found some preliminary support for this suggestion. Goodwin et al. (2004) found that the relationship between asthma and depression or anxiety disorder in a birth cohort of adolescents was explained by childhood adversity and other shared risk factors. In a further study, Goodwin, Wamboldt, and Pine (2003) found an association between retrospectively reported childhood abuse and lung disease–mental disorder comorbidity experienced in adulthood (age 18–54 years). However, the latter study was limited by lack of information on the age of onset (AOO) of either lung disease or mental disorders (making the temporal sequence between onset of abuse, lung disease, and mental disorders unclear) and by single-item assessment of child abuse.

In sum, prior research suggests that childhood adversity may be associated with asthma, especially among children but even among adults, and moreover, childhood adversity has been suggested to account for the relationship between mental disorders and asthma. Investigation of this topic has been fairly limited to date, however. The advantages that the WMH Surveys offer are that they provide information on mental disorders together with asthma diagnosis, on age of onset of both asthma and mental disorders, and on the experience of a wide range of childhood family adversities. AOO information allows us to disentangle some of the possible temporal relationships between childhood adversity, mental disorders, and asthma.

In this study of 10 of the WMH countries there were three aims: (1) to investigate whether childhood adversity predicts adult-onset (>21 years of age) asthma (with and without adjustment for current anxiety or depressive disorder to control for mood-congruent recall bias); (2) to investigate whether early-onset (prior to age 21) depressive/anxiety disorders predict adult-onset asthma; (3) to investigate whether childhood adversity and early-onset depressive/anxiety disorders predict adult-onset asthma independently of each other. If early-onset depressive/anxiety disorders do not predict adult-onset asthma independently of childhood adversity, this would be supportive of the suggestion from prior research that the mental disorder–asthma relationship is a function of a shared background of childhood adversity.

Why did we focus on adult onset of asthma given that we had the option of investigating childhood onset of asthma through AOO information? Essentially, we chose to focus only on adult-onset cases to minimize the possibility that inaccuracies in retrospectively reported AOO could bias conclusions about the temporal sequencing of the predictor (childhood adversity and early-onset mental disorder) and outcome (asthma) variables.

8.2. APPROACH

The following description of the approach to this study of asthma is generic to the analysis of the other physical and pain conditions included in this section (with the exception of the analysis approach for obesity). Aspects of the methods that are specific to a given condition (such as the ascertainment of the condition) are described in the relevant chapters.

The study was based on surveys carried out in the Americas (Colombia, Mexico, and the United States), Europe (Belgium, France, Germany, Italy, the Netherlands, and Spain), and Asia (Japan). The mental disorders included were anxiety disorders (generalized anxiety disorder, panic disorder and/or agoraphobia, posttraumatic stress disorder, and social phobia) and depressive disorders (dysthymia and major depressive disorder). The childhood family adversities included were physical abuse, sexual abuse, neglect, parental death, parental divorce, other parental loss, parental mental disorder, parental substance use, parental criminal behavior, family violence, and family economic adversity. Those respondents who reported that the experience occurred before the age of 18 and met the criteria specified for a given adversity were coded as having experienced childhood adversity (see Chapter 4).

In a series of questions about chronic conditions adapted from the U.S. Health Interview Survey, respondents were asked about the lifetime presence of selected chronic conditions. Respondents were asked, "Did a doctor or other health professional ever tell you that you had any of the following illnesses... asthma?" Respondents were also asked how old they were when the condition was first diagnosed. Clinical guidelines for diagnosis of asthma such as those issued by the American Thoracic Society recommend a combination of methods including a medical history, physical examination, and respiratory function tests (Goodwin et al. 2003; Pearce et al. 2000), but such methods are not feasible in large epidemiology surveys, and indeed the international asthma prevalence surveys such as the European Community Respiratory Health Survey have used self-reported symptoms of asthma to determine the condition (Burney et al. 1996; Pearce et al. 2000). An investigation of the correspondence of self-reported chronic conditions in the U.S. National Health Interview Survey with medical records abstracted in the prior 3 years found self-reported current asthma to be in fairly good agreement with medical record, though underreported by 20–30% (National Center of Health Studies 1994). The definition of asthma used in this survey was self-report of a diagnosis of asthma, not simply self-report of asthma, so it is likely to correspond more closely to actual medical records.

The association of childhood adversities and early-onset mental disorders with adult-onset asthma (or other conditions) was studied with survival analyses, using retrospectively reported AOO (age of diagnosis) of asthma (reported in whole years). The start of the period at risk of adult-onset asthma was set at age 20. Persons who had not developed asthma were censored at their current age. Persons who reported that asthma developed before age 21 were excluded. Cox proportional hazards models estimated risk of adult-onset asthma as a function of number and type of childhood adversities and early-onset (<21 years of age) depressive/anxiety disorder status while adjusting for potential confounders (sex, current age, and for asthma and heart disease, smoking status: current/ever/never). Country was included in the analyses as a stratifying variable, which allows each country to have a unique hazard function. The associations are expressed as hazard ratios measuring relative risk. Childhood adversities were analyzed in four categories of number of adversities – none, one, two, and three or more – with no adversities as the reference group. Childhood adversities and early-onset mental disorders were included in the models both separately and simultaneously.

To account for the possibility of differential recall of childhood adversities among those with a current mood or anxiety disorder, we performed an additional analysis that adjusted for current (12-month) mood or anxiety disorder. We also performed an additional analysis adjusting for educational attainment (above/below the

Psychosocial Predictors of Adult-Onset Asthma

Table 8.1. Characteristics of total and adult-onset asthma samples

	Total cross-national sample (N = 18,303)		Adult-onset asthma (≥21 years) sample (N = 649)
	Unweighted N	Weighted %	Weighted %
Age (21–98 years)			
21–44	9,538	51.9	29.1
>45	8,765	48.1	70.9
Female	10,909	52.7	66.0
Education (above median)[a]	10,270	48.3	43.4
Adult-onset asthma (>21 years)	649	3.0	100.0
Current smoker	4,969	25.1	23.6
Country			
Colombia	2,104	11.5	2.7
Belgium	980	5.3	4.0
France	1,326	7.2	5.7
Germany	1,283	7.1	7.5
Italy	1,698	9.4	9.1
The Netherlands	1,017	5.3	6.8
Spain	2,006	10.8	10.3
Japan	856	4.7	4.5
Mexico	2,064	11.3	2.7
United States	4,969	27.3	46.8

[a] Educational attainment measured as years of education: percentages in table represent those above the country-specific median (weighted).

median education level for each country). Because the inclusion of education in the models made virtually no difference to the results, however, we have reported the results unadjusted for education. (Education data were not collected in France for legal reasons, so to have reported all results adjusting for education would have meant excluding France from the data set.) We screened for interaction of childhood adversities with early-onset depressive/anxiety disorders in predicting asthma onset, but the interaction was nonsignificant, so only main effects are reported in this chapter. (This applies to all the physical and pain conditions included in this section.)

The assumption of proportional hazards was assessed by inspecting log-minus-log plots of the survival functions. Statistical significance was set at 0.05 for a two-sided test. The analyses were performed using the SURVIVAL procedure in SUDAAN statistical software to account for the complex survey design.

8.3. FINDINGS

8.3.1. Sample Characteristics and Disorder/Adversity Prevalence

The characteristics of the total cross-national sample and of the sample of those with adult-onset asthma are compared in Table 8.1. Those with adult-onset asthma are more likely to be female, consistent with other research (Melgert et al. 2007), and older than 45 years. It is clear that higher proportions of those with adult-onset asthma (relative to the total sample) experienced early-onset depressive/anxiety disorders and childhood adversities. Table 8.2 provides the prevalence of individual

Table 8.2. Percent with early-onset depressive/anxiety disorders and childhood adversities in total and adult-onset asthma samples

	Weighted %	
	Total cross-national sample ($N = 18{,}303$)	Adult-onset asthma (≥ 21 years) sample ($N = 649$)
Early-onset (prior to age 21) mental disorders		
Any depressive/anxiety disorder	10.1	16.4
Major depressive disorder	4.4	8.1
Generalized anxiety disorder	1.3	2.2
Social phobia	4.8	6.7
Posttraumatic stress disorder	1.7	4.0
Panic disorder/agoraphobia	1.8	3.7
Number of childhood adversities		
None	56.2	50.5
One	25.7	26.9
Two	10.0	11.8
Three or more	8.2	10.9
Type of childhood adversity		
Physical abuse	9.7	12.6
Sexual abuse	2.5	4.2
Neglect	6.6	6.2
Parental death	12.9	16.0
Parental divorce	9.6	11.1
Other loss of parent	5.2	6.7
Parental mental disorder	7.0	10.2
Parental substance-use disorder	5.0	6.5
Violence in family	9.3	11.2
Parental criminal behavior	3.3	4.2
Family economic adversity	5.7	5.9

mental disorders and specific types of childhood adversities in the total and adult-onset asthma samples. All mental disorders and all but one of the childhood adversities are overrepresented in the adult-onset asthma sample.

8.3.2. Association of Childhood Adversity with Adult-Onset Asthma

After adjustment for age, sex, smoking status, and country, two or more childhood adversities significantly predicted the onset of asthma among those 21 years and older (Table 8.3), with increasing risk with a greater number of childhood adversities experienced. With additional adjustment for current (12-month or 1-month) depressive/anxiety disorder status, the association of childhood adversities with asthma onset reduced slightly but remained significant. This indicates that the relationship between childhood adversities and asthma onset is not just a function of current mood, which might be biasing recall of adversities.

8.3.3. Association of Early-Onset Mental Disorders and Specific Childhood Adversities with Adult-Onset Asthma

Early-onset depressive/anxiety disorders also predicted adult-onset asthma after adjustment

Table 8.3. Effect of childhood adversity on risk of adult-onset asthma (21 years and older), with and without adjustment for current (12-month or 1-month) depressive/anxiety disorders

Number of childhood adversities	Hazard ratios (95% CI) for adult-onset asthma (adjusted for age, sex, smoking status, and country)		
	Without adjustment for current (12-month) depressive/anxiety disorder	With adjustment for current (12-month) depressive/anxiety disorder	With adjustment for current (1-month) depressive/anxiety disorder
One	1.24 (0.98, 1.57)	1.21 (0.96, 1.53)	1.23 (0.97, 1.55)
Two	1.49 (1.07, 2.09)*	1.42 (1.02, 1.97)*	1.45 (1.04, 2.03)*
Three or more	1.71 (1.12, 2.61)*	1.50 (1.01, 2.22)*	1.60 (1.06, 2.43)*

* $p < .05$.

for age, sex, smoking status, and country (Table 8.4). The individual disorders that were significantly related to asthma onset were major depressive disorder, posttraumatic stress disorder, and panic disorder and/or agoraphobia. Of the individual childhood adversities, physical abuse, parental death, parental mental disorder, and family violence significantly predicted adult-onset asthma.

8.3.4. Independent Associations of Childhood Adversity and Mental Disorder with Adult-Onset Asthma

When childhood adversities and early-onset mental disorders were entered into the same model, both childhood adversities (two or more) and early-onset mental disorders independently predicted adult-onset asthma (Table 8.5). The hazard ratio for three or more childhood adversities reduced from 1.71 (shown in Table 8.3) to 1.55 (Table 8.5) once controlling for early-onset depressive/anxiety disorder. A very similar magnitude reduction is evident in the hazard ratio for any depressive/anxiety disorder of 1.67 prior to adjustment for childhood adversity (Table 8.4) reducing to 1.54 (Table 8.5) after adjustment for adversity. These results suggest that only a portion of the relationship between early-onset mental disorder and adult-onset asthma is accounted for by childhood adversity.

8.4. DISCUSSION

Three interesting findings emerged from this study: First, the experience of two or more childhood adversities predicted adult-onset asthma, with increasing strength with a greater number of adversities. The relationship between two or more childhood adversities and adult-onset asthma occurred independently of current depressive/anxiety disorders, and also independently of early-onset depressive/anxiety disorders. Second, depressive and anxiety disorders occurring prior to adulthood predicted adult-onset asthma. Third, childhood adversity explained only a portion of the sequential comorbidity between early-onset depressive/anxiety disorders and adult-onset asthma.

These findings confirm the few prior reports of an association between childhood adversity and adult-onset asthma, and extend them by demonstrating this relationship independently of depressive and anxiety disorders (early onset or current), and in adults spanning the full age range. Given the many cases of childhood adversity and adult-onset asthma that were excluded in the current study, which probably have stronger

Table 8.4. Effect of early-onset (prior to age 21) depressive/anxiety disorders and specific childhood adversities on risk of adult-onset asthma (≥21 years of age)

	Hazard ratios (95% CI) for adult-onset asthma (adjusted for age, sex, smoking status, and country)
Early-onset (prior to age 21) mental disorders	
Any depressive/anxiety disorder	1.67 (1.23, 2.28)*
Major depressive disorder	2.11 (1.51, 2.93)*
Generalized anxiety disorder	1.46 (0.89, 2.38)
Social phobia	1.19 (0.85, 1.67)
Posttraumatic stress disorder	1.95 (1.07, 3.58)*
Panic disorder/agoraphobia	2.06 (1.34, 3.18)*
Childhood adversities	
Physical abuse	1.92 (1.32, 2.81)*
Sexual abuse	1.26 (0.84, 1.82)
Neglect	1.02 (0.70, 1.49)
Parental death	1.34 (1.01, 1.77)*
Parental divorce	1.23 (0.84, 1.82)
Other loss of parent	1.36 (0.94, 1.97)
Parental mental disorder	1.50 (1.05, 2.17)*
Parental substance-use disorder	1.28 (0.83, 1.97)
Violence in family	1.51 (1.05, 2.17)*
Criminal behavior in family	1.37 (0.82, 2.31)
Family economic adversity	0.90 (0.61, 1.33)

* $p < .05$.

connections with childhood adversity than adult-onset cases (Chida et al. 2008), these findings can be considered a conservative test of the relationship between childhood adversity and asthma onset.

These results are particularly intriguing in light of a recent prospective study on a New Zealand birth cohort which found that childhood maltreatment predicted adult inflammation (indexed by C-reactive protein) independently of major depressive disorder (Danese et al. 2007). That finding suggests that the stress associated with childhood adversity can affect immune system function, increasing inflammation; this then may have implications for conditions such as asthma. Exactly how stress dysregulates immune function is not completely understood. It may decrease the responsiveness of the hypothalamic–pituitary–adrenal (HPA) axis, reducing cortisol secretion, which in turn may lead to increased production of proinflammatory cytokines (Wright 2005). Alternatively, prolonged exposure to cortisol via HPA axis activation has been suggested to trigger a counterregulatory response in white blood cells, making them more resistant to the anti-inflammatory properties of cortisol (Miller, Cohen, & Ritchey 2002). Alterations in a range of other neuroendocrine mediators (such as substance P) and neurotransmitters likely also play a part in immune regulation and inflammatory responses in the lung (Wright 2005).

One thing that is reasonably clear is that the developing stress response and immune systems are particularly susceptible to disruption in early life (Wright 2005), as discussed in Chapter 7. Such neuroimmunologic disruption, in interaction with genetic factors and particular environmental exposures, may then create the basis for an influence of childhood adversity on asthma (Wright 2005). Moreover, early adverse environments can shape behavioral responses and subsequent environmental exposures in a way that may increase risk of disease development in adulthood (see Chapter 7).

The other key finding in the current study is that early-onset depressive/anxiety disorders were associated with subsequent asthma onset independently of childhood adversity.

Psychosocial Predictors of Adult-Onset Asthma

This does not support the suggestion from prior research that childhood adversity accounts for the relationship between mental disorders and asthma. This finding is consistent with two possibilities.

The first possibility is that the relationship observed here between early-onset depressive/anxiety disorders on adult-onset asthma is noncausal, but rather than being a function primarily of childhood adversity, it may be a function of other common risk factors not measured in this study, such as genetic factors (Wamboldt et al. 2000), or perinatal problems (Nomura et al. 2007). Some evidence for this possibility is provided by Goodwin et al. (2004), who found that while childhood adversity accounted for some of the association between mental disorders and asthma, other unspecified shared risk factors accounted for the remainder of the association, though that study was not able to provide information on what those risk factors might be.

The second possibility is that early-onset depressive/anxiety disorders have a causal effect on risk of asthma onset. This could occur through behavioral pathways whereby health risk behaviors associated with mental disorders may increase risk of atopic disease in vulnerable individuals (Chida et al. 2008), though smoking status was controlled for in this study. Biological pathways have also been suggested, from panic disorder to asthma through the effect of chronic hyperventilation (Hasler et al. 2005; Rietveld, Everaerd, & Creer 2000) and from depression to asthma through depression-associated abnormalities in inflammatory and atopic processes (Cohen et al. 1998; Irwin & Miller 2007).

Table 8.5. Independent effects of childhood adversity and early-onset depressive/anxiety disorders on risk of adult-onset asthma (each controlling for the effect of the other, plus age, sex, smoking, and country)[a]

	Hazard ratios (95% CI) for adult-onset asthma (adjusted for age, sex, smoking status, and country)
Number of childhood adversities	
One	1.21 (0.96, 1.54)
Two	1.43 (1.04, 1.98)*
Three or more	1.55 (1.06, 1.28)*
Early-onset (prior to age 21) mental disorders	
Any depressive/anxiety disorder	1.54 (1.17, 2.03)*
Major depressive disorder	1.91 (1.38, 2.63)*
Generalized anxiety disorder	1.26 (0.76, 2.08)
Social phobia	1.08 (0.78, 1.49)
Posttraumatic stress disorder	1.70 (0.96, 2.98)
Panic disorder/agoraphobia	1.86 (1.20, 2.91)*

[a] The effect of the individual depressive/anxiety disorders is not adjusted for the other depressive/anxiety disorders.
* $p < .05$.

If increased inflammation is associated with both childhood adversity and depression, how can it be that these two factors apparently have independent pathways to asthma onset, as this study suggests? This will require further research to clarify, but one possibility is that early-onset mental disorders may constitute a source of additional chronic stress, further taxing a stress system disrupted by early adversity, in keeping with the concept of allostatic load (McEwen 2003). Another possibility is that biological pathways may primarily link either childhood adversity or early-onset mental disorders with asthma, while behavioral pathways may mediate the influence of the other factor.

This study had some notable limitations. In contrast to the detailed assessment of both mental disorders and childhood adversity, asthma was assessed by the questions only about lifetime diagnosis (asthma status) and age at which the diagnosis was made. With regard to asthma status, it has been suggested that it is unlikely that healthy subjects will respond affirmatively to a question on the presence of asthma (Pattaro et al. 2007), and this is supported by research showing that asthma was underestimated by self-report in comparison with medical records (National Center for Health Status 1994). The current study used self-report of diagnosis, so the discrepancy between self-report and medical record is likely to be less. The use of self-reported diagnosis versus self-reported symptoms to ascertain asthma status is both a weakness, in that it may not accurately pinpoint symptom onset, and a strength, in that while depression has been found to bias the self-report of physical symptoms, it has not been found to bias the self-report of diagnosed physical conditions (Kolk et al. 2002; Vassend & Skrondal 1999).

With regard to retrospectively reported AOO of asthma, recent studies have found it to be accurate (Toren et al. 2006) to show excellent reliability over repeat assessments (Pattaro et al. 2007) and for reliability to be unaffected either by the age at onset or by the difference between the age at onset and the age at interview (Pattaro et al. 2007). This study used the age of asthma diagnosis, which, as noted previously, may lag behind symptom onset, so it is possible that in a small proportion of cases there may have been some overlap between the timing of predictors and asthma symptom onset. It is also a limitation that there were no measures of asthma severity, nor of asthma medication use. The associations reported are therefore averaged across the full spectrum of asthma severity, and as such may underestimate the magnitude of the relationships between childhood adversity early-onset depressive/anxiety disorders, and severe asthma.

The other important limitation is that the report of childhood adversities was also retrospective. The possibility of mood-congruent recall bias was addressed in the analyses: the predictive effect of two or more childhood adversities on risk of adult-onset asthma was found to be robust to adjustment for current mood. Note that this is likely to be an overadjustment because (1) it controls for both anxiety and depression, though only depression has been reliably associated with mood-congruent recall (Williams et al. 1997); and (2) it removes from the association of adversity with subsequent asthma the influence of the association between adversity, current mood, and asthma. In so doing, it controls for the possibility of bias in recall, but some of the real relationship between adversity and asthma is lost since those with current depressive/anxiety disorder not only are more likely to recall adverse experiences, but are more likely to have experienced them (Edwards et al. 2003; Maughan & McCarthy 1997).

None of this addresses the generic under-recall that occurs as a function of the time lag between the childhood experience of adversity and the assessment of it in adulthood (Hardt and Rutter, 2004)). We do not consider this to be a major threat to validity, however, as the detailed nature of the assessment for childhood adversity would have mitigated against underrecall somewhat, and any general underreporting of childhood adversity would not have determined the pattern of results obtained, though again it may mean that the size of the effects observed is somewhat underestimated.

There is no disputing that the ideal study for this topic is prospective in design, but the desirability of investigating adult chronic disease outcomes in a sample spanning the full adult age range makes prospective collection of data a very long term proposition. In the interim, this kind of study using retrospective reports of adversities and condition onsets offers noteworthy preliminary results, which need to be confirmed in more definitive designs.

In conclusion, this study finds that both childhood adversity and early-onset depressive/anxiety disorders independently predict adult-onset asthma, suggesting that the sequential comorbidity between early-onset mental disorder and adult-onset asthma is not primarily a function of a shared background of childhood adversity. This does not rule out other possible noncausal models of mental disorder–asthma comorbidity. The predictive associations between childhood adversity, early-onset mental disorder, and adult-onset asthma are plausible in light of other research linking these variables with dysregulation of neuroendocrine and immunologic pathways that results in increased inflammation.

ACKNOWLEDGMENT

Some material in this chapter appeared in Scott et al. (2008). This material is reprinted with the permission of the copyright owner, Lippincott Williams & Wilkins.

REFERENCES

Afari, N., Schmaling, K. B., Barnhart, S., & Buchwald, D. (2001). Psychiatric comorbidity and functional status in adult patients with asthma. *Journal of Clinical Psychology in Medical Settings*, **8**, 245–52.

Brown, E., Khan, D., & Mahadi, S. (2000). Psychiatric diagnosis in inner city outpatients with moderate to severe asthma. *International Journal of Psychiatry in Medicine*, **30**, 295–7.

Burney, P. G. J., Chinn, S., Jarvis, D., Luczynska, C., & Lai, E. (1996). Variations in the prevalence of respiratory symptoms, self-reported asthma attacks, and use of asthma medication in the European Community Respiratory Health Survey (ECRHS). *European Respiratory Journal*, **9**, 687–95.

Chida, Y., Hamer, M., & Steptoe, A. (2008). A bidirectional relationship between psychosocial factors and atopic disorders: A systematic review and meta-analysis. *Psychosomatic Medicine*, **70**, 102–16.

Cohen, P., Pine, D. S., Must, A., Kasen, S., & Brook, J. (1998). Prospective associations between somatic illness and mental illnesss from childhood to adulthood. *American Journal of Epidemiology*, **147**, 232–9.

Danese, A., Pariante, C. M., Caspi, A., Taylor, A., & Poulton, R. (2007). Childhood maltreatment predicts adult inflammation in a life-course study. *Proceedings of the National Academy of Sciences*, **104**, 1319–24.

Edwards, V. J., Holden, G. W., Felitti, V. J., & Anda, R. F. (2003). Relationship between multiple forms of childhood maltreatment and adult mental health in community respondents: Results from the adverse childhood experiences study. *American Journal of Psychiatry*, **160**, 1453–60.

Goldney, R. D., Ruffin, R., Fisher, L. J., & Wilson, D. H. (2003). Asthma symptoms associated with depression and lower quality of life: A population survey. *Medical Journal of Australia*, **178**, 437–41.

Goodwin, R. D., & Eaton, W. W. (2003). Asthma and the risk of panic attacks among adults in the community. *Psychological Medicine*, **33**, 879–85.

Goodwin, R. D., Fergusson, D. M., & Horwood, L. J. (2004). Asthma and depressive and anxiety disorders among young persons in the community. *Psychological Medicine*, **34**, 1465–74.

Goodwin, R. D., Jacobi, F., & Thefeld, W. (2003). Mental disorders and asthma in the community. *Archives of General Psychiatry*, **60**, 1125–30.

Goodwin, R. D., Olfson, M., Shea, S., Lantigua, R. A., Carrasquilo, O., Gameroff, M. J., & M. Weissman, M. (2003). Asthma and mental disorders in primary care. *General Hospital Psychiatry*, **25**, 479–83.

Goodwin, R. D., Wamboldt, M. Z., & Pine, D. S. (2003). Lung disease and internalizing disorders. Is childhood abuse a shared etiologic factor? *Journal of Psychosomatic Research*, **55**, 215–19.

Hardt, J. & Rutter, M. (2004). Validity of adult retrospective reports of adverse childhood experiences: Review of the evidence. *Journal of Child Psychology and Psychiatry*, **45**, 260–73.

Hasler, G., Gergen, P. J., Kleinbaum, D. G., Ajdacic, V., Gamma, A., Eich, D., Rossler, W., & Angst, J. (2005). Asthma and panic in young adults.

American Journal of Respiratory and Critical Care Medicine, **171**, 1224–30.

Irwin, M. R., & Miller, A. H. (2007). Depressive disorders and immunity: 20 years of progress and discovery. *Brain, Behavior and Immunity*, **21**, 374–83.

Janson, C., Bjornsson, E., Hetta, J., & Boman, G. (1994). Anxiety and depression in relation to respiratory symptoms and asthma. *American Journal of Respiratory Critical Care Medicine*, **149**, 930–4.

Jenkins, M. A., Hopper, J. L., Bowes, G., Carlin, J. B., Flander, L. B., & Giles, G. G. (1994). Factors in childhood as predictors of asthma in adult life. *British Medical Journal*, **309**, 90–3.

Kolbe, J., Fergusson, W., Vamos, M., & Garrett, J. (2002). Case-control study of severe life threatening asthma (SLTA) in adults: Psychological factors. *Thorax*, **57**, 317–22.

Kolk, A. M., Hanewald, G. J., Schagen, S., & Gijsbers van Wijk, C. M. (2002). Predicting medically unexplained physical symptoms and health care utilization. A symptom-perception approach. *Journal of Psychosomatic Research*, **52**, 35–44.

Maughan, B., & McCarthy, G. (1997). Childhood adversities and psychosocial disorders. *British Medical Bulletin*, **53**, 156–69.

McEwen, B. S. (2003). Mood disorders and allostatic load. *Biological Psychiatry*, **54**, 200–7.

Melgert, B. N., Ray, A., Hylkema, M. N., Timens, W., & Postma, D. S. (2007). Are there reasons why adult asthma is more common in females? *Current Allergy and Asthma Reports*, **7**, 143–50.

Miller, G. E., Cohen, S., & Ritchey, A. K. (2002). Chronic psychological stress and the regulation of pro-inflammatory cytokines: A glucocorticoid resistance model. *Health Psychology*, **21**, 536–41.

Nascimento, I., Nardi, A. E., Valenca, A. M., Lopes, F. L., Mezzasalma, M. A., Nascentes, R., & Zin, W. A. (2002). Psychiatric disorders in asthmatic outpatients. *Psychiatry Research*, **110**, 73–80.

National Center for Health Studies. (1994). Evaluation of National Health Interview Survey diagnostic reporting. *Vital and Health Statistics 2*, **120**, 1–116.

Nomura, Y., Brooks-Gunn, J., Davey, C., Ham, J., & Fifer, W. P. (2007). The role of perinatal problems in risk of co-morbid psychiatric and medical disorders in adulthood. *Psychological Medicine*, **37**, 1323–34.

Pattaro, C., Locatelli, F., Sunyer, J., & de Marco, R. (2007). Using the age at onset may increase the reliability of longitudinal asthma assessment. *Journal of Clinical Epidemiology*, **60**, 704–11.

Pearce, N., Douwes, J., & Beasley, R. (2000). The rise and rise of asthma: A new paradigm for the new millennium? *Journal of Epidemiology and Biostatistics*, **5**, 5–16.

Perna, G., Bertani, A., Politi, E., Columbo, G., & Bellodi, L. (1997). Asthma and panic attacks. *Biological Psychiatry*, **42**, 625–30.

Rietveld, S., Everaerd, W., & Creer, T. L. (2000). Stress-induced asthma: A review of research and potential mechanisms. *Clinical and Experimental Allergy*, **30**, 1058–66.

Romans, S., Belaise, C., Martin, J., Morris, E., & Raffi, A. (2002). Childhood abuse and later medical disorders in women. *Psychotherapy & Psychosomatics*, **71**, 141–50.

Scott, K. M., Von Korff, M., Alonso, J., Angermeyer, M. C., Benjet, C., Bruffaerts, R., de Girolamo, G., Haro, J. M., Kessler, R. C., Kovess, V., Ono, Y., Ormel, J., & Posada-Villa, J. (2008). Childhood adversity, early-onset depressive/anxiety disorders, and adult-onset asthma. *Psychosomatic Medicine*, **70(9)**, 1035–43.

Scott, K. M., Von Korff, M., Ormel, J., Zhang, M.-Y., Bruffaerts, R., Alonso, J., Kessler, R., Tachimori, H., Karam, E., Levinson, D., Bromet, E., Posada-Villa, J., Gasquet, I., Angermeyer, M., Borges, G., de Girolamo, G., Herman, A., & Haro, J. M. (2007). Mental disorders among adults with asthma: Results from the World Mental Health Survey. *General Hospital Psychiatry*, **29**, 123–33.

Shavitt, R. G., Gentil, V., & Mandetta, R. (1992). The association of panic/agoraphobia and asthma. Contributing factors and clinical implications. *General Hospital Psychiatry*, **14**, 420–3.

Toren, K., Palmqvist, M., Lowhagen, O., Balder, B., & Tunsater, A. (2006). Self-reported asthma was biased in relation to disease severity while reported year of asthma onset was accurate. *Journal of Clinical Epidemiology*, **59**, 90–3.

Vassend, O., & Skrondal, A. (1999). The role of negative affectivity in self-assessment of health. *Journal of Health Psychology*, **4**, 465–82.

von Behren, J., Kreutzer, R., & Hernandez, A. (2002). Self-reported asthma prevalence in adults in California. *Journal of Asthma*, **39**, 429–40.

Wainwright, N. W., Surtees, P. G., Wareham, N. J., & Harrison, B. D. W. (2007). Psychosocial factors and incident asthma hospital admissions in the EPIC-Norfolk cohort study. *Allergy*, **62**, 554–60.

Wamboldt, M. Z., Hewitt, F. K., Schmitz, S., Wamboldt, F. S., Rasanen, M., Koskenvuo, M., Romanov, K., Varjonen, J., & Kaprio, J. (2000). Familial association between allergic disorders and depression in adult Finnish twins. *American Journal of Medical Genetics*, **96**, 146–53.

Williams, J. M. G., Watts, F. N., MacLeod, C., & Mathews, A., eds. (1997). *Cognitive Psychology and Emotional Disorders*, 2nd ed. Chichester, England: John Wiley & Sons.

Wright, R. J. (2005). Stress and atopic disorders. *Journal of Allergy and Clinical Immunology*, **116**, 1301–6.

Yellowlees, P. M., Alpers, J. H., Bowden, J. J., Bryant, G. D., & Ruffin, R. E. (1987). Psychiatric morbidity in patients with chronic airflow obstruction. *Medical Journal of Australia*, **146**, 305–7.

Yellowlees, P. M., Haynes, S., Potts, N., & Ruffin, R. (1988). Psychiatric morbidity in patients with life-threatening asthma: Initial report of a controlled study. *Medical Journal of Australia*, **149**, 246–9.

9 Childhood Adversities, Mental Disorders, and Heart Disease

HUIBERT BURGER

9.1. INTRODUCTION

By 2030, ischemic heart disease and depression are projected to be among the top three causes of life-years lost in good health worldwide (Mathers & Loncar 2006). It is well established that these disorders tend to co-occur in the same individual (Rudisch & Nemeroff 2003). For these reasons, identification of mechanisms that can explain the co-occurrence of depression and heart disease has high public health significance. Although there is abundant evidence that depression predicts heart disease and vice versa (Thomas, Kalaria, & O'Brien 2004), the association may also be indirect, resulting from factors that increase the risk of both conditions; that is, they are shared risk factors.

Childhood adversities may constitute shared risk factors for both depression and heart disease as they have repeatedly been shown to predict psychiatric disorders and also physical disorders (Arnow 2004). For example, in a recent study, child abuse and neglect that was substantiated and recorded at the time it had occurred was associated with a 51% higher risk of major depressive disorder in young adulthood as compared to those without abuse or neglect (Widom, DuMont, & Czaja 2007). Findings from the National Comorbidity Survey showed that childhood sexual abuse was associated with an almost four times higher risk of cardiac disease (Goodwin & Stein 2004). For these reasons, childhood adversities may explain the co-occurrence of depression and heart disease, at least partly. Research on this topic is sparse, however.

Previous studies that have linked childhood adversities to both mental and physical outcomes in the same persons have typically focused on just physical symptoms (Brown, Berenson, & Cohen 2005; Martin et al. 2000; McCauley et al. 1997; Walker et al. 1999) or on indirect measures of health, like health care utilization (Chartier, Walker, & Naimark 2007; Walker et al. 1999), rather than on specific physical diseases. There are also studies in which childhood adversities were related to depression and "cardiac disease" (Goodwin & Stein 2004), ischemic heart disease (Dong et al. 2004), and cardiovascular diseases as a group (Batten et al. 2004). However, these studies have reported conflicting results. Except for the study by Dong et al. (2004), these studies assessed a limited set of childhood adversities, focusing on sexual abuse, physical abuse, and neglect. Interestingly, the question whether the number of adversities experienced in childhood is associated with heart disease and depression has not been addressed to date.

In the present study we examined the association of childhood adversities and early-onset common mental disorders, that is, depression and anxiety before the age of 21, with adult-onset heart disease. If childhood adversities are associated with both common mental disorders and increased risks of developing heart disease in the same persons,

Childhood Adversities, Mental Disorders, and Heart Disease

this might partially explain the well-known and scientifically established co-occurrence of depression and heart disease in adulthood. Therefore, we additionally analyzed to what extent the associations of childhood adversities with adult-onset heart disease and early-onset common mental disorders were independent of each other. Finally, we determined whether specific individual adversities differed in their association with adult-onset heart disease.

9.2. APPROACH

Cox proportional hazards models estimated risk of adult-onset heart disease as a function of number and type of childhood adversities and early-onset depressive/anxiety disorder status while adjusting for potential confounders. Ascertainment of heart disease was with the following question: "Did a medical doctor or other health professional ever tell you that you had heart disease?" Respondents were also asked how old they were when the condition was first diagnosed. Self-report measures of heart disease have been used previously in epidemiological research on heart disease and psychopathology (Stansfeld et al. 2002). However, the potential errors that can result from using self-report of medically recognized heart disease need to be considered in interpreting the results of the World Mental Health (WMH) Surveys.

Kaplan–Meier curves were constructed for graphical comparison of increasing proportion of respondents reporting onset of heart disease with age between three categories of number of childhood adversities: none, one, and two or more adversities. Kaplan–Meier curves were also used to compare onset of heart disease for persons with and without early-onset depressive and/or anxiety disorder. See Chapter 4 (4.5.5) for further description of the methods, which were generic across

Table 9.1. Demographic characteristics of the study population

Number	18,303
Female gender (%)	52.8
Age (mean; SD)	45.7 (16.5)
Ever smoking (%)	46.4
Completed secondary education (%)	61.3

Note: Persons with heart disease onset before the age of 21 were excluded from the sample. Percentages and mean are weighted.
SD, standard deviation.

the physical condition and pain condition outcomes included in this section.

9.3. FINDINGS

Demographic characteristics of the study population are shown in Table 9.1. A little more than half the sample was female, the average age was about 46 years, and 61% had completed secondary education. The frequency of individual childhood adversities, as well as the distribution of the number of adversities reported by respondents, is given in Table 9.2. The most common childhood adversities had a frequency in the order of 10% and concerned adversities such as parental death or divorce, as well as events such as physical abuse and family violence. The lowest frequency rate was observed for sexual abuse with 2.6%. A little more than half reported none of the childhood adversities that we asked about, whereas around 10% of the respondents reported two or more. About 10% of the respondents reported onset of a depressive or anxiety disorder prior to age 21, while an ample 4% reported heart disease that developed after age 21 (Table 9.3).

Throughout adult life (Figure 9.1), respondents who reported two or more childhood adversities experienced increased risk of developing heart disease after the age of 21 when compared to persons with no childhood adversities. Persons with a history of

Table 9.2. Frequency of childhood adversities and the distribution of number of adversities within respondents

	Unweighted N	Weighted %
Childhood adversities		
Neglect	1,549	6.5
Physical abuse	2,430	9.7
Sexual abuse	747	2.6
Parental death	2,416	12.9
Parental divorce	2,006	9.9
Other parental loss	1,178	5.3
Parental mental disorder	1,883	7.2
Parental substance abuse	1,232	5.0
Family violence	2,250	9.5
Parental crime	828	3.4
Economic adversity	1,199	5.9
Number of adversities		
None	9,392	56.0
One	4,723	25.6
Two	2,126	10.0
Three or more	2,062	8.3

only one childhood adversity also showed a slight increase in risk of adult-onset heart disease, but the increased risk was evident only after the age of 65 (see Figure 9.1).

A strong and graded positive association or dose–response relation was observed between the grouped number of childhood adversities and the relative risk of adult-onset heart disease as indicated by the hazard ratios in Table 9.4. Compared to respondents without a history of childhood adversities, those reporting two or more childhood adversities experienced about a 60% increase in risk of adult-onset heart disease. Persons reporting only one childhood adversity experienced about a 20% increase in risk, which was statistically non-significant. Persons with three or more childhood adversities showed a more than twofold increase in risk of adult-onset heart disease. These relative risk estimates remained unaltered when we adjusted for current (12-month) anxiety or mood disorder. Among respondents with early-onset depressive/anxiety disorder, the risk of adult-onset heart disease was doubled compared to those without, an excess risk that was highly statistically significant as evident from the narrow 95% confidence interval.

When childhood adversities and early-onset mental disorders were analyzed with mutual adjustment (Model 2 in Table 9.4), their associations with heart disease hardly attenuated, indicating that the associations were largely independent. Adjustment for educational attainment did not markedly affect these results (Model 3 in Table 9.4). The relative risk estimates for the interaction between two or more adversities and early-onset mental disorders was small and not statistically significant (1.34; 95% CI = 0.87–2.19).

Analyses with individual adversities adjusted for age, gender, and ever smoking indicated that the associations with adult-onset heart disease were strongest for physical abuse, sexual abuse, parental mental disorder, and parental substance abuse with hazard ratios (95% CI) of 1.82 (1.37–2.43), 3.91 (2.40–6.39), 1.58 (1.18–2.12), and 1.75 (1.18–2.60), respectively. The hazard ratios associated with the remaining adversities

Table 9.3. Percent with early-onset mental disorders and adult-onset heart disease

	Unweighted N	Weighted %
Early-onset mental disorders[a]		
Major depressive disorder	1,719	4.6
Major depressive or anxiety disorder	3,537	10.3
Adult-onset heart disease[b]	914	4.2

[a] Onset before the age of 21.
[b] Onset after the age of 20.

Childhood Adversities, Mental Disorders, and Heart Disease

Table 9.4. Relative risk of heart disease associated with early-onset mental disorders and childhood adversities

	Model 1	Model 2	Model 3
Number of childhood adversities			
One	1.24 (1.00–1.55)	1.23 (0.98–1.52)	1.21 (0.96–1.51)
Two	1.60 (1.22–2.09)	1.55 (1.19–2.03)	1.61 (1.22–2.11)
Three or more	2.40 (1.75–3.28)	2.19 (1.59–3.01)	1.82 (1.34–2.47)
Early-onset mental disorders	1.91 (1.48–2.46)	1.66 (1.26–2.18)	1.77 (1.34–2.33)

Notes: Values are hazard ratios (95% confidence interval).
Reference category is no childhood adversities.
Early-onset mental disorders are depression and/or anxiety before the age of 21.
Model 1 adjusted for age, sex, and ever smoking status.
Model 2 adjusted for age, sex, and ever smoking status; adversities and mental disorders were adjusted for each other.
Model 3 adjusted for age, sex, ever smoking status, and educational attainment. Adversities and mental disorders were adjusted for each other.

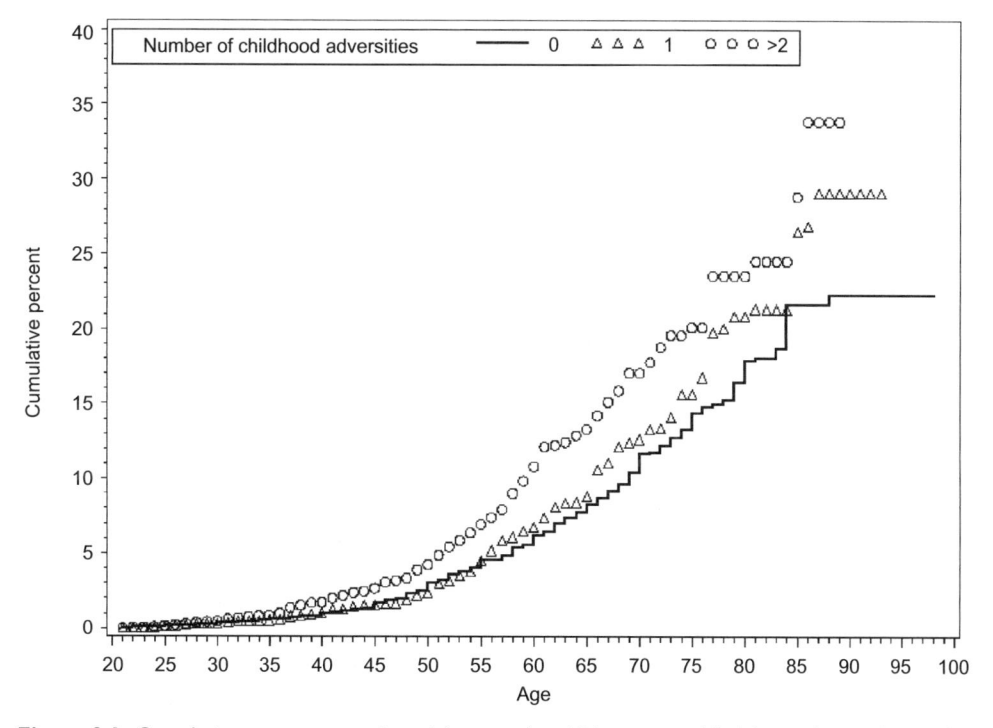

Figure 9.1. Cumulative percent reporting adult-onset (aged 21 years or older) heart disease by number of childhood adversities.

were either smaller than 1.5 or not statistically significant, or both.

9.4. DISCUSSION

9.4.1. Main Findings

The present study shows strong associations of childhood adversities in the context of the family and early-onset common mental disorders with adult-onset heart disease. The analyses were carried out using self-report data from the populations of 10 countries around the world. The risk of heart disease showed a dose–response relationship with increasing number of childhood adversities. In the presence of a history of three or more adversities, the risk of heart disease more than doubled. Out of the childhood adversities assessed, sexual abuse and physical abuse were most strongly associated with adult-onset heart disease. Yet, because the individual adversities were not adjusted for each other and were likely correlated, we cannot state with certainty which adversities were independently from the other adversities associated with heart disease. Still, the association of number of adversities with risk of developing heart disease suggests that the possibility that the diversity of exposure to childhood adversities may be more important than the specific kinds of adversities. If this is the case, the fact that prior research has assessed a limited range of adversities is a significant limitation.

Early-onset anxiety/depressive disorder was associated with an approximately twofold higher risk of heart disease. The associations of childhood adversities and early-onset mental disorders with heart disease appeared to be largely independent of each other; that is, these associations must have existed in different persons. Variation in educational attainment between individuals did not explain these results.

9.4.2. Limitations

One may question the validity of self-report heart disease. However, in studies comparing medical record and patient data, the concordance has generally been good for myocardial infarction and, in men, also for angina when asked for doctor-diagnosed disease (Lampe et al. 1999). In addition, given the fairly low overall frequency of a report of heart disease in our study (4.2%), it is unlikely that respondents reported atypical chest pain that may mimic the symptoms of genuine ischemic heart disease. Furthermore, the occurrence of heart disease in the WMH Surveys conformed to expected demographic variation, with increasing frequency rates with age, lower frequency rates in relatively poor countries, and existing more often in males than in females (Ormel et al. 2007).

It is in our view unlikely that respondents with a report of doctor-diagnosed heart disease are inclined to systematically over- or underreport childhood adversities as compared to those without. If this is the case, then risk estimates would not be different from the true but unknown risks. Further, because adjustment for current (12-month) anxiety or mood disorder did not alter the risk estimates for childhood adversities, systematic error in recall related to present mental state is not likely to explain the observed associations. In any case, reliance on self-reported heart disease is a significant limitation. We propose that the initial findings here should be replicated in prospective research with objective assessment of heart disease status.

It should be noted that the frequency of self-reported adult-onset heart disease cannot be interpreted as the true risk of heart disease from age 20 because, inherent to the survey design, the total population from which the cases of heart disease arose has not been enumerated. Therefore, the denominator for the risk estimate is not exactly known. Further, self-reported heart disease necessarily excludes fatal heart disease.

9.4.3. Implications for Research and Clinical Practice

The present study confirms that childhood adversities and depression or anxiety are each associated with heart disease (Arnow 2004; Thomas et al. 2004). Contrary to expectation, however, these associations were independent of each other. Therefore, the data indicate that childhood adversities cannot explain the established co-occurrence of depression and adult-onset heart disease. In other words, childhood adversities may not be shared risk factors for depression and heart disease in adulthood. Rather, the associations of childhood adversities and early-onset mental disorders with heart disease may be independent, for example, acting in different individuals. One of the implications is that other mechanisms account for the co-occurrence of ischemic heart disease and depressive disorders. For instance, a common genetic vulnerability to depression and cardiovascular disease has been suggested as a contributing factor (McCaffery et al. 2006).

There are three previous studies that have specifically addressed the role of depression in the relationship between childhood adversity and heart disease (Batten et al. 2004; Dong et al. 2004; Goodwin & Stein 2004). These studies showed different results. Goodwin and Stein (2004) and Dong et al. (2004) observed substantial decreases in relative risk estimates when they adjusted for depressive or anxiety disorder and psychological risk factors, respectively. In contrast, the results in Batten et al.'s study (2004) showed no evidence of such decreases when accounting for lifetime diagnosis of depressive disorder with adult onset. Because it was unknown in these studies whether the psychiatric disorders and psychological risk factors actually preceded development of heart problems it is uncertain whether the analyses really addressed the question whether childhood adversities lead to depression and depression in turn promotes heart disease. Alternatively, the depressive or anxiety disorders may have resulted from heart disease in these studies, which could have decreased the relative risks as well. In this context, because we restricted mental disorders to those with early onset, our finding that depressive or anxiety disorder does not seem to be part of the route from childhood adversities to adult-onset heart disease may be an important addition to the literature. Although in a recent study significant associations of childhood physical abuse were observed with "heart trouble," symptoms of depression, anger, and anxiety, no analysis controlling these variables for each other was presented, leaving the question of independence unanswered (Springer et al. 2007).

Mechanistic pathways cannot be elucidated with the data in either of these studies. A retrospective study design has the potential problem of systematic error in recall. Future studies on mental and physical consequences of childhood adversities therefore need to be prospective and should include detailed measurements of behavioral, psychological, or biological parameters. An example of a pathway could be that adversities in childhood increase the likelihood of engaging in an unhealthy lifestyle, including smoking, obesity, and low levels of physical activity, all of which may, in turn, increase the risk of ischemic heart disease. Future research on pathways of childhood adversities to ischemic heart disease may consider measurement of subclinical atherosclerosis that has shown to be predictive of later heart disease and can already be noninvasively assessed in childhood or adolescence by ultrasonic measurement of the intima-media thickness of the carotid wall (Sabri & Kelishadi 2007).

Our finding that the association of childhood adversities with heart disease was most strongly associated with sexual abuse and physical abuse concurs with findings by Goodwin and Stein (2004), who also observed strongest associations for sexual abuse followed by physical abuse and no association for child neglect. Yet, there is evidence that other adversities occurring in the context of the family, such as serious conflicts, may precipitate heart disease as well (Sumanen et al. 2005). Collectively, these findings point to the importance of assessing a wide range of childhood adversities when assessing the impact of childhood adversities on risk of developing heart disease.

In conclusion, childhood adversities were associated with self-reported adult-onset heart disease independently of early-onset depressive/anxiety disorder. This suggests that the established co-occurrence of depression and heart disease in adulthood may not be explained by childhood adversities. Prospective studies of the association of diverse childhood adversities with risk of developing (objectively ascertained) heart disease are needed.

REFERENCES

Arnow, B. (2004). Relationships between childhood maltreatment, adult health and psychiatric outcomes, and medical utilization. *Journal of Clinical Psychiatry*, **65**, 10–15.

Batten, S. V., Aslan, M., Maciejewski, P. K., & Mazure C. M. (2004). Childhood maltreatment as a risk factor for adult cardiovascular disease and depression. *Journal of Clinical Psychiatry*, **65**, 249–54.

Brown, J., Berenson, K., & Cohen, P. (2005). Documented and self-reported child abuse and adult pain in a community sample. *Clinical Journal of Pain*, **21**, 374–7.

Chartier, M. J., Walker, J. R., & Naimark, B. (2007). Childhood abuse, adult health, and health care utilization: Results from a representative community sample. *American Journal of Epidemiology*, **165**, 1031–8.

Dong, M., Anda, R. F., Dube, S. R., Giles, W. H., & Felitti, V. J. (2004). Insights into causal pathways for ischemic heart disease: Adverse childhood experiences study. *Circulation*, **110**, 1761–6.

Goodwin, R. D., & Stein, M. B. (2004). Association between childhood trauma and physical disorders among adults in the United States. *Psychological Medicine*, **34**, 509–20.

Lampe, F. C., Walker, M., Lennon, L. T., Whincup, P. H., & Ebrahim, S. (1999). Validity of a self-reported history of doctor-diagnosed angina. *Journal of Clinical Epidemiology*, **52**, 73–81.

Martin, L., Rosen, L. N., Durand, D. B., Knudson, K. H., & Stretch, R. H. (2000). Psychological and physical health effects of sexual assaults and nonsexual traumas among male and female United States Army soldiers. *Behavioral Medicine*, **26**, 23–33.

Mathers, C. D., & Loncar, D. (2006). Projections of global mortality and burden of disease from 2002 to 2030. *PLoS Medicine*, **3**, e442.

McCaffery, J. M., Frasure-Smith, N., Dube, M. P., Théroux, P., Rouleau, G. A., Duan, Q., & Lespérance, F. (2006). Common genetic vulnerability to depressive symptoms and coronary artery disease: A review and development of candidate genes related to inflammation and serotonin. *Psychosomatic Medicine*, **68**, 187–200.

McCauley, J., Kern, D. E., Kolodner, K., Dill, L., Schroeder, A. F., DeChant, H. K., Ryden, J., Derogatis, L. R., & Bass, E. B. (1997). Clinical characteristics of women with a history of childhood abuse: Unhealed wounds. *The Journal of the American Medical Association*, **277**, 1362–8.

Ormel, J., Von Korff, M., Burger, H., Scott, K. M., Demyttenaere, K., Huang, Y. Q., Posada-Villa, J., Pierre Lepine, J., Angermeyer, M. C., Levinson, D., de Girolamo, G., Kawakami, N., Karam, E., Medina-Mora, M. E., Gureje, O., Williams, D., Haro, J. M., Bromet, E. J., Alonso, J., & Kessler, R. C. (2007). Mental disorders among persons with heart disease – Results from World Mental Health Surveys. *General Hospital Psychiatry*, **29**, 325–34.

Rudisch, B., & Nemeroff, C. B. (2003). Epidemiology of comorbid coronary artery disease and depression. *Biological Psychiatry*, **54**, 227–40.

Sabri, M. R., & Kelishadi, R. (2007). The thickness of the intimal and medial layers of the carotid arteries, and the index of left ventricular mass, in children of patients with premature coronary arterial disease. *Cardiology in the Young,* **17,** 609–16.

Springer, K. W., Sheridan, J., Kuo, D., & Carnes, M. (2007). Long-term physical and mental health consequences of childhood physical abuse: Results from a large population-based sample of men and women. *Child Abuse & Neglect,* **31,** 517–30.

Stansfeld, S. A., Fuhrer, R., Shipley, M. J., & Marmot, M. G. (2002). Psychological distress as a risk factor for coronary heart disease in the Whitehall II Study. *International Journal of Epidemiology,* **31,** 248–55.

Sumanen, M., Koskenvuo, M., Sillanmaki, L., & Mattila, K. (2005). Childhood adversities experienced by working-aged coronary heart disease patients. *Journal of Psychosomatic Research,* **59,** 331–5.

Thomas, A. J., Kalaria, R. N., & O'Brien, J. T. (2004). Depression and vascular disease: What is the relationship? *Journal of Affective Disorders,* **79,** 81–95.

Walker, E. A., Gelfand, A., Katon, W. J., Koss, M. P., Von Korff, M., Bernstein, D., & Russo, J. (1999). Adult health status of women with histories of childhood abuse and neglect. *American Journal of Medicine,* **107,** 332–9.

Widom, C. S., DuMont, K., & Czaja, S. J. (2007). A prospective investigation of major depressive disorder and comorbidity in abused and neglected children grown up. *Archives of General Psychiatry,* **64,** 49–56.

10 Early Child Adversity and Later Hypertension

DAN J. STEIN, KATE M. SCOTT, AND MICHAEL R. VON KORFF

10.1. INTRODUCTION

Recent research has found that psychosocial factors, in particular depression, anxiety, and anger, contribute to the etiology of hypertension (Kaplan & Nunes 2003; Rutledge & Hogan 2002). Psychological trauma has been hypothesized to be a particularly important contributor to hypertension (Mann & Delon 1995). Such a relationship would be consistent with research that has found chronic adverse psychobiological sequelae of early childhood adversity (Felitti et al. 1998; Gluckman & Hanson 2004) and with an increasingly sophisticated and integrative approach to understanding mental–physical comorbidity (Evans et al. 2005).

Nevertheless, studies on psychosocial contributors to hypertension have important limitations (Kaplan & Nunes 2003; Rutledge & Hogan 2002). Most of these studies have been conducted in only a few countries. The relationship between childhood adversity and hypertension has received relatively little attention, with little data available on the contribution of different childhood adversities. Further, despite evidence that childhood adversities are a risk factor for depression and anxiety disorders (Heim & Nemeroff 2001), there has been no research assessing whether the association of depression and anxiety with subsequent hypertension might be explained by exposure to childhood adversities.

Using data from cross-national population surveys, this chapter reports on the relationship between early-onset depression–anxiety disorders, childhood adversities, and adult-onset hypertension. On the basis of prior research, we hypothesized that exposure to significant childhood adversities is associated with adult-onset hypertension. To assess the potential mediation of early-onset depression–anxiety disorders of the association between childhood adversities and hypertension, we assessed whether such early-onset mental disorders are associated with increased risk of adult-onset hypertension and whether childhood adversity and early-onset depression–anxiety disorders predict adult-onset hypertension independently of each other.

10.2. APPROACH

Cox proportional hazards models estimated risk of adult-onset hypertension as a function of number and type of childhood adversities and early-onset depression–anxiety disorder status while adjusting for potential confounders. Ascertainment of hypertension was with the following question: "Did a doctor or other health professional ever tell you that you had any of the following illnesses ... hypertension?" Respondents were also asked how old they were when the condition was first diagnosed. Kaplan–Meier curves were developed for graphical comparison of the age-specific cumulative proportion of respondents reporting onset of hypertension, comparing three categories of number of

Table 10.1. Characteristics of total and adult-onset hypertension samples

	Total cross-national sample (N = 18,600)		Adult-onset hypertension (>21 years) sample (N = 3,215)
	Unweighted N	Weighted %	Weighted %
Age (21–98 years)			
21–44	9,827	52.5	18.0
>45	8,803	47.5	82.0
Female	11,092	52.8	55.6
Adult-onset hypertension (>21 years)	18,600	3215	17.3
Country			
Colombia	2,122	11.5	8.0
Belgium	989	5.3	4.6
France	1,359	7.3	6.4
Germany	1,273	6.9	7.9
Italy	1,699	9.1	6.8
The Netherlands	1,052	5.6	5.2
Spain	2,015	10.8	9.6
Japan	873	4.7	4.4
Mexico	2,059	11.0	6.6
United States	5,189	27.8	23.6

childhood adversities: none, one, and two or more adversities. Kaplan–Meier curves were also used to compare onset of hypertension for persons with and without early-onset depression–anxiety disorder. See Chapter 4 (4.5.5) for further description of the methods that were generic across the physical condition and pain condition outcomes included in this section.

10.3. FINDINGS

Characteristics of the sample are presented in Table 10.1, and prevalence of self-reported adult-onset hypertension, childhood adversities, and early-onset depression–anxiety disorders are presented in Table 10.2. Overall, 17.3% of the respondents reported hypertension, 48.6% (almost half) noted a history of childhood adversity, and about 18.5% (one-fifth) were found to have early onset of depression–anxiety disorder. Prevalence of childhood adversity varied across countries, ranging from 30% in Spain to 65% in Colombia.

Kaplan–Meier curves for the cumulative percent of hypertension by age for persons with zero, one, or two or more childhood adversities (Figure 10.1) and for persons with versus without early-onset depression–anxiety disorders (Figure 10.2) were plotted, and they indicate associations between hypertension and both multiple childhood adversity and early-onset depression–anxiety disorders. In these unadjusted analyses, early-onset depression–anxiety disorders appeared more strongly associated with adult-onset hypertension than having two or more childhood adversities, particularly after the age of 60.

Table 10.3 provides hazard ratios for the relationship between childhood adversities, early-onset depression–anxiety disorder, and adult-onset hypertension. The unadjusted hazard ratio for adult-onset hypertension for

Table 10.2. Percent with early-onset depressive–anxiety disorders and childhood adversities in total and adult-onset hypertension samples

	Weighted %	
	Total cross-national sample (N = 18,600)	Adult-onset hypertension (>21 years) sample (N = 3,215)
Early-onset (prior to age 21) mental disorders		
Any depressive/anxiety disorder	10.2	18.5
Major depressive disorder	4.5	9.0
Generalized anxiety disorder	1.3	2.5
Social phobia	4.8	8.3
Posttraumatic stress disorder	1.7	2.7
Panic disorder/agoraphobia	1.8	3.3
Number of childhood adversities		
None	56.1	51.4
One	25.6	25.8
Two	10.0	11.6
Three or more	8.3	11.2
Type of childhood adversity		
Physical abuse	9.6	12.9
Sexual abuse	2.6	3.9
Neglect	6.5	8.2
Parental death	12.8	12.7
Parental divorce	9.8	10.6
Other loss of parent	5.3	6.2
Parental mental disorder	7.2	10.0
Parental substance-use disorder	5.0	6.5
Violence in family	9.4	11.9
Parental criminal behavior	3.3	4.4
Family economic adversity	5.8	6.3

persons with early-onset depression–anxiety disorder (relative to those without) was 1.34 ($p < .001$). After adjusting for number of childhood adversities, this hazard ratio was essentially unchanged (HR = 1.29, $p < .001$). Unadjusted hazard ratios for number of childhood adversities (relative to persons with no childhood adversities) were 1.03 for persons with one adversity ($p = $ ns), 1.19 for persons with two adversities ($p < .01$), and 1.28 for persons with three or more adversities ($p < .001$) prior to adjusting for early-onset depression–anxiety disorder status. After adjusting for depression–anxiety disorder status, the hazard ratios for number of childhood adversities were somewhat reduced, but remained significantly greater than 1.0 for persons with three or more adversities ($p < .01$), as given in the second column of Table 10.2. Adjusting for current depression–anxiety disorder status rather than early-onset depression–anxiety disorder status changed the hazard ratios for number of childhood adversities only slightly, suggesting that effects of current mood on recall of childhood adversities or hypertension status do not explain their association.

Hazard ratios for each of the specific childhood adversities, adjusted for gender, age, and country, are provided in Table 10.4.

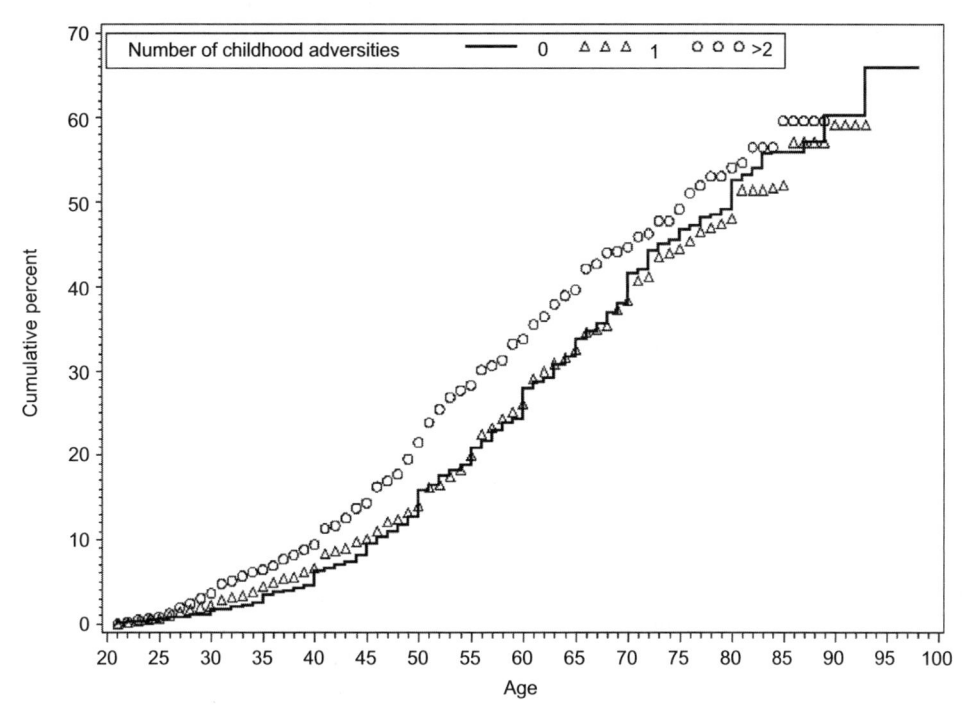

Figure 10.1. Kaplan–Meier curve for the cumulative percent of hypertension by age for persons with no, one, or two or more childhood adversities.

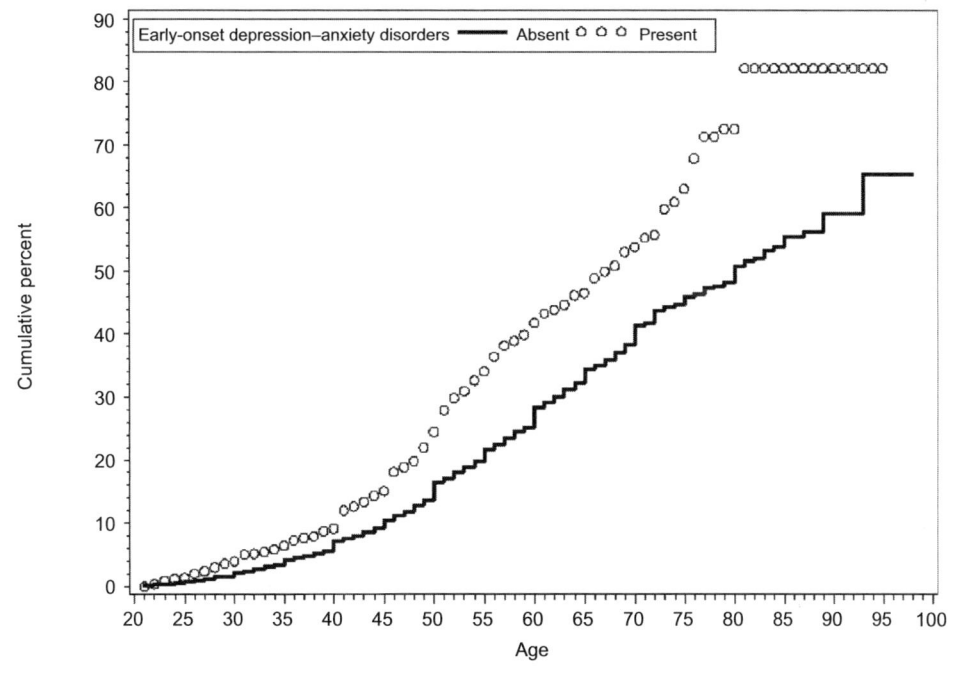

Figure 10.2. Kaplan–Meier curve for the cumulative percent of hypertension by age for persons with versus without early-onset depression–anxiety disorders.

Table 10.3. Association between early-onset depression–anxiety disorders, childhood adversities, and depression

Risk factor	Main effect for hypertension	Adjusted for early-onset depression–anxiety disorders	Adjusted for current depression/anxiety
Depression/anxiety onset before age 21	1.34***		
Number of childhood adversities			
One	1.03 (ns)	1.03 (ns)	1.02 (ns)
Two	1.19*	1.17 (ns)	1.17**
Three or more	1.28**	1.22*	1.21***

* $p < .05$.
** $p < .01$.
*** $p < .001$.

Of the 11 childhood adversities ascertained, 6 of them were significantly associated with adult-onset hypertension (with ORs ranging from 1.17 to 1.55). Among the five specific *Diagnostic and Statistical Manual of Mental Disorders, Fourth Edition* (DSM-IV) mental disorders assessed, early-onset social phobia and panic disorder/agoraphobia were significantly associated with increased risk of adult-onset hypertension, while early-onset depression, generalized anxiety, and posttraumatic stress disorder were not (Table 10.3).

10.4 DISCUSSION

It is important to emphasize several limitations of this study. Blood pressure levels can be directly measured in epidemiological studies, but the current study relied on self-report and provided only a categorical measure of hypertension. At the same time, epidemiological studies of hypertension are rarely able to obtain detailed data on mental illness and psychological stressors. Partial reassurance is obtained from data that self-reported hypertension is moderately associated with objective data on hypertensive status (Alonso et al. 2005; Tormo et al. 2000). It is also important to note that the self-report in the current study was of a doctor's diagnosis of hypertension. Nevertheless, although estimates of sensitivity of self-report of hypertension range from 64 to 91% in several Western countries, it may be lower in other locations (Goldman et al. 2003). A second crucial limitation is that the focus here was on childhood family adversity rather than on a range of other possible early traumas, and the reliance on retrospective reports of childhood stressors. False-negative reports of childhood reports may lead to an underestimation of associated effects. Some reassurance is obtained from a recent review of the validity of retrospective report of childhood adversities, which found that although false-negative reports are common, false-positive reports are rare and which concluded that retrospective case-control studies of major, easily defined adversities are potentially valid (Hardt & Rutter 2004). Finally, retrospective reports of age of onset of both hypertension and mental disorders are subject to bias.

Given these limitations we view the results reported in this chapter as exploratory findings that would need to be replicated with more rigorous ascertainment of hypertension

Table 10.4. Effect of early-onset (prior to age 21) depressive–anxiety disorders and specific childhood adversities on adult-onset hypertension (aged 21 years and older)

	Hazard ratios (95% CI) for adult-onset hypertension (adjusted for age, sex, and country)
Early-onset (prior to age 21) mental disorders	
Major depressive disorder	1.17 (ns)
Generalized anxiety disorder	1.17 (ns)
Social phobia	1.38***
Posttraumatic stress disorder	1.17 (ns)
Panic disorder/agoraphobia	1.55***
Childhood adversities	
Physical abuse	1.23*
Sexual abuse	1.14 (ns)
Neglect	1.10
Parental death	1.02 (ns)
Parental divorce	0.96 (ns)
Other loss of parent	1.26*
Parental mental disorder	1.29**
Parental substance-use disorder	1.30**
Violence in family	1.17*
Criminal behavior in family	1.33**
Family economic adversity	1.03 (ns)

* $p < .05$.
** $p < .01$.
*** $p < .001$.

and hypertension onset and with prospective studies of subjects exposed to early adversity. The main findings of the current study were that (1) the presence of two or more early childhood adversities was significantly associated with adult-onset hypertension; (2) early-onset depression–anxiety disorder was also significantly associated with increased risk of hypertension; and (3) in multivariate analyses, three or more childhood adversities, as well as early-onset depression–anxiety disorder, continued to be significantly associated with increased risk of hypertension and the strength of the association of each factor was undiminished by controlling for the other.

The observed hazard ratios suggest a "dose–response" relationship between early childhood adversity and subsequent hypertension. The extent and number of childhood adversities may be more important than the specific type of adversity experienced. There was no increased risk of adult-onset hypertension among persons who reported only one childhood adversity, and the hazard ratios for the relationship between early adversity and subsequent hypertension were relatively low. Given that 22.8% of the respondents experienced two or more childhood adversities, however, the potential impact of these exposures on hypertension risks has the potential to be important.

Although childhood adversities are associated with increased risk of early-onset depression–anxiety disorders, controlling for number of childhood adversities did not explain the association of early-onset depression–anxiety disorders with adult-onset hypertension. Additional work is needed to understand the specific psychobiological mechanisms that mediate the relationships between childhood adversity, early-onset depression–anxiety disorders, and subsequent adult-onset hypertension. Effect sizes for the association of psychosocial factors and hypertension are modest, and empirical support for theoretical models emphasizing cardiovascular reactivity to stress, altered central nervous system control of baroreceptor function, and risk behavior is relatively sparse (Rutledge & Hogan 2002).

Research documenting how both early trauma and depression–anxiety disorders alter the autonomic system, potentially contributing to increased allostatic load (Bedi & Arora 2007; Evans et al. 2007; Grippo et al. 2007; Heim & Nemeroff 2001), may be particularly relevant in this regard. Genetic, early environmental, and later environmental effects on hypertension and other cardiovascular conditions require further delineation (Dong et al. 2004; Eisen et al. 1998). Effects sizes for behavioral treatments for hypertension are quite variable (Linden & Moseley 2006), and this is another area of research requiring additional attention.

In conclusion, the World Mental Health Surveys provide a unique opportunity to assess the relationship between childhood adversities, early-onset depression–anxiety disorders, and adult-onset hypertension in a large multinational sample. The data are consistent with a prior literature on the role of psychosocial factors in the pathogenesis of hypertension, and call attention to the potential role of both early childhood adversities and early-onset depression–anxiety disorders as risk factors for hypertension. These exploratory results suggest the need for prospective studies assessing the independent and joint effects of childhood adversities and early-onset emotional disorders in influencing risks of developing hypertension as an adult.

ACKNOWLEDGMENT

Some material in this chapter appeared in Stein et al. (in press). This material is reprinted with the permission of the American Academy of Clinical Psychiatrists.

REFERENCES

Alonso, A., Beunza, J. J., Delgado-Rodriguez, M., & Martinez-Gonzalez, M. A. (2005). Validation of self reported diagnosis of hypertension in a cohort of university graduates in Spain. *BMC Public Health*, **5**, 94.

Bedi, U. S., & Arora, R. (2007). Cardiovascular manifestations of posttraumatic stress disorder. *Journal of the National Medical Association*, **99**, 642–9.

Dong, M., Giles, W. H., Felitti, V. J., Dube, S. R., Williams, J. E., Chapman, D. P., & Anda, R. F. (2004). Insights into causal pathways for ischemic heart disease: Adverse childhood experiences study. *Circulation*, **110**, 1761–6.

Eisen, S. A., Neuman, R., Goldberg, J., True, W. R., Rice, J., Scherrer, J. F., & Lyons, M. J. (1998). Contribution of emotionally traumatic events and inheritance to the report of current physical health problems in 4042 Vietnam era veteran twin pairs. *Psychosomatic Medicine*, **60**, 533–9.

Evans, D. L., Charney, D. S., Lewis, L., Golden, R. N., Gorman, J. M., Krishnan, K. R. R., Nemeroff, C. B., Bremner, J. D., Carney, R. M., Coyne, J. C., Delong, M. R., Frasure-Smith, N., Glassman, A. H., Gold, P. W., Grant, I., Gwyther, L., Ironson, G., Johnson, R. L., Kanner, A. M., Katon, W. J., Kaufmann, P. G., Keefe, F. J., Ketter, T., Laughren, T. P., Leserman, J., Lyketsos, C. G., McDonald, W. M., McEwen, B. S., Miller, A. H., Musselman, D., O'Connor, C., Petitto, J. M., Pollock, B. G., Robinson, R. G., Roose, S. P., Rowland, J., Sheline, Y., Sheps, D. S., Simon, G., Spiegel, D., Stunkard, A., Sunderland, T., Tibbits, J., & Valvo, W. J. (2005). Mood disorders in the medically ill: Scientific review and recommendations. *Biological Psychiatry*, **58**, 175–89.

Evans, G. W., Kim, P., Ting, A. H., Tesher, H. B., & Shannis, D. (2007). Cumulative risk, maternal responsiveness, and allostatic load among young adolescents. *Developmental Psychology*, **43**, 341–51.

Felitti, V. J., Anda, R. F., Nordernberg, D., Willimason, D. F., Spitz, A. M., Edwards, V., Koss, M. P., & Marks, J. S. (1998). Relationship of child abuse to many of the leading causes of death in adults: The adverse childhood experiences (ACE) study. *American Journal of Preventive Medicine*, **14**, 245–8.

Gluckman, P. D., & Hanson, M. A. (2004). Living with the past: Evolution, development, and patterns of disease. *Science*, **305**, 1733–6.

Goldman, N., Lin, I.-F., Weinstein, M., & Lin, Y.-H. (2003). Evaluating the quality of self-reports of hypertension and diabetes. *Journal of Clinical Epidemiology*, **56**, 148–54.

Grippo, A. J., Lamb, D. G., Carter, C. S., & Porges, S. W. (2007). Social isolation disrupts autonomic regulation of the heart and influences negative affective behaviors. *Biological Psychiatry*, **62**, 1162–70.

Hardt, J., & Rutter, M. (2004). Validity of adult retrospective reports of adverse childhood experiences: Review of the evidence. *Journal of Child Psychology and Psychiatry*, **45**, 260–73.

Heim, C., & Nemeroff, C. B. (2001). The role of childhood trauma in the neurobiology of mood and anxiety disorders: Preclinical and clinical studies. *Biological Psychiatry*, **49**, 1023–9.

Kaplan, M. S., & Nunes, A. (2003). The psychosocial determinants of hypertension. *Nutrition, Metabolism and Cardiovascular Diseases*, **13**, 52–9.

Linden, W., & Moseley, J. V. (2006). The efficacy of behavioral treatments for hypertension. *Applied Psychophysiology and Biofeedback*, **31**, 51–63.

Mann, S. J., & Delon, M. (1995). Improved hypertension control after disclosure of decades-old trauma. *Psychosomatic Medicine*, **57**, 501–5.

Rutledge, T., & Hogan, B. E. (2002). A quantitative review of prospective evidence linking psychological factors with hypertension development. *Psychosomatic Medicine*, **64**, 758–66.

Stein, D. J., Scott, K. M., & Von Korff, M. (In press). Early childhood adversity and later hypertension: Data from the World Mental Health Survey. *Annals of Clinical Psychiatry*.

Tormo, M. J., Navarro, C., Chirlaque, M. D., Barber, X., & the EPIC Group of Spain. (2000). Validation of self diagnosis of high blood pressure in a sample of the Spanish EPIC cohort: Overall agreement and predictive values. *Journal of Epidemiology and Community Health*, **54**, 221–6.

11 Early-Life Psychosocial Factors and Adult-Onset Diabetes

CARMEN LARA

11.1. INTRODUCTION

Diabetes mellitus affects almost 6% of the world's population (Adeghate, Schattner, & Dunn 2006) and its prevalence is increasing rapidly (Townsend 2000). The number of diabetes patients worldwide is projected to reach 300 million by 2025 (International Diabetes Federation 2003). Type 2 diabetes is associated with both nonmodifiable (heredity and aging) and modifiable risk factors. The association of genetic factors with type 2 diabetes is well established (Bell 1991). However, genetic factors may need to be modified by nongenetic (environmental and individual) factors for diabetes mellitus to become overt (Adeghate et al. 2006; Ge et al. 2006). Such factors may include obesity, low levels of physical activity, high dietary fat intake, and low fiber intake. Recently, several studies have demonstrated the importance of residence on the prevalence of diabetes mellitus. Its prevalence is higher in urban than rural populations (Aekplakorn et al. 2007; Kim et al. 2006).

There has also been interest in psychosocial factors as possible contributors to diabetes development. A proposed relationship between diabetes and stress has a long history. In 1935, after studying 22 patients, Menninger wrote, "The evidence gained from this study indicates that diabetes is the direct result of psychological disturbances. Conservatively, five of the cases show such an origin of the diabetes, and several others suggest the possibility of such a causal relationship" (Menninger 1935). Although present-day researchers would be unlikely to be quite so conclusive about the role of psychological disturbance, there are plausible biological links between stress and diabetes. These may occur through autonomic nervous system and hypothalamic–pituitary–adrenal (HPA) axis–mediated persistent elevations in blood glucose, leading to insulin insensitivity over time (Huang, Cabanela, & Howell 1997; Mooy et al. 2000; Norberg et al. 2007). Additionally, studies have consistently observed a relationship between stress and poor glycemic control in various populations of type 2 diabetes patients (Surwit et al. 2002).

Mooy et al. (2000) in a cross-sectional study found that the number of major stressful life events experienced during the past 5 years was positively associated with the prevalence of hitherto undetected diabetes. They point out that their findings are partially consistent with Bjorntorp's theory that stressful life events, indicative of chronic psychological stress, are associated with undetected type 2 diabetes and visceral adiposity (Bjorntorp 1995). However, in the white middle-aged population that Mooy et al. (2000) studied, visceral adiposity did not seem to be the main link between stress and diabetes. This work has several limitations: they included only middle-aged women and the investigators asked only about the past 5-year period.

There have been few longitudinal studies that link stressful events to diabetes onset.

Although Räikkönen et al. (2007) investigated metabolic syndrome rather than diabetes, the relationship between diabetes and metabolic syndrome makes their research relevant. Among women who did not have the metabolic syndrome at baseline, the risk of developing metabolic syndrome 15 years later was 1.21- to 2.12-fold greater among those with more severe depressive symptoms or very stressful life event(s). The other important study of relevance here is the Adverse Childhood Experiences (ACE) Study, which found that when persons with four or more categories of childhood adversity exposure were compared to those with none, the odds ratio for the presence of diabetes was 1.6 (Felitti et al. 1998).

In considering a possible etiologic role of psychosocial stress in diabetes development, the role of mental disorders such as depression must also be considered since depression has a well-established link to diabetes (Engum 2007; Talbot & Nouwen 2000). Cross-sectional studies have reported a higher prevalence of depression among persons with diabetes compared to controls (Anderson et al. 2001). More recently, the World Mental Health Surveys have confirmed a modest relationship between diabetes and both depressive and anxiety disorders (Lin et al. 2008; Scott et al. 2007). In addition, Knol et al. (2006) reviewed nine longitudinal studies and concluded that depressed adults have a 37% increased risk of developing type 2 diabetes mellitus.

The particular advantage of the World Mental Health Surveys is that they included information on both mental disorders and childhood adversity stressors, together with self-report of diabetes and its year of onset. This allows us to investigate the possible role of early-life psychosocial factors (childhood adversity and early-onset mental disorders) in increasing risk of diabetes development among adults.

11.2. APPROACH

Cox proportional hazards models estimated risk of adult-onset diabetes as a function of number and type of childhood adversities and early-onset depression/anxiety disorder status while adjusting for potential confounders. Ascertainment of diabetes was with the following question: "Did a medical doctor or other health professional ever tell you that you had diabetes?" Respondents were also asked how old they were when the condition was first diagnosed. Information on the validity of self-report of diabetes is discussed in Chapter 4 (4.5.5). Kaplan–Meier curves were constructed for graphical comparison of increasing proportion of respondents reporting onset of diabetes with age between four categories of number of childhood adversities: none, one, two, and three or more adversities. See Chapter 8 for further description of the methods that were generic across the physical condition and pain condition outcomes included in this section.

11.3. FINDINGS

The percent of the combined cross-national sample reporting that they had diabetes was 5.3%, 53.5% of whom were female and 84% of whom were older than 45 years (Table 11.1). The cross-national prevalence rates of diabetes are provided in Table 11.1. They are, for the most part, comparable with other cross-national estimates of the prevalence of diabetes (Wild et al. 2004).

Early-onset depressive/anxiety disorders were not more prevalent in the adult-onset diabetes sample relative to the total sample (Table 11.2). Three or more childhood adversities however, and some specific childhood adversities, were associated with increased risk of adult-onset diabetes. The Kaplan–Meier curves show that risk for diabetes becomes elevated among those with three

Table 11.1. Characteristics of total and adult-onset diabetes sample

	Total cross-national Sample (N = 18,303)		Adult-onset diabetes (>21 years) sample (N = 649)
	Unweighted N	Weighted %	Weighted %
Age (21–98 years)			
21–44	9,992	52.4	15.7
>45	8,961	47.6	84.4
Female	11,287	52.8	53.5
Education (above median)[a]	8,521	48.7	32.6
Adult-onset diabetes (>21 years)	1,005	5.3	100.0
Country[b]			
Colombia	2,151	11.4	2.9
Belgium	1,010	5.3	3.5
France	1,377	7.3	4.1
Germany	1,307	7.0	4.8
Italy	1,724	9.2	3.3
The Netherlands	1,065	5.4	7.2
Spain	2,047	10.7	5.7
Japan	883	4.7	6.6
Mexico	2,092	11.1	4.7
United States	5,297	28.0	7.0

[a] Educational attainment measured as years of education: percentages in table represent those above the country-specific median (weighted).

[b] The first two columns of country-specific data describe the number and percent of the sample from each country; the third column describes the percent in each country with diabetes.

or more adversities from around 45 years of age.

The association of multiple childhood adversities with adult-onset diabetes is considered further in Table 11.3. The risk of diabetes onset was increased among persons with multiple childhood adversities after adjustment for depressive/anxiety (early-onset or prior 12-month) disorders and educational attainment. The specific adversities that were associated with elevated risk of adult-onset diabetes were physical abuse, divorce of parents, other loss of parent, criminal behavior in the family, and family economic adversity (Table 11.4). Early-onset mental disorders were not associated with increased risk of adult-onset diabetes (Table 11.4).

11.4. DISCUSSION

Three or more childhood family adversities significantly increased the risk of developing diabetes in adulthood. This finding adds to the limited prior literature on the relationship between early childhood stressors and later diabetes onset. Interestingly, we found no relationship between early-onset depressive/anxiety disorders and adult-onset diabetes. This is despite the fact that the World Mental Health Surveys have documented a relationship between 12-month depressive and anxiety disorders and diabetes (Lin et al. 2008; Scott et al. 2007). The time course of the relationship between depression and diabetes has not been sufficiently explored to draw firm conclusions about our null finding

Table 11.2. Percent with early-onset depressive/anxiety disorders and childhood adversities in total and adult-onset diabetes samples

	Weighted %	
	Total cross-national sample (N = 18,303)	Adult-onset diabetes (>21 years) sample (N = 649)
Early-onset (prior to age 21) mental disorders		
Any depressive/anxiety disorder	10.4	9.4
Major depressive disorder	4.6	3.3
Generalized anxiety disorder	1.4	1.1
Social phobia	4.9	4.6
Posttraumatic stress disorder	1.7	1.5
Panic disorder/agoraphobia	1.8	1.9
Number of childhood adversities		
None	56.1	52.4
One	25.6	26.0
Two	10.0	10.9
Three or more	8.4	10.8
Type of childhood adversity		
Physical abuse	9.7	12.6
Sexual abuse	2.5	2.3
Neglect	6.6	6.7
Parental death	12.9	14.1
Parental divorce	9.9	10.3
Other loss of parent	5.2	8.2
Parental mental disorder	7.2	6.6
Parental substance-use disorder	5.0	6.3
Violence in family	9.5	9.8
Parental criminal behavior	3.4	5.1
Family economic adversity	5.9	8.1

in this study, but it may suggest that depression that occurs in temporal proximity to diabetes onset is more influential than earlier depressive episodes, as has been suggested for the depression–heart disease relationship (Steptoe 2007).

The connection we observed between childhood adversity and adult risk of diabetes could be mediated by biological mechanisms associated with the stress response. Physiological adaptation to stressful events includes activation of neural, neuroendocrine, and immune mechanisms. Biological responses to stressful challenges have been termed "allostasis" (McEwen & Stellar 1993). "Allostatic load" has been conceptualized as a cumulative biological burden imposed on the body through attempts to adapt to daily physical and emotional stress (McEwen & Seeman 1999). When people experience greater than average levels of stress through their life, resulting allostatic load has been hypothesized to contribute to an excess observed risk for a variety of health conditions. Childhood adversities may therefore lead to HPA axis–mediated sensitivity manifested in exaggerated stress-related sympathetic and neuroendocrine responses in adulthood, resulting in an enhanced risk of disorders such as depression (Korkeila et al. 2005), insulin resistance, obesity, and

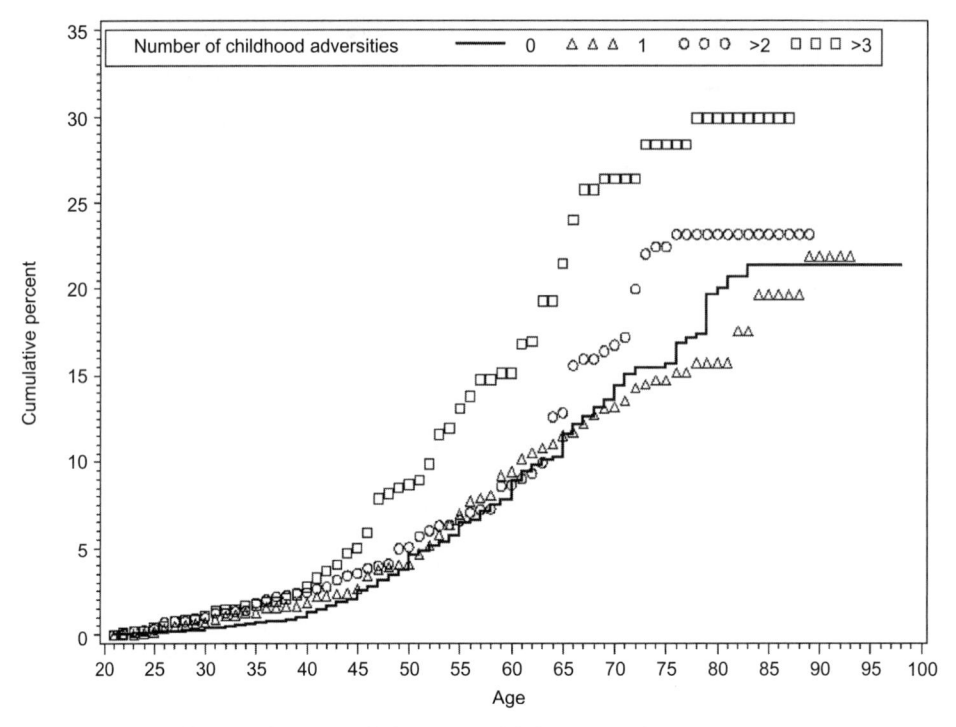

Figure 11.1. Age of adult onset of diabetes cumulative percent.

diabetes (Roland 2003). For example, it has been proposed that Pima Indians, who are known for their high prevalence of type 2 diabetes, may have exaggerated sensitivity to adrenergic stimulation (Tataranni et al. 1999). These results need to be considered in the context of the study limitations. Diabetes was ascertained by self-report of physician diagnosis, rather than direct metabolic and somatometry measures. It is likely to be a reasonable estimate of diagnosed diabetes (Okura et al. 2004), but it may underestimate the occurrence of diabetes in the population since a number of people do not realize they have diabetes in the early stages. An additional limitation is that we relied on self-report of childhood adversities, likely resulting in underreporting of childhood adversity

Table 11.3. Hazard ratios (95% CIs) showing effect of number of childhood adversities on risk of adult-onset diabetes (aged 21 years and older)

Number of childhood adversities	With adjustment for early-onset (<21 years) depressive/anxiety disorder	With adjustment for current (12-month) depressive/anxiety disorder	With adjustment for educational attainment
One	1.06 (0.84, 1.34)	1.06 (0.84, 1.34)	1.06 (0.83, 1.35)
Two	1.19 (0.88, 1.62)	1.18 (0.87–1.61)	1.05 (0.79, 1.41)
Three or more	1.59 (1.20, 2.09)*	1.54 (1.16, 2.04)*	1.44 (1.07, 1.92)*

* $p < .05$.

Table 11.4. Hazard ratios showing effect of early-onset (prior to age 21) depressive/anxiety disorders and specific childhood adversities on risk of adult-onset diabetes (aged 21 years and older)

	Hazard ratios (95% CI) for adult-onset diabetes (adjusted for age, sex, and country)
Early-onset (prior to age 21) mental disorders	
Any depressive/anxiety disorder	1.17 (0.95, 1.44)
Major depressive disorder	1.14 (0.88, 1.47)
Generalized anxiety disorder	0.96 (0.80, 1.16)
Social phobia	0.96 (0.80, 1.16)
Posttraumatic stress disorder	0.96 (0.80, 1.16)
Panic disorder/agoraphobia	0.96 (0.80, 1.16)
Childhood adversities	
Physical abuse	1.52 (1.16, 2.00)*
Sexual abuse	0.99 (0.63, 1.55)
Neglect	1.02 (0.74, 1.42)
Parental death	0.91 (0.71, 1.18
Parental divorce	1.37 (1.01, 1.86)*
Other loss of parent	1.58 (1.12, 2.23)*
Parental mental disorder	1.04 (0.74, 1.47)
Parental substance-use disorder	1.30 (0.92, 1.84)
Violence in family	1.16 (0.87, 1.55)
Criminal behavior in family	1.81 (1.26, 2.59)*
Family economic adversity	1.44 (1.04, 1.98)*

* $p < .05$.

experience, although false-positive reports are rare (Hardt & Rutter 2004).

In conclusion, the evidence from this study suggests that childhood adversities may play a role in modifying risks of diabetes. Multiple childhood adversities increased the risk of diabetes onset in adulthood, but early-onset depressive/anxiety disorders did not. These retrospective analyses suggest the need for prospective evaluation of the association of childhood adversities with risks of developing diabetes in adulthood.

REFERENCES

Adeghate, E., Schattner, P., & Dunn, E. (2006). An update on the etiology and epidemiology of diabetes mellitus. *Annals of the New York Academy of Sciences*, **1084**, 1–29.

Aekplakorn, W., Abbott-Klafter, J., Premgamone, A., Dhanamun, B., Chaikittiporn, C., Chongsuvivatwong, V., Suwanprapisa, T., Chaipornsupaisan, W., Tiptaradol, S., & Lim, S. S. (2007). Prevalence and management of diabetes and associated risk factors by regions of Thailand. Third National Health Examination Survey 2004. *Diabetes Care*, **30**, 2007–12.

Anderson, R. J., Freedland, K. E., Clouse, R. E., & Lustman, P. J. (2001). The prevalence of comorbid depression in adults with diabetes: A meta-analysis. *Diabetes Care*, **24**, 1069–78.

Bell, G. I., & Polonsky, K. S. (2001). Diabetes mellitus and genetically programmed defects in beta-cell function. *Nature*, **414**, 788–91.

Bjorntorp, P. (1995). Endocrine abnormalities of obesity. *Metabolism: Clinical & Experimental*, **44**, 21–3.

Engum, A. (2007). The role of depression and anxiety in onset of diabetes in a large population-based study. *Journal of Psychosomatic Research*, **62**, 31–8.

Felitti, V. J., Anda, R. F., Nordenberg, D., Williamson, D. F., Spitz, A. M., Edwards, V., Koss, M. P., & Marks, J. S. (1998). Relationship of childhood abuse and household dysfunction to many of the leading causes of death in adults. The Adverse Childhood Experiences (ACE) Study. *American Journal of Preventive Medicine*, **14**, 245–58.

Ge, D., Dong, Y., Wang, X., Treiber, F. A., & Snieder, H. (2006). The Georgia Cardiovascular Twin Study: Influence of genetic predisposition and chronic stress on risk for cardiovascular disease and Type 2 diabetes. *Twin Research & Human Genetics: The Official Journal of the International Society for Twin Studies*, **9**, 965–70.

Hardt, J., & Rutter, M. (2004). Validity of adult retrospective reports of adverse childhood experiences: Review of the evidence. *Journal of Child Psychology and Psychiatry*, **45**, 260–73.

Huang, Z., Cabanela, V., & Howell, T. (1997). Stress, bottlefeeding, and diabetes. *Lancet*, **350**, 889.

Hypponen, E., Power, C., & Smith, G. D. (2003). Prenatal Growth, BMI, and risk of type 2 diabetes by early midlife. *Diabetes Care*, **26**, 2512–17.

International Diabetes Federation. (2003). *Diabetes Atlas*. Brussels, Belgium: International Diabetes Federation. Also available at www.eatlas.idf.org.

Kim, S., Lee, J., Lee, J., Na, J., Han, J., Yoon, D., Baik, S., Choi, D., & Choi, K. (2006). Prevalence of diabetes and impaired fasting glucose in Korea. *Diabetes Care*, **29**, 226–31.

Knol, M. J., Twisk, J. W., Beekman, A. T., Heine, R. J., Snoek, F. J., & Pouwer, F. (2006). Depression as a risk factor for the onset of type 2 diabetes mellitus: A meta-analysis. *Diabetologia*, **49**, 837–45.

Korkeila, K., Korkeila, J., Vahtera, J., Kivimäki, M., Kivelä, S. L., Sillanmäki, L., & Koskenvuo, M. (2005). Childhood adversities, adult risk factors and depressiveness: A population study. *Social Psychiatry and Psychiatric Epidemiology*, **40**, 700–6.

Lin, E. H., Korff, M. V., Alonso, J., Angermeyer, M. C., Anthony, J., Bromet, E., Bruffaerts, R., Gasquet, I., de Girolamo, G., Gureje, O., Haro, J. M., Karam, E., Lara, C., Lee, S., Levinson, D., Ormel, J. H., Posada-Villa, J., Scott, K., Watanabe, M., & Williams, D. (2008). Mental disorders among people with diabetes: Results from the World Mental Health Surveys. *Journal of Psychosomatic Research*, **65**, 571–80.

McEwen, B. S., & Seeman, T. (1999). Protective and damaging effects of mediators of stress. Elaborating and testing the concepts of allostasis and allostatic load. *Annals of the New York Academy of Sciences*, **896**, 30–47.

McEwen, B. S., & Stellar, E. (1993). Stress and the individual. Mechanisms leading to disease. *Archives of Internal Medicine*, **153**, 2093–101.

Menninger, W. C. (1935). The interrelationships of mental disorders and diabetes mellitus. *Journal of Mental Science*, **81**, 332–57.

Mooy, J. M., de Vries, H., Grootenhuis, P. A., Bouter, L. M., & Heine, R. J. (2000). Major stressful life events in relation to prevalence of undetected type 2 diabetes: The Hoorn Study. *Diabetes Care*, **23**, 197–201.

Norberg, M., Stenlund, H., Lindahl, B., Andersson, C., Eriksson, J. W., & Weinehall, L. (2007). Work stress and low emotional support is associated with increased risk of future type 2 diabetes in women. *Diabetes Research & Clinical Practice*, **76**, 368–77.

Okura, Y., Urban, L. H., Mahoney, D. W., Jacobsen, S. J., & Rodeheffer, R. J. (2004). Agreement between self-report questionnaires and medical record data was substantial for diabetes, hypertension, myocardial infarction and stroke but not for heart failure. *Journal of Clinical Epidemiology*, **57**, 1096–103.

Raikkonen, K., Matthews, K. A., & Kuller, L. H. (2007). Depressive symptoms and stressful life events predict metabolic syndrome among middle-aged women: A comparison of World Health Organization, Adult Treatment Panel III, and International Diabetes Foundation definitions. *Diabetes Care*, **30**, 872–7.

Rosmond, R. (2003). Stress-induced disturbances of the HPA axis: A pathway to Type 2 diabetes? *Medical Science Monitor*, **9**, RA35–9.

Scott, K. M., Bruffaerts, R., Stang, A., Ormel, J., Alonso, J., Angermeyer, M. C., Benjet, C., Bromet, E., de Girolamo, G., de Graaf, R., Gasquet, I., Gureje, O., Haro, J. M., He, Y., Kessler, R. C., Levinson, D., Mneimneh, Z. N., Oakley Browne, M. A., Posada-Villa, J., Stein, D. J., Takeshima, T., & Von Korff, M. (2007). Depression-anxiety relationships with chronic physical conditions: Results from the World Mental Health Surveys. *Journal of Affective Disorders*, **103**, 113–20.

Steptoe, A., Strike, P. C., Perkins-Porras, L., McEwan, J. R., & Whitehead, D. L. (2006).

Acute depressed mood as a trigger of acute coronary syndromes. *Biological Psychiatry*, **60**, 837–42.

Surwit, R. S., van Tilburg, M. A., Zucker, N., McCaskill, C. C., Parekh, P., Feinglos, M. N., Edwards, C. L., Williams, P., & Lane, J. D. (2002). Stress management improves long-term glycemic control in type 2 diabetes. *Diabetes Care*, **25**, 30–4.

Talbot, F., & Nouwen, A. (2000). A review of the relationship between depression and diabetes in adults. Is there a link? *Diabetes Care*, **23**, 1556–62.

Tataranni, P. A., Cizza, G., Snitker, S., Gucciardo, F., Lotsikas, A., Chrousos, G. P., & Ravussin, E. (1999). Hypothalamic-pituitary-adrenal axis and sympathetic nervous system activities in Pima Indians and Caucasians. *Metabolism: Clinical & Experimental*, **48**, 395–9.

Townsend, T. (2000). A decade of diabetes research and development. *International Journal of Diabetes and Metabolism*, **8**, 88–92.

Wild, S., Roglic, G., Green, A., Sicree, R., & King, H. (2004). Global prevalence of diabetes: Estimates for the year 2000 and projections for 2030. *Diabetes Care*, **27**, 1047–53.

12 Psychosocial Stressors in Childhood and Adult-Onset Arthritis

MICHAEL R. VON KORFF

12.1. INTRODUCTION

Osteoarthritis is a common cause of pain and disability among older adults (Brooks 2002; Leigh, Seavey, & Leistikow 2001; Reginster 2002; Simon 1999). The prevalence of osteoarthritis increases from about 5% for persons aged 15–44 years, to 25–30% for persons aged 45–64 years, to more than 60% among persons aged 65 years or older (Dieppe 1995; Elders 2000; Felson 1995). The World Mental Health Surveys found that 10–29% of household-residing adults in developed countries reported arthritis, as did 6–20% of adults in developing countries (He 2008). These surveys found that arthritis was consistently associated with depressive and anxiety disorders in both developed and developing countries. In common with other chronic physical diseases, there is evidence that symptom severity is greater among persons with arthritis who have a comorbid psychological disorder, after taking into consideration objective indicators of disease severity (Katon, Lin, & Kroenke, 2007). Osteoarthritis has significant implications for quality of life, as it is associated not only with emotional distress, but also with work loss, interference with daily activities, sleep disturbance, and increased use of health care services (Grotle et al. 2008; Yelin & Callahan 1995). The importance of recognizing and treating comorbid depressive illness is underscored by results of a large randomized controlled trial that showed significant reductions in arthritis pain and pain-related interference with activities among persons with arthritis who received enhanced depression care relative to controls who received care as usual (Lin et al. 2003).

Although emotional distress is a likely and understandable consequence of chronic arthritis pain, it is also possible that psychological disorder and exposure to chronic psychosocial stress increase risks of developing arthritis. Although the course of osteoarthritis is highly variable, it is a progressive chronic disease that results from a combination of risk factors including genetic factors, acute and/or chronic trauma, and inflammatory processes (Krasnokutsky, Samuels, & Abramson 2007). There is increasing interest in whether proinflammatory cytokines, acting as negative regulatory signals, play a pathogenic role in diverse chronic physical diseases, including arthritis (O'Connor et al. 2008). Allostatic load is the burden placed on homeostatic systems repeatedly activated and deactivated in response to chronic psychosocial, psychological, and physical stressors (McEwen 1998a, 1998b). Chronic effects of allostatic load on neural, endocrine, and immune stress mediators are hypothesized to have potentially pathogenic effects. Adverse effects of allostatic load may increase risks of developing chronic diseases such as arthritis if chronic psychosocial stressors are present over long time periods (McEwen & Stellar 1993). Cross talk between the brain and the immune system through the hypothalamic–pituitary–adrenal (HPA) axis may play an etiologic role in the development of inflammatory arthritis (Vassiloupoulos & Mantzoukis 2006).

Thus, exposure to chronic psychosocial stressors may increase risks of developing arthritis. Chronic psychosocial stress can be endogenous (e.g., chronic mood/anxiety disorder due to genetic factors), exogenous (e.g., exposure to significant childhood adversities), or both. While there are no prospective studies assessing whether depression is a risk factor for onset of osteoarthritis, prospective studies have found that psychological distress is associated with increased risk of developing back and neck pain (Linton 2000). For example, Carroll, Cassidy, and Cote (2004) found that persons with high levels of depression had a fourfold increased risk of developing troublesome back or neck pain over a 12-month follow-up period, and Linton (2005) reported similar results in a prospective cohort study. Based on these results, and cross-sectional studies showing that mood and anxiety disorders are more common among persons with osteoarthritis, research assessing whether pre-existing psychological disorder is associated with increased risk of developing arthritis is needed.

There have been several studies of psychosocial stressors and risk of developing arthritis. In an uncontrolled qualitative study of 23 women with osteoarthritis, 4 identified stress as a cause of their arthritis and 13 reported that their arthritis symptoms started after a period of stressful life events or depression (Okma-Keulen & Hopman-Rock 2001). A prospective cohort study found that 21,062 parents who experienced the death of a child before age 18 were no more likely than parents matched on family structure ($N = 293,745$) who did not experience the death of a child to develop rheumatoid arthritis (Li, Schiottz-Christensen, & Olsen 2005). In this study, onset of rheumatoid arthritis was ascertained only for hospitalized cases, and death of a child was the only psychosocial stressor assessed. Kopec and Sayre (2004) found that in cohort of 9,159 persons without arthritis at baseline, multiple childhood adversities were associated with increased risk of developing arthritis over a 4-year follow-up period. They found that the presence of two or more childhood adversities was associated with a hazard ratio (HR) of 1.27, with confidence intervals of 0.99–1.62 – an increase of borderline statistical significance. Spending 2 or more weeks in a hospital (HR = 1.33) and being very scared in childhood (HR = 1.29) were significantly associated with increased risk of arthritis onset. Given uncertainty in how to interpret these results, there is a need to further assess whether endogenous and exogenous stressors are associated with increased risk of developing arthritis.

In this chapter, we employ data from 10 countries participating in the World Mental Health Surveys to assess whether adult onset of arthritis is associated with early onset of psychological disorder and with exposure to multiple childhood adversities.

12.2. APPROACH

Cox proportional hazards models estimated risk of adult-onset arthritis as a function of number and type of childhood adversities and early-onset depression/anxiety disorder status while adjusting for potential confounders. Ascertainment of arthritis was assessed by asking respondents whether they had had arthritis or rheumatism in the past 12 months and, if they had arthritis, they were asked their age when they developed arthritis initially. Kaplan–Meier curves were developed for graphical comparison of the age-specific cumulative proportion of respondents reporting onset of arthritis comparing three categories of number of childhood adversities, none, one, and two or more adversities, and comparing onset of arthritis for persons with and without early-onset depression/anxiety disorder. See Chapter 4 (4.5.5) for further description of the methods that were generic across the physical condition and pain condition outcomes included in this section.

12.3. FINDINGS

Across all 10 surveys, 18,309 World Mental Health Survey respondents were included in analyses assessing the association of childhood psychosocial stressors with risk of developing arthritis after age 21. The demographic characteristics of the sample, and weighted population estimates of the frequency of childhood adversities and early-onset mood/anxiety disorder, are shown in Table 12.1. In the combined populations, the most common childhood adversities in the surveyed populations were parental death (12.8%), parental divorce (9.8%), physical abuse as a child (9.6%), and family violence (9.4%). Almost half the surveyed populations reported at least one childhood adversity, while 18.1% reported two or more childhood adversities. About 10% of the population reported early-onset mood/anxiety disorder, while 17.6% reported adult-onset arthritis.

There was considerable cross-national variability in the prevalence of multiple childhood adversities and there was also cross-national variability in the prevalence of adult-onset arthritis (Table 12.2). To control for possible ecological correlation of childhood adversities and arthritis, the survival analyses were stratified by country so that a unique hazard function was estimated for each country, with hazard ratio estimates aggregated across country strata to provide pooled estimates.

The risk of developing adult-onset arthritis was substantially higher among persons who reported onset of a mood/anxiety disorder prior to age 21, as shown by the Kaplan–Meier curves in Figure 12.1. By age 65, the risk of developing arthritis by age 65 was around 60% for those with early-onset psychological disorder, whereas it was less than 40% for those without. It should be noted that these estimates of lifetime risk of arthritis onset exclude persons with arthritis onset before age 21.

While there was essentially no difference in risk of adult-onset arthritis between persons with no childhood adversities and those reporting a single childhood adversity. There was increased risk of arthritis among persons reporting two or more childhood adversities (see Figure 12.2). The risk of developing arthritis began to diverge for persons with multiple childhood adversities only after the age of 35. By age 65, about 45% of persons with

Table 12.1. Sample characteristics (*N* = 18,309), weighted estimates

Mean age	45.5 (SD = 16.2)
Female	52.5%
Completed secondary education	61.6%
Childhood adversities	
Parental death	12.8%
Parental divorce	9.8%
Other parental loss	5.3%
Physical abuse as a child	9.6%
Family violence	9.4%
Parental mental disorder	7.1%
Neglect as a child	6.5%
Family economic adversity	5.8%
Family criminal behavior	3.3%
Parental substance abuse	5.0%
Sexual abuse as a child	2.5%
Number of childhood adversities	
None	56.3%
One	25.6%
Two	9.8%
Three or more	8.3%
Early-onset mood/anxiety disorder	10.2%
Adult-onset arthritis	17.6%

Psychosocial Stressors in Childhood and Adult-Onset Arthritis

Table 12.2. Percent with two or more childhood adversities and early-onset mood/anxiety disorder by country, weighted estimates and unweighted sample size

	Two or more childhood adversities (%)	Adult-onset arthritis (%)	N unweighted
Colombia	35.7	6.1	2,140
Belgium	11.3	17.5	970
France	15.2	27.2	1,281
Germany	8.3	10.4	1,284
Italy	6.7	23.6	1,614
The Netherlands	13.0	10.7	1,054
Spain	5.2	20.0	1,937
Japan	11.3	7.4	855
Mexico	25.5	5.9	2,032
United States	24.3	26.7	5,139

multiple childhood adversities had developed arthritis, while about 35% of those without multiple childhood adversities had developed arthritis.

As shown in Table 12.3, an initial multivariate analysis assessed whether the number of childhood adversities was associated with differences in risk of developing arthritis during adulthood. This initial analysis (see Model One in Table 12.3) controlled for age, sex, and country, but did not control for mental disorder status. Persons who reported two childhood adversities (relative to those with no childhood adversities) were at significantly increased risk of adult-onset arthritis (HR = 1.31), while persons reporting three or more childhood adversities were at still higher risk (HR = 1.53). This suggests a dose–response relationship between number of childhood adversities and risk of adult-onset arthritis. Consistent with the descriptive

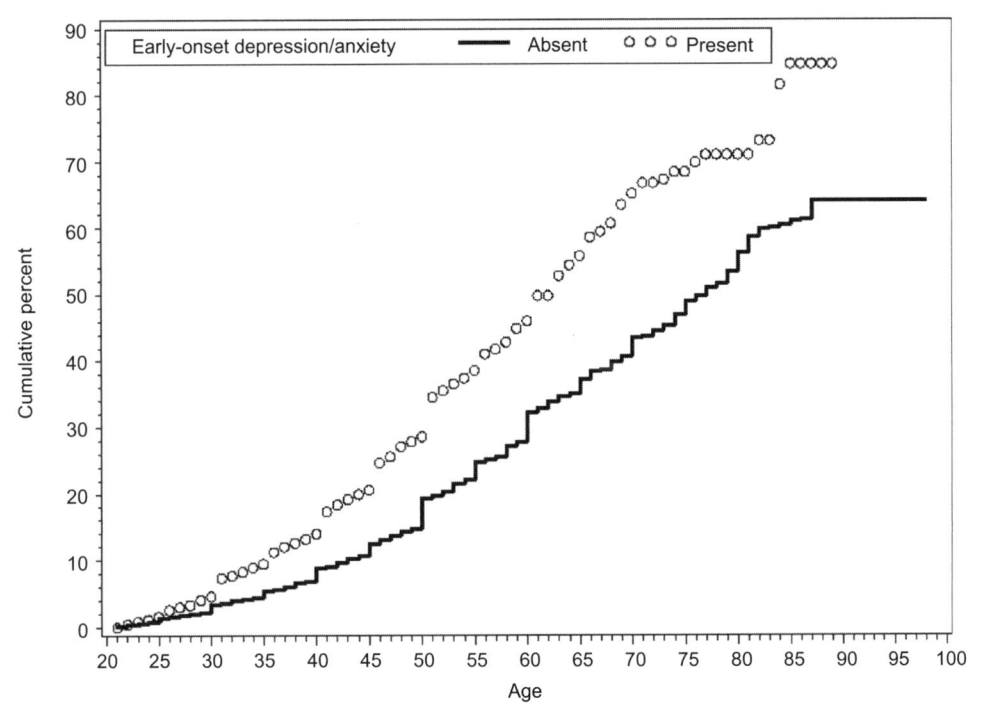

Figure 12.1. Cumulative percent with adult-onset arthritis by presence or absence of early-onset mood/anxiety disorder (persons reporting arthritis onset prior to age 21 excluded).

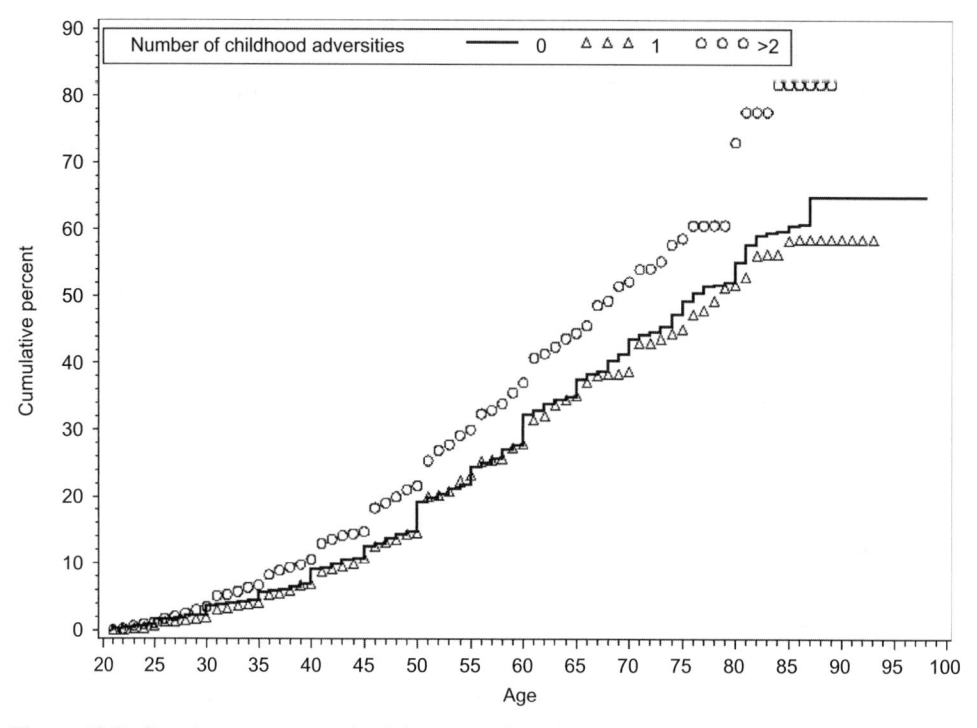

Figure 12.2. Cumulative percent with adult-onset arthritis by number of childhood adversities (persons reporting arthritis onset prior to age 21 excluded).

analysis shown in Figure 12.2, the presence of a single childhood adversity was not associated with increased risk of developing arthritis in adulthood.

An important methodological question is whether the association of childhood adversities and arthritis may be explained by the higher prevalence of mood/anxiety disorder among persons with arthritis. If mood disturbance resulted in increased likelihood of recalling negative childhood experiences, this could affect retrospective evaluation of the association of childhood adversities and risk of developing arthritis. We addressed this issue in a survival analysis controlling for current (12-month) mood/anxiety disorder (see Model Two in Table 12.3). After controlling for current mood/anxiety disorder, the HR estimates did not differ appreciably from estimates not controlling for current mood/anxiety disorder (Model One).

We evaluated whether early-onset psychological disorder and exposure to multiple childhood adversities were independently associated with risk of adult-onset arthritis. As shown in the survival analyses estimating effects of both early-onset psychological disorder and childhood adversities (see Model Three in Table 12.3), early-onset depression/anxiety disorder was associated with increased risk of developing arthritis (HR = 1.43) after controlling for childhood adversities. Likewise, the presence of multiple childhood adversities was associated with increased risk of adult-onset arthritis after controlling for early-onset psychological disorder.

Survival analyses that estimated the risk of developing arthritis as a function of early-onset psychological disorder that did not control for childhood adversities did not appreciably alter the HR estimates (Model Four compared to Model Three in Table 12.3).

Table 12.3. Survival analyses estimating HRs (and 95% confidence intervals) for adult-onset arthritis with stratification by country

	Early-onset mood disorder/ childhood adversities				Current mood/anxiety disorder		Anxiety disorder	
	None	One	Two	Three or more	Absent	Present	Absent	Present
Model One: Effect of childhood adversities without controlling for mood/anxiety disorder	1.00	1.02 [.89, 1.16]	1.31 [1.12, 1.54]	1.53 [1.31, 1.78]				
Model Two: Effect of childhood adversities controlling for current mood/anxiety disorder	1.00	1.01 [.88, 1.15]	1.28 [1.09, 1.50]	1.43 [1.24, 1.60]			1.00	1.43 [1.29, 1.57]
Model Three: Effect of childhood adversities and early-onset mood/anxiety disorder	1.00	1.00 [.88, 1.14]	1.27 [1.08, 1.50]	1.44 [1.24, 1.67]	1.00	1.43 [1.28, 1.61]		
Model Four: Effect of early-onset mood/anxiety disorder without controlling for childhood adversities					1.00	1.52 [1.36, 1.70]		

Notes: All models control for sex and current age and are stratified by country. Interaction of early-onset mood disorder and presence of multiple childhood adversities was nonsignificant.

Table 12.4. Hazard ratios (and 95% confidence intervals) for adult-onset arthritis for specific childhood adversities and specific early-onset psychological disorders

	Hazard ratio	95% confidence interval
Sexual abuse as a child	1.64	(1.28, 2.09)
Physical abuse as a child	1.42	(1.22, 1.66)
Family violence	1.39	(1.16, 1.67)
Parental substance abuse	1.38	(1.14, 1.67)
Family criminal behavior	1.36	(1.07, 1.71)
Neglect as a child	1.29	(1.08, 1.55)
Parental mental disorder	1.27	(1.07, 1.51)
Other parental loss	1.26	(1.04, 1.54)
Family economic adversity	1.08	(0.93, 1.26)
Parental death	1.02	(0.89, 1.18)
Parental divorce	1.02	(0.86, 1.22)
Posttraumatic stress disorder	1.91	(1.50, 2.43)
Generalized anxiety disorder	1.69	(1.32, 2.17)
Panic disorder/agoraphobia	1.68	(1.38, 2.03)
Major depression	1.53	(1.26, 1.85)
Social phobia	1.54	(1.34, 1.76)

Note: All models control for sex and current age and are stratified by country.

This suggests that early-onset psychological disorder exerts its effect on risk of developing arthritis independently of the association of childhood adversities and early-onset psychological disorder. Similarly, a survival analysis including number of childhood adversities but not early-onset psychological disorder (Model One in Table 12.3) yielded HR estimates that were quite similar to those that controlled for early-onset psychological disorder (Model Three in Table 12.3). Overall, these analyses suggest that early-onset psychological disorder and exposure to multiple childhood adversities are independently associated with risk of developing arthritis in adulthood. The estimates reported in Table 12.3 control for age and sex, and are stratified by country, but do not control for education. Replication of these analyses controlling for education (excluding the French sample) yielded very similar results (data not shown). A survival analysis was also carried out estimating the interaction effect of multiple childhood adversities and early-onset mood disorder on risk of adult-onset arthritis. The interaction effects were nonsignificant (data not shown).

We examined which childhood adversities and which early-onset psychological disorders were associated with increased risk of adult-onset arthritis (see Table 12.4). The survival analyses for these HR estimates controlled for age and sex, and were stratified by country. Each of the childhood adversities was associated with increased risk of arthritis onset except for parental death, parental divorce, and family economic adversity. Sexual abuse as a child was associated with the highest arthritis risk, while the HRs for the other childhood adversities were similar to each other. Each of the early-onset psychological disorders (major depression, generalized anxiety disorder, social phobia, posttraumatic stress disorder, and panic disorder/agoraphobia) was associated with increased risk of adult-onset arthritis. Posttraumatic stress disorder had the highest HR for adult-onset arthritis.

12.4. DISCUSSION

The World Mental Health Survey estimates concerning increased risk of developing arthritis among persons with multiple childhood adversities are strikingly similar to those reported by the Kopec and Sayre (2004) prospective study. The fact that risk of adult-onset arthritis increases with number of childhood adversities suggests the importance of assessing multiple adversities, rather than a single adversity evaluated in isolation. For example, parental death and parental divorce, two of the most common childhood adversities, were not associated with increased risk of adult-onset arthritis. The HR estimates for multiple childhood adversities were not affected by controlling for the presence of a current mood/anxiety disorder, suggesting that the observed results may not be explained by mood-biased recall of unpleasant life experiences.

It is of interest that early-onset psychological disorder was an independent risk factor for adult-onset arthritis. This suggests that major childhood adversities may influence disease risks even when the life event does not produce a diagnosable psychological disorder. There are, of course, significant limits on what can be confidently inferred from a retrospective study that relies on recall of the age of onset of psychological disorder, on recall of childhood adversities, and on self-report of arthritis. There is evidence, however, supporting the validity of retrospective recall of major childhood adversities (Hardt & Rutter 2004).

The limitations of this research include the reliance on self-report ascertainment of arthritis, and recall of the age of onset of arthritis, as well as retrospective recall of childhood adversities and the age of onset of lifetime psychological disorders. The value of this research is to motivate future prospective studies, rather than provide a conclusive answer to the question of whether psychosocial stressors increase the risks of developing arthritis. The complexities of carrying out a valid prospective study to address this question, however, would be substantial. The results reported here suggest that ascertainment of focal childhood adversities may not be sufficient, since disease risk was most strongly associated with multiple childhood adversities. For this reason, ascertainment of focal childhood adversities from archival records of a child welfare agency may not be adequate to assess adversity exposure. The increment in risk of multiple childhood adversities was moderate, so large sample sizes may be needed to provide adequate statistical power. For a disease as common as arthritis, a moderate increase in the HR could be associated with a large difference in the chances of developing the disease over the life span. An additional complexity is the long latency between exposure to childhood adversities and onset of arthritis. A true prospective study in which both exposure and outcome were measured directly from subjects might take 20–30 years or more to complete. The Kopec and Sayre (2004) study, for example, relied on retrospective recall of childhood adversities and then followed participants prospectively for 4 years to ascertain onsets of arthritis, so only case ascertainment, not assessment of exposure, was fully prospective in their study.

The robust association of early-onset psychological disorder with adult-onset arthritis may offer an avenue for testing whether exposure to psychosocial stress in childhood increases risks of developing arthritis in adulthood. For example, large integrated health plans in the United States have treatment records for psychological disorders among children that could be used in a nonconcurrent prospective design. Such health plans are also able to ascertain cases of arthritis that are treated, making a record-based study potentially feasible. A difficulty would be to identify sufficient numbers of individuals enrolled in the same health plan from childhood through older ages when arthritis incidence rates are highest. These considerations suggest the difficulties in executing a definitive study of whether exposure to psychosocial stressors in childhood is associated with increased risks of adult onset of a chronic physical disease such as arthritis. Feasible research designs are likely to have significant limitations. Determining whether childhood psychosocial stressors increase disease risks may depend on the accumulation of evidence from diverse studies, each with particular limitations and strengths.

If childhood adversities and early-onset psychological disorders are, in fact, broad-spectrum risk factors (see Chapter 1) for onset of multiple chronic physical diseases in later life, then it may be possible to organize research that assesses the contribution of childhood psychosocial stressors to risks of multiple physical disease endpoints. If exposure to major chronic psychosocial stressors in childhood increases risk of chronic physical disease across the adult life span, as suggested by research by Felitti et al. (1998) and others, it would have significant public health implications. The fact that rates of exposure to multiple childhood adversities differed markedly across the 10 countries included in this research offers the possibility that social environments might be modified to protect children from experiencing at least some adversities. Although the results reported here are provocative, albeit inconclusive, they underscore the importance of future research that addresses the role of childhood adversities and early-onset psychological disorder in the development of arthritis and other chronic diseases that may result from chronic exposure to psychosocial stressors and associated allostatic load.

In conclusion, this retrospective analysis of data from 10 countries participating in the World Mental Health Surveys found that exposure to multiple childhood adversities and early-onset depression/anxiety disorders were both independently associated with increased risk of adult-onset arthritis. The results point to the need for further research to assess the role of exposure to multiple childhood adversities and early-onset mood/anxiety disorder in subsequent risks of developing arthritis, as well as other chronic physical diseases whose risks may be influenced by chronic psychosocial stress.

ACKNOWLEDGMENT

Some material in this chapter appeared in Von Korff et al. (2009). This material is reprinted with the permission of the International Association for the Study of Pain.

REFERENCES

Brooks, P. M. (2002). Impact of osteoarthritis on individuals and society: How much disability? Social consequences and health economic implications. *Current Opinion in Rheumatology*, **14**, 573–7.

Carroll, L. J., Cassidy, J. D., & Cote, P. (2004). Depression as a risk factor for onset of an episode of troublesome neck and low back pain. *Pain*, **107**, 134–9.

Dieppe, P. (1995). The classification and diagnosis of osteoarthritis. In *Osteoarthritis Disorders*, ed. K. E. Kuettner & V. M. Goldberg, pp. 5–12. Rosemont, IL: American Academy of Orthopedic Surgeons.

Elders, M. J. (2000). The increasing impact of arthritis on public health. *The Journal of Rheumatology*, **60**, 6–8.

Felitti, V. J., Anda, R. F., Nordenberg, D., Williamson, D. F., Spitz, A. M., Edwards, V., Koss, M. P., & Marks, J. S. (1998). Relationship of childhood abuse and household dysfunction to many of the leading causes of death in adults: The Adverse Childhood Experiences (ACE) Study. *American Journal of Preventive Medicine*, **14**, 245–58.

Felson, D. T. (1995). The epidemiology of osteoarthritis: Prevalence and risk factors. In *Osteoarthritis Disorders*, ed. K. E. Kuettner & V. M. Goldberg, pp. 13–24. Rosemont, IL: American Academy of Orthopedic Surgeons.

Grotle, M., Hagen, K. B., Natvig, B., Dahl, F. A., & Kvien, T. K. (2008). Prevalence and burden of osteoarthritis: Results from a population survey in Norway. *The Journal of Rheumatology*, **35**, 677–84.

Hardt, J., & Rutter, M. (2004). Validity of adult retrospective reports of adverse childhood experiences: Review of the evidence. *Journal of Child Psychology and Psychiatry*, **45**, 260–73.

He, Y. L., Zhang, M., Lin, E. H. B., Bruffaerts, R., Posada-Villa, P., Andemeyer, M. C., Levinson, D., de Girolamo, G., Uda, H., Mneimneh, Z., Benjet, C., de Graaf, R., Scott, K. M., Gureje, O., Seedat, S., Haro, J. M., Bromet, E. J., Alonso,

J., Von Korff, M., & Kessler, R. (2008). Mental disorders among persons with arthritis – Results from the World Mental Health Surveys. *Psychological Medicine*, **38**, 1639–50.

Katon, W., Lin, E. H., & Kroenke, K. (2007). The association of depression and anxiety with medical symptom burden in patients with chronic medical illness. *General Hospital Psychiatry*, **29**, 147–55.

Kopec, J. A., & Sayre, E. C. (2004). Traumatic experiences in childhood and the risk of arthritis: A prospective cohort study. *Canadian Journal of Public Health*, **95**, 361–5.

Krasnokutsky, S., Samuels, J., & Abramson, S. B. (2007). Osteoarthritis in 2007. *Bulletin of the NYU Hospital for Joint Diseases*, **65**, 222–8.

Leigh, J. P., Seavey, W., & Leistikow, B. (2001). Estimating the costs of job related arthritis. *The Journal of Rheumatology*, **28**, 1647–54.

Li, J., Schiottz-Christensen, B., & Olsen, J. (2005). Psychological stress and rheumatoid arthritis in parents after death of a child: A national follow-up study. *Scandinavian Journal of Rheumatology*, **34**, 448–50.

Lin, E. H. B., Katon, W., Von Korff, M., Tang, L., Williams, J. W., Kroenke, K., Hunkeler, E., Harpole, L., Hegel, M., Arean, P., Hoffing, M., Penna, R. D., Langston, C., & Unutzer, J. (2003). Effect of improving depression care on pain and functional outcomes among older adults with arthritis: A randomized controlled trial. *The Journal of the American Medical Association*, **290**, 2428–34.

Linton, S. J. (2000). A review of psychological risk factors in back and neck pain. *Spine*, **25**, 1148–56.

Linton, S. J. (2005). Do psychological factors increase the risk for back pain in the general population in both a cross-sectional and prospective analysis? *European Journal of Pain*, **9**, 355–61.

McEwen, B. S. (1998a). Stress, adaptation, and disease: Allostasis and allostatic load. *Annals of the New York Academy of Science*, **840**, 33–44.

McEwen, B. S. (1998b). Protective and damaging effects of stress mediators. *New England Journal of Medicine*, **338**, 171–9.

McEwen, B. S., & Stellar, E. (1993). Stress and the individual: Mechanisms leading to disease. *Archives of Internal Medicine*, **153**, 2093–101.

O'Connor, J. C., McCusker, R. H., Strle, K., Johnson, R. W., Dantzer, R., & Kelley, K. W. (2008). Regulation of IGF-I function by proinflammatory cytokines: At the interface of immunology and endocrinology. *Cell Immunology*, **252**, 91–110.

Okma-Keulen, P., & Hopman-Rock, M. (2001). The onset of generalized osteoarthritis in older women: A qualitative approach. *Arthritis and Rheumatism*, **45**, 183–90.

Reginster, J. Y. (2002). The prevalence and burden of arthritis. *Rheumatology (Oxford, England)*, **41**, 3–6.

Simon, L. S. (1999). Osteoarthritis: A review. *Clinical Cornerstone*, **2**, 26–37.

Vassiloupoulos, D., & Mantzoukis, D. (2006). Dialogue between the brain and the immune system in inflammatory arthritis. *Annals of the New York Academy of Science*, **1088**, 132–8.

Von Korff, M., Alonso, J., Ormel, J., Angermeyer, M., Bruffaerts, R., Fleiz, C., de Girolamo, G., Kessler, R. C., Kovess-Masfety, V., Posada-Villa, J., Scott, K. M., & Uda, H. (2009). Childhood psychosocial stressors and adult onset arthritis: Broad spectrum risk factors and allostatic load. *Pain*, **143**, 76–83.

Yelin, E., & Callahan, L. F. (1995). The economic cost and social and psychological impact of musculoskeletal conditions. National Arthritis Data Work Groups. *Arthritis and Rheumatism*, **38**, 1351–62.

13 The Role of Childhood Adversities in Adult-Onset Spinal Pain

RONNY BRUFFAERTS AND KOEN DEMYTTENAERE

13.1. INTRODUCTION

In both population and clinical studies, and in both developed and developing countries, a significant association between spinal (back or neck) pain and anxiety and depressive disorders has been a consistent observation. In a World Health Organization study carried out among primary care patients in Asia, Africa, Europe, and the Americas, one in three of those with persistent pain met the International Classification of Mental and Behavioural Disorders (ICD-10) definition of anxiety or depression compared with about one in ten of those without persistent pain (Gureje et al. 1998). Reporting data from the National Comorbidity Survey – Replication, Von Korff et al. (2005) found that respondents with spinal pain were more likely to suffer from comorbid depressive disorders compared to persons without back or neck pain (with odds ratios ranging between 1.6 and 2.3). Also in cross-national and cross-cultural research, there has been evidence for a similar association between spinal pain and not only depressive disorders, but also anxiety and alcohol disorders (Demyttenaere et al. 2007; Scott et al. 2007). Hotopf et al. (1998) showed evidence for a bidirectionality between pain and psychiatric symptoms. Persons with mental disorders had a three- to sevenfold increase in reporting physical symptoms 7 years later. Similarly, they also found that having physical symptoms at age 37 was associated with increased risk of reporting psychiatric symptoms at age 43. Mental disorders could thus develop after the onset of the back or neck pain, as a response to living with chronic pain. Mental disorders may also precede the onset of chronic pain, particularly in light of the tendency of mood and anxiety disorders to onset during adolescence (Kessler et al. 2007).

From both clinical and epidemiological samples, mental disorders have been commonly observed among survivors of childhood abuse (Anda et al. 2002; Edwards et al. 2003; Molnar, Buka, & Kessler 2001; Turner & Muller 2004; Wilsnack et al. 1997). This association has been explained in terms of increased sensitivity to stress (Heim et al. 2001), negative attribution styles (Sachs-Ericsson, Kendall-Tackett, & Hernandez 2007), or decreased social support from friends or family (Golding, Wilsnack, & Cooper 2002). A history of childhood adversities has also been linked to the presence of pain symptoms, such as generalized pain, back pain, headache, and musculoskeletal pain (Davis, Luecken, & Zautra 2005; Kendall-Tackett, Marshall, & Ness 2003; Sachs-Ericsson et al. 2007). This relationship has largely been observed in clinical samples, generally among patients treated for pain symptoms. In their review of both case-control and population-based epidemiological studies, Raphael, Chandler, and Cicccone (2004) concluded that findings regarding the link between childhood adversities and pain were mixed. One prospective study by Raphael, Widom, and Lange (2001) did not find increased reporting among persons with a documented history of child abuse or neglect, whereas an association was found among persons who retrospectively reported a history of abuse or neglect. In contrast, Kopec and Sayre (2004) found, in a prospective follow-up study, that onset rates of arthritis pain were higher among persons who reported a history of childhood psychological trauma at baseline than among persons without.

All in all, available studies suggest that childhood adversities may be implicated in the relationship between mental disorders and chronic pain, but this question is far from settled. Existing literature on this question has three important limitations: First, to our knowledge, mostly clinical studies have investigated either the relationship between childhood adversities and either mental disorders (mostly depression) or pain problems. Population-based studies that investigate the relationship between childhood adversities, a broad range of mental disorders, and the adult onset of back or neck pain are nonexistent. Second, population-based and clinical studies have often assessed only a limited number of childhood adversities. The effects of a broad range of adversities on adult-onset spinal pain have not been investigated. Third, little is known about the association of childhood adversities, mental disorders, and the adult onset of spinal pain in general population samples with marked differences in culture, language, and level of socioeconomic development.

In this chapter we use data from the World Mental Health Surveys to investigate these questions. Information was also collected on back or neck pain, on age of onset of both back or neck pain and anxiety or depressive disorders, as well as on the experience of childhood adversities. The aims of this study were to investigate (1) whether the experience of childhood adversities predict adult-onset back or neck pain (age >20), with and without adjusting for current mental disorder (in order to control for mood-congruent recall bias); (2) whether early-onset anxiety or depressive disorders (age <21) predict adult-onset back or neck pain; and (3) whether childhood adversities and early-onset depressive or anxiety disorders predict adult-onset back or neck pain independently of each other.

13.2. APPROACH

Cox proportional hazards models estimated risk of adult-onset spinal pain as a function of number and type of childhood adversities and early-onset depression or anxiety disorder status while adjusting for potential confounders. Ascertainment of spinal pain was with a question about whether the respondent had chronic back or neck pain during the past 12 months, and a further question about how old they were the first time they had back or neck pain.

Kaplan–Meier curves were developed for graphical comparison of the age-specific cumulative proportion of respondents reporting onset of spinal pain comparing three categories of number of childhood adversities: none, one, and two or more adversities. Kaplan–Meier curves were also used to compare onset of spinal pain for persons with and without early-onset depression and/or anxiety disorder. See Chapter 4 (4.5.5) for further description of the methods that were generic across the physical condition and pain condition outcomes included in this section.

13.3. FINDINGS

13.3.1. Sample Characteristics and the Prevalence of Mental Disorders and Childhood Adversities

The characteristics of the total cross-national sample and the sample of those with

Table 13.1. Characteristics of the total and adult-onset spinal pain sample

	Unweighted N	Weighted %	
	Total cross-national sample (N = 17,331)	Total cross-national sample (N = 17,331)	Adult-onset spinal pain sample (N = 4,717)
Age (21–98 years)			
21–45	8,933	51.3	34.8
>45	8,398	48.7	65.2
Female	10,291	52.6	56.6
Completed secondary education	9,771	60.9	
Onset of mental disorder before 21 years	3,081	9.8	12.1
Adult-onset spinal pain	4,717	23.5	–
Number of childhood adversities			
None	9,613	60.2	57.5
One	4,118	23.2	23.0
Two	1,839	8.9	10.2
Three or more	1,761	7.7	9.2
Country			
Colombia	2,028	11.8	6.9
Belgium	936	5.2	5.4
France	1,206	7.0	9.2
Germany	1,200	7.0	6.9
Italy	1,480	8.6	15.9
The Netherlands	989	5.5	4.9
Spain	1,931	10.9	9.3
Japan	821	4.8	4.2
Mexico	1,922	11.2	9.0
United States	4,818	28.0	28.3

adult-onset spinal pain are provided in Table 13.1. Respondents with adult-onset spinal pain were slightly more likely to be female and older than 45 years. Somewhat higher proportions of those with adult-onset spinal pain (compared to the total sample) met criteria for early-onset depression or anxiety disorders and reported childhood adversities. Moreover, all mental disorders and childhood adversities were more common in the adult spinal pain sample than in the total cross-national sample (Table 13.2).

13.3.2. Effect of Childhood Adversity on Adult-Onset Spinal Pain

After adjustment for age, sex, and country, childhood adversities were associated with increased risk of onset of chronic spinal pain after age 20, with an increasing risk depending on the number of adversities experienced (Table 13.3). Survival curves for the cumulative percentage of reporting back or neck pain by age for respondents with childhood adversities are shown in Figure 13.1. Additional adjustments for either current (i.e., in the past 12 months prior to the interview) or early-onset (i.e., before the age of 21) *Diagnostic and Statistical Manual of Mental Disorders, Fourth Edition* (DSM-IV) depressive or anxiety disorders yielded similar results. Adjusted hazard ratios (HRs) range between 1.13 and 1.15 for one childhood adversity, between 1.34 and 1.39 for two, and between 1.57 and 1.72 for three or more adversities. This implies that the link between childhood adversity and

The Role of Childhood Adversities in Adult-Onset Spinal Pain

Table 13.2. Early-onset mood or anxiety disorders and childhood adversities in the total and adult-onset spinal pain samples

	Weighted %	
	Total cross-national sample ($N = 17,331$)	Adult-onset spinal pain sample ($N = 4,717$)
Early-onset (prior to age 21) mental disorders		
Major depressive disorder	4.2	4.8
Generalized anxiety disorder	1.2	1.8
Social phobia	4.7	5.7
Posttraumatic stress disorder	1.6	2.7
Panic/agoraphobia	1.7	2.2
Type of childhood adversity		
Neglect	7.0	9.8
Physical abuse	9.4	11.4
Sexual abuse	2.4	3.3
Parental death	13.1	14.7
Parental divorce	11.5	11.4
Other parent loss	5.2	5.9
Parental mental disorder	6.9	8.5
Parental substance-use disorder	5.0	5.7
Violence in family	9.2	10.2
Criminal behavior in family	3.2	3.4
Family economic adversity	5.7	6.1

adult-onset spinal pain is not simply a function of those with either a current or early-onset depressive or anxiety disorder.

Analyses of the specific adversities that exert an influence on adult-onset spinal pain showed that all but two adversities were significantly associated with adult-onset spinal pain (Figure 13.2). Nine out of eleven adversities yielded significant HRs between 1.16 (for parental divorce) and 1.62 (for having experienced sexual abuse). The two adverse experiences that were not associated with adult-onset back or neck pain were the experience of family economic adversity (HR = 1.13) and having experienced the death of a parent (HR = 1.08).

Table 13.3. Effects of childhood adversities on adult-onset spinal pain

Number of childhood adversities	No adjustment for depressive or anxiety disorders	With adjustment for current (12-month) depressive or anxiety disorders	With adjustment for early-onset depressive or anxiety disorders
None	1.00	1.00	1.00
One	1.15 (1.04–1.27)*	1.13 (1.02–1.25)*	1.13 (1.02–1.25)*
Two	1.39 (1.21–1.59)**	1.35 (1.17–1.55)**	1.34 (1.17–1.54)**
Three or more	1.72 (1.50–1.98)**	1.57 (1.36–1.80)**	1.59 (1.36–1.82)**

* $p < .01$.
** $p < .001$.

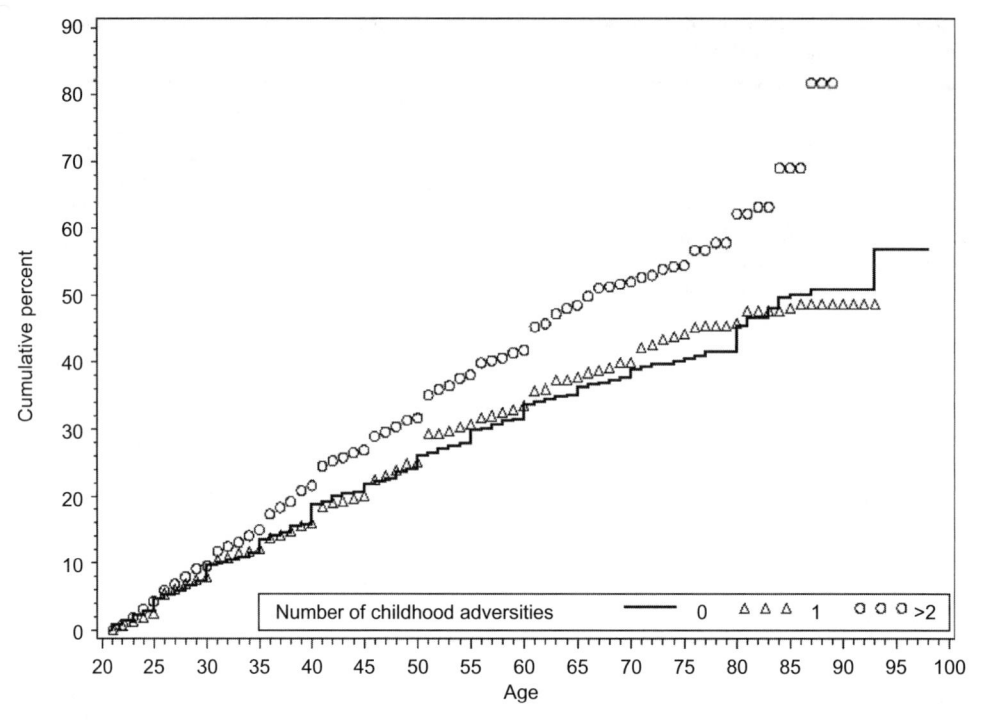

Figure 13.1. Survival curves for the cumulative percentage of reporting back or neck pain in respondents with none, one, and two or more childhood adversities.

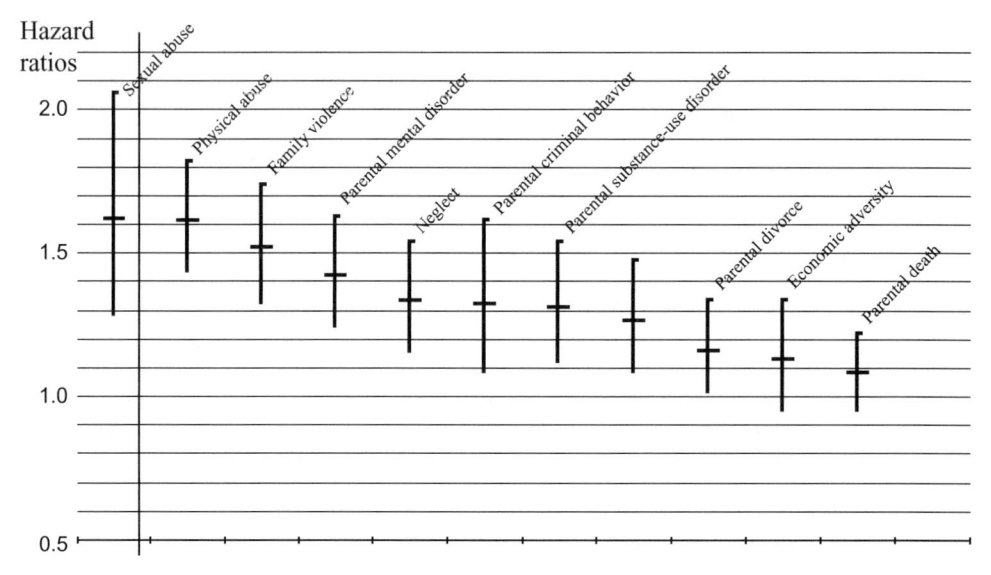

Figure 13.2. Effects of specific childhood adversities on adult-onset spinal pain.

The Role of Childhood Adversities in Adult-Onset Spinal Pain

Table 13.4. Effects of early-onset anxiety or depressive disorders on adult-onset spinal pain

	HRs for adult-onset spinal pain (adjusted for age, sex, and country)
Any depression or anxiety disorder onset (<21 years)	1.56 (1.40–1.73)*
Major depression episode onset (<21 years)	1.59 (1.37–1.85)*
Generalized anxiety disorder onset (<21 years)	2.01 (1.64–2.45)*
Social phobia onset (<21 years)	1.52 (1.34–1.73)*
Posttraumatic stress disorder onset (<21 years)	2.27 (1.76–2.92)*
Panicagoraphobia onset (<21 years)	1.62 (1.32–1.99)*

* $p < .001$.

13.3.3. Effect of Early-Onset Mental Disorder on Adult-Onset Spinal Pain

We also found effects of early-onset anxiety or depressive disorders on adult-onset back or neck pain, as shown in Figure 13.3. Table 13.4 shows the effects of specific early-onset anxiety or depressive disorders with adult-onset spinal pain. Early-onset anxiety or depressive disorders were found to predict adult-onset spinal pain after adjustment for age, sex, and country. HRs for all anxiety or depressive disorders were significant, ranging between 1.59 (for early-onset major depressive disorder) and 2.27 (for early-onset posttraumatic stress disorder).

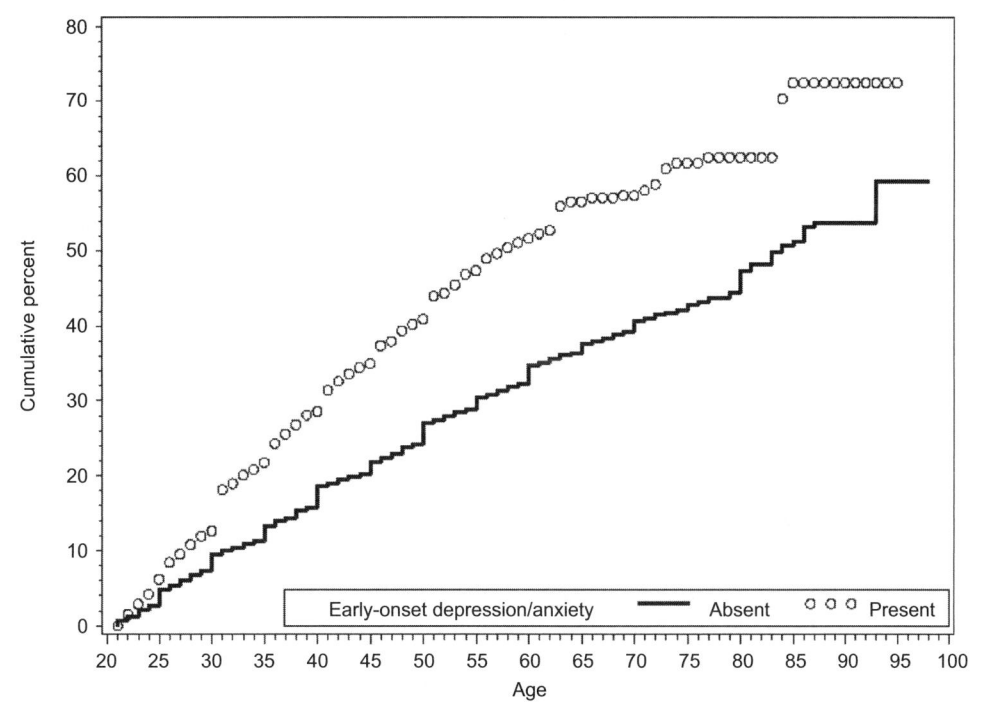

Figure 13.3. Survival curves for the cumulative percentage of reporting back or neck pain in respondents with early-onset anxiety or depressive disorders.

13.3.5. Independent Effects of Adversity and Mental Disorder on Adult-Onset Spinal Pain

When childhood adversities and early-onset anxiety or depressive disorders were entered into the same statistical model (together with age, sex, and country), both childhood adversity and early-onset mental disorder independently predicted adult-onset spinal pain. Even after adjusting for the potential influence of current or early-onset anxiety or depressive disorders on adult-onset spinal pain, the HRs remained consistently significant (Table 13.3). HRs for one childhood adversity were reduced from 1.15 to 1.13 after adjusting for either current or early-onset anxiety or depressive disorders. Similar results were found for two adversities on adult-onset spinal pain, with decreased HRs from 1.39 to 1.35 (after adjusting for current anxiety or depressive disorders) and from 1.39 to 1.34 (after adjusting for early-onset anxiety or depressive disorders), respectively. Finally, HRs for the influence of three or more adversities were 1.72 (prior to adjustment for the influence of anxiety or depressive disorders), 1.57 (adjusted for the potential influence of current anxiety or depressive disorders), and 1.59 (adjusted for the potential influence of early-onset anxiety or depressive disorders), respectively. These results suggest that childhood adversities are associated with increased risks of adult onset of back pain both in the presence and in the absence of early-onset psychological illness.

We also investigated the independent effects of early-onset anxiety or depressive disorders on adult-onset back or neck pain. Unadjusted HR for early-onset anxiety or depressive disorder was 1.68 (95% CI = 1.51–1.87). After adjustment for childhood adversities, HRs remained significant, ranging between 1.43 (95% CI = 1.21–1.68) and 1.50 (95% CI = 1.31–1.71). Similarly, these results suggest only minimal influence of childhood adversities on adult-onset spinal pain when respondents met criteria for an early-onset anxiety or depressive disorder. Analyses were also undertaken to assess whether there was a statistical interaction between childhood adversities and early-onset anxiety or depressive disorders in predicting the risk of adult-onset spinal pain. We could not find interaction effects (all p-values $>.05$).

13.4. DISCUSSION

There are three important findings from this study: First, the experience of at least one childhood adversity (before the age of 18) predicts increased risk of onset of back or neck pain after the age of 20. This relationship is independent of age, sex, country, or prior (i.e., before the age of 21) or current anxiety or depressive disorders. Second, the existence of anxiety or depressive disorders prior to the age of 21 predicts the onset of back or neck pain after the age of 21. Similarly, this relationship is independent of age, sex, country, or prior experiences of childhood adversities (before the age of 18). Third, there is no interaction between early-onset anxiety or depressive disorders in the relation studied. Similarly, we found no interaction effects of childhood adversities in the relationship between early-onset anxiety or depressive disorders and adult-onset back or neck pain.

That early-onset depressive disorders predict adult-onset back or neck pain independent of childhood adversities is in line with recent previous reports (Bair et al. 2003). We may add to existing literature that early-onset anxiety disorders predict adult-onset back or neck pain as the scientific interest in the link between anxiety disorders and chronic pain is of a recent nature (Demyttenaere et al. 2006). What our study also confirms is previous data showing that childhood adversities predict adult-onset back or neck pain (Sachs-Ericsson et al. 2007). Our study adds to previous findings in that we used a comprehensive assessment of both mental (i.e., anxiety and depressive) disorders and a broad range of childhood adversities. Moreover, we point to the temporal relationship between the occurrence of childhood adversities and subsequent onset of either back or neck pain.

There was a clear and direct dose–response relationship between the number of childhood experiences and adult-onset back or neck pain: respondents with one childhood adverse experience had a 15% increase, those with two a 39% increase, and those with three or more up to a 72% increase of spinal pain in adulthood. Even after adjustment for either past or current anxiety or depressive disorders, these associations remained pretty stable and robust. These findings suggest that the impact of childhood adversities is cumulative and relatively independent of mental disorder history.

A wide range of childhood adversities predicted adult-onset back or neck pain. Persons who had experienced either sexual or physical abuse or violence in the family were, generally speaking, more than 50% more likely to have spinal pain in adulthood. These findings are consistent with previous research showing that the experience of either sexual or physical abuse increases the likelihood of developing spinal (Davis et al. 2005; Nickel, Egle, & Hart 2002) or arthritic pain in adult life (Kopec & Sayre 2004). To the best of our knowledge, the present study is the first one comparing consequences of more violent versus less violent childhood adversities in a general population sample. Most interestingly though, sexual or physical abuse in particular, or the experience of family violence, seems to yield the highest risk of developing back or neck problems in adult life. These findings are consistent with clinical evidence that pain, as well as depression, can be thought of as a function of "introjected aggression" (Longstreth et al. 1998). Moreover, our findings also fit well with neurobiological evidence that aggressive early childhood adversities result in endocrine changes in adulthood which are linked to both anxiety or depression and pain (McEwen 2003; Heim et al. 2001; Heim & Nemeroff 2001).

Our findings contradict those of Raphael et al. (2001). Although their measures of association were roughly in the same range as ours, they did not find a significant association between the reporting of spinal pain and a history of sexual or physical abuse or neglect in childhood. But if we take a closer look at their results, their negative findings could be explained by respondents' young age at follow-up (i.e., 29 years). Indeed, if we look at the survival curves at age 30 in our study (Figure 13.1), there is a remarkable similarity: there are no discernable differences in cumulative onset rates between respondents with and without childhood adversities. This suggests that the sample of the Raphael et al. study may have been too young to detect differences in the onset of pain.

Our data suggest that early-onset anxiety or depressive disorders directly predicted adult-onset back or neck pain, even after adjustment for the presence of childhood adversities. This confirms the commonly reported link between pain and psychological illness. Indeed, both anxiety and depressive disorders were found to be significantly associated with chronic spinal pain, in both clinical (Haggman, Maher, & Refshauge 2004;) and general population samples (Bair et al. 2003; Currie & Wang 2004; Demyttenaere et al. 2007). In addition, the findings reported here suggest that early-onset mental disorder predicts subsequent onset of back or neck pain. Prospective studies have yielded similar results. For example, in the prospective general population study ($N = 7,669$) from

Croft et al. (2001), even the presence of mild anxiety or depressive symptoms (as measured with a General Health Questionnaire [GHQ-12] score ≥12) was predictive for a higher risk of back pain onset 12 months after the initial interview.

The results of this study should be interpreted in light of its limitations. In contrast to the detailed assessment of both mental disorders and childhood adversities, spinal pain was assessed by a question only about lifetime and 12-month status, and one question regarding age of onset. In the context of the World Mental Health Surveys, primarily concerned with assessing mental health status, it was not feasible to include a more comprehensive assessment of back or neck pain. Notwithstanding, there is evidence that self-report methods show moderate agreement with medical records data (National Center for Health Statistics 1994) and that self-reported pain episodes even tend to be underestimated (Biering-Sorenson & Hilden 1984; Jamison et al. 2006). A second limitation is that there were no measures of back or neck pain severity. Therefore, the associations in this study are averaged across the full spectrum of back or neck pain severity. A third limitation is the retrospective report of childhood adversities. It has been shown that recall bias may affect the accuracy of the adversity recall: rates of forgetting to report abusive experiences have been estimated in the 20–33% range (Elliot & Briere 1995; Wilsnack et al. 2002), but there is also evidence for the validity of the recall of childhood adversities (Hardt & Rutter 2004).

In conclusion, retrospective report of childhood adversities and early-onset psychological disorder were independently associated with increased risk of adult back or neck pain. Further research is needed to determine whether these associations can be replicated in prospective designs.

REFERENCES

Anda, R. F., Whitfield, C. L., Felitti, V. J., Chapman, D. J., Edwards, V. J., Dube, S. R., & Williamson, D. F. (2002). Adverse childhood experiences, alcoholic parents, and later risk of alcoholism and depression. *Psychiatric Services*, 53, 1001–9

Bair, M. J., Robinson, R. L., Katon, W., & Kroenke, K. (2003). Depression and comorbidity: A literature review. *Archives of Internal Medicine*, 163, 2433–55.

Biering-Sorensen, F., & Hilden, J. (1984). Reproductivity of the history of low back trouble. *Spine*, 9, 280–6.

Croft, P., Lewis, M., Papageorgiou, A. C., Thomas, E., Jayson, M. I. V., MacFarlane, G. J., & Silman, A. J. (2001). Risk factors for neck pain: A longitudinal study in the general population. *Pain*, 93, 317–25.

Currie, S. R., & Wang, J. (2004). Chronic back pain and major depression in the general Canadian population. *Pain*, 107, 54–60.

Davis, D. A., Luecken, L. J., & Zautra, A. J. (2005). Are reports of childhood abuse related to the experience of chronic pain in adulthood? A meta-analytic review of the literature. *Clinical Journal of Pain*, 21, 398–405.

Demyttenaere, K., Bonnewyn, A., Bruffaerts, R., Brugha, T., De Graaf, R., & Alonso, J. (2006). Comorbid painful physical symptoms and anxiety disorders: Prevalence, work loss, and help seeking. *Journal of Affective Disorders*, 92, 264–72.

Demyttenaere, K., Bruffaerts, R., Lee, S., Posada-Villa, J., Kovess, V., Angermeyer, M. C., Levinson, D., de Girolamo, G., Nakane, H., Mneimneh, Z., Lara, C., de Graaf, R., Scott, K. M., Gureje, O., Stein, D. J., Haro, J. M., Bromet, E. J., Kessler, R. C., Alonso, J., & Von Korff, M. (2007). Mental disorders among persons with chronic back or neck pain: Results from the World Mental Health Surveys. *Pain*, 129, 332–42.

Edwards, V. J., Holden, G. W., Felitti, V. J., & Anda, R. F. (2003). Relationship between multiple forms of childhood maltreatment and adult mental health in community respondents: Results from the adverse childhood experiences study. *American Journal of Psychiatry*, 160, 1453–60.

Elliot, D. M., & Briere, J. (1995). Posttraumatic stress associated with delayed recall of sexual abuse: A general population study. *Journal of Traumatic Stress*, **8**, 629–47.

Golding, J., Wilsnack, S., & Cooper, M. (2002). Sexual assault and social support: Six general population studies. *Journal of Trauma*, **15**, 187–97.

Gureje, O., Von Korff, M., Simon, G. E., & Gater, R. (1998). Persistent pain and well-being. A World Health Organization Study in Primary Care. *The Journal of the American Medical Association*, **280**, 147–51.

Haggman, S., Maher, C. G., & Refshauge, K. M. (2004). Screening for symptoms of depression by physical therapists managing low back pain. *Physical Therapy*, **84**, 1157–66.

Hardt, J., & Rutter, M. (2004). Validity of adult retrospective reports of adverse childhood experiences: Review of the evidence. *Journal of Child Psychology and Psychiatry*, **45**, 260–73.

Heim, C., & Nemeroff, C. B. (2001). The role of childhood trauma in the neurobiology of mood and anxiety disorders: Preclinical and clinical studies. *Biological Psychiatry*, **49**, 1023–39.

Heim, C., Newport, D. J., Bonsall, R., Miller, A. H., & Nemeroff, C. B. (2001). Altered pituitary-adrenal axis responses to provocative challenge tests in adult survivors of childhood abuse. *American Journal of Psychiatry*, **158**, 575–81.

Hotopf, M., Mayou, R., Wadsworth, M., & Wessely, S. (1998). Temporal relationships between physical symptoms and psychiatric disorder. Results from a national birth cohort. *British Journal of Psychiatry*, **173**, 255–61.

Jamison, R. N., Raymond, S. A., Slawsby, E. A., McHugo, G. J., & Baird, J. C. (2006). Pain assessment in patients with low back pain: Comparison of weekly recall and momentary electronic data. *Journal of Pain*, **7**, 192–9.

Kendall-Tackett, K. A., Marshall, R., & Ness, K. E. (2003). Chronic pain syndromes and violence against women. *Women and Therapy*, **26**, 45–56.

Kessler, R. C., Angermeyer, M., Anthony, J. C., de Graaf, R., Demyttenaere, K., Gasquet, I., de Girolamo, G., Gluzman, S., Gureje, O., Haro, J. M., Kawakami, N., Karam, A., Levinson, D., Medina Mora, M. E., Oakley Browne, M. A., Posada-Villa, J., Stein, D. J., Tsang, C. H. A., Aguilar-Gaxiola, S., Alonso, J., Lee, S., Heeringa, S., Pennell, B.-E., Berglund, P. A., Gruber, M., Petukhova, M., Chatterji, S., & Ustun, T. B. (2007). Lifetime prevalence and age-of-onset distributions of mental disorders in the WHO World Mental Health (WMH) Surveys. *World Psychiatry*, **6**, 168–76.

Kopec, J. A., & Sayre, E. C. (2004) Traumatic experiences in childhood and the risk of arthritis: A prospective cohort study. *Canadian Journal of Public Health*, **95**, 361–5.

Longstreth, G. F., Mason, C., Schreiber, I. G., & Tsao-Wei, D. (1998). Group psychotherapy for women molested in childhood: Psychological and somatic symptoms and medical visits. *International Journal of Group Psychotherapy*, **48**, 533–41.

McEwen, B. S. (2003). Mood disorders and allostatic load. *Biological Psychiatry*, **54**, 200–7.

Molnar, B., Buka, S., & Kessler, R. (2001). Child sexual abuse and subsequent psychopathology: Results from the National Comorbidity Survey. *American Journal of Public Health*, **91**, 753–60.

Nickel, E., Egle, U. T., & Hardt, J. (2002). Are childhood adversities relevant in patients with low back pain? *European Journal of Pain*, **6**, 221–8.

Raphael, K. G., Chandler, H. K., & Ciccone, D. S. (2004). Is childhood abuse a risk factor for chronic pain in adulthood? *Current Pain and Headache Reports*, **8**, 99–110.

Raphael, K. G., Widom, C. S., & Lange, G. (2001). Childhood victimization and pain in adulthood: A prospective investigation. *Pain*, **92**, 283–93.

Sachs-Ericsson, N., Kendall-Tackett, K., & Hernandez, A. (2007). Childhood abuse, chronic pain, and depression in the National Comorbidity Survey. *Child Abuse and Neglect*, **31**, 531–47.

Scott, K. M., Bruffaerts, R., Tsang, A., Ormel, J., Alonso, J., Angermeyer, M. C., Benjet, C., Bromet, E., de Girolamo, G., de Graaf, R., Gasquet, I., Gureje, O., Haro, J. M., He, Y., Kessler, R. C., Levinson, D., Mneimneh, Z. N., Oakley Browne, M. A., Posada-Villa, J., Stein, D. J., Takeshima, T., & Von Korff, M. (2007). Depression-anxiety relationships with chronic physical conditions: Results from the World Mental Health surveys. *Journal of Affective Disorders*, **103**, 113–20.

Turner, H. A., & Muller, P. A. (2004). Long-term effects of child corporal punishment on depressive symptoms in young adults: Potential moderators and mediators. *Journal of Family Issues*, **25**, 761–82.

Von Korff, M., Crane, P., Lane, M., Miglioretti, D. L., Simon, G., Suanders, K., Stang, P.,

Brandenburg, N., & Kessler, R. (2005). Chronic spinal pain and physical-mental comorbidity in the United States: Results from the national comorbidity survey replication. *Pain*, **115**, 331–9.

Wilsnack, S. C., Vogeltanz, N. D., Klassen, A. D., & Harris, T. R. (1997). Childhood sexual abuse and women's substance abuse: National survey findings. *Journal of Studies on Alcohol*, **58**, 264–71.

Wilsnack, S. C., Wonderlich, S. A., Kristjanson, A. F., Vogeltanz-Holm, N. D., & Wilsnack, R. (2002). Self-reports of forgetting and remembering childhood sexual abuse in a nationally representative sample of US women. *Child Abuse and Neglect*, **26**, 139–47.

14 Childhood Adversities and Adult Obesity

RONNY BRUFFAERTS AND KOEN DEMYTTENAERE

14.1. INTRODUCTION

Obesity presents significant public health challenges in the twenty-first century on a worldwide basis (World Health Organization 2004). Recent studies show that obesity (defined as a body mass index (BMI) of more than 30 kg/m^2) is a common condition: between 22 and 35% of the adult population in the United States and between 10 and 23% of the adult population in Europe meet criteria for obesity (Bruffaerts et al. 2008; Maillard et al. 1999; Neovius, Janson, & Rössner 2006; Scott et al. 2008). Obesity is associated with diverse adverse health effects including increased mortality and chronic somatic diseases (e.g., hypertension, diabetes mellitus, coronary heart disease, and congestive heart failure) (Flegal et al. 2005; Kress, Hartzel, & Peterson 2005; Pi-Sunyer, 1993, 2003; Salahudeen et al. 2004). Obesity is also related to a wide range of emotional problems, especially anxiety and depression. Compared to normal-weight persons (with a BMI between 18.5 and 25 kg/m^2), obese persons were up to two times more likely to meet criteria for a *Diagnostic and Statistical Manual of Mental Disorders, Fourth Edition* (DSM-IV) depressive or anxiety disorder in the past year (Scott et al. 2008; Simon et al. 2006; Stunkard, Faith, & Allison 2003). This is a finding that has shown to be consistent among populations from different cultures (Scott et al. 2008) and among both community and clinical samples (Guallar-Castillón et al. 2002). The high prevalence and increasing incidence of obesity, and its significant comorbidity with somatic and mental health, have led to increased empirical attention to the role of psychological and environmental factors in influencing risks of obesity.

The causes of obesity are believed to be multifactorial, including genetic, environmental, and individual factors. Whereas the heritability of obesity has been estimated to be in the 40–70% range (Comuzzie & Allison 1998; Devlin, Yanovski, & Wilson 2000), behavioral factors are undoubtedly important determinants of recent increases in the incidence of obesity. For example, obesity is associated with higher access to calorie-rich foods (Pereira 2006) and reduced levels of physical activity (Hill & Peters 1998). There is also evidence that obesity is more common among persons who have experienced childhood sexual abuse. The Adverse Childhood Experiences (ACE) Study ($N = 17{,}421$) has convincingly shown that a broad range of psychological, physical, and sexual adversities in childhood affected adult health decades later (Felitti et al. 1998). Research suggests that the relationship between childhood sexual abuse and obesity may be stronger for those persons who experienced more severe forms of abuse (Gustafson & Sarwer 2004).

Prior research on childhood adversities and adult obesity has several limitations. Although particular childhood adversities may be significantly related to adult obesity, this has not been extensively studied. Most studies have investigated the relationship between a limited set of childhood adversities (typically sexual and physical abuse), mental disorders (typically depression), and obesity. We are not aware of studies that have investigated the relationship between a broad range of childhood adversities and adult obesity. Most research has employed clinical samples, raising questions regarding the generalizability of their findings. Depressive and anxiety disorders often have an early age of onset (Kessler et al. 2007). The association between obesity and mental disorders (Scott et al. 2008) suggests the possibility that the relationship between childhood adverse experiences and obesity in adulthood could be mediated by early-onset mental disorders.

The aims of the study reported in this chapter were to investigate whether (1) obese respondents were more likely to have experienced childhood adversities, with and without adjusting for current mental health; (2) early-onset anxiety/depressive disorders (age <21) were more common among obese respondents; and (3) childhood adversities and early-onset depressive/anxiety disorders were independently associated with adult obesity.

14.2. APPROACH

Obesity ascertainment was based on self-report of height and weight, from which BMI was calculated. Consistent with recommendations of previous population research (Seidel & Flegal 1997), we used cutpoints to define BMI categories: underweight (BMI < 18.5 kg/m^2), normal weight (BMI between 18.5 and 24.9 kg/m^2), overweight (BMI between 25.0 and 29.9 kg/m^2), and obesity (BMI ≥ 30 kg/m^2). In this study, underweight respondents were excluded from the analyses. Two main categories were retained: obese and nonobese (normal-weight and overweight) respondents.

Multivariate logistic regression analysis estimated the odds ratio (ORs) of obesity as a function of number of childhood adversities and early-onset depression/anxiety disorder status while adjusting for potential confounders (sex, current age, and country). The associations are expressed in odds ratios (ORs) with 95% confidence intervals (95% CI). Childhood adversities were analyzed in four categories of number of adversities (none, one, two, and three or more), with no adversities as reference group. Childhood adversities and early-onset mental disorders were included in the models both separately and simultaneously. We screened for interaction of childhood adversities and early-onset depression/anxiety disorder, but the interaction was nonsignificant, so only main effects are reported in this chapter. In order to account for the possibility of differential recall of childhood adversities among those with a current anxiety or depressive disorder, an additional analysis was performed, adjusting for this current disorder. See Chapter 4 (4.5.5) for further description of the methods.

14.3. FINDINGS

14.3.1. Sample Characteristics and the Prevalence of Mental Disorders and Childhood Adversities

The characteristics of the total cross-national sample ($N = 18,207$) and of the sample of respondents who met criteria for obesity ($N = 3,126$) are provided in Table 14.1. Obese respondents were slightly more likely to be female and older than 45 years. Childhood adversities were common: one in four (i.e., 25.5%) of the respondents reported one adverse experience prior to the age of 18, one in ten (i.e., 10.0%) reported two, and a slightly lower proportion (i.e., 8.3%) reported three or more. Death of one of the parents, parental divorce, physical abuse, family violence, and economic adversities were the most common adversities before the age of

Childhood Adversities and Adult Obesity

Table 14.1. Characteristics of the total and obesity sample

	Total cross-national sample (N = 18,207)		Adult obesity sample (N = 3,126)
	Unweighted N	Weighted %	Weighted %
Age (years)			
21–45	9,536	51.9	43.5
>45	8,671	48.1	56.5
Female	7,559	48.6	51.6
Body mass index >30 kg/m²	3,126	16.1	100.0
Onset of anxiety/depressive disorder before 21 years	3,394	10.3	12.4
Number of childhood adversities			
None	9,378	56.2	51.5
One	4,684	25.5	25.6
Two	2,101	10.0	12.1
Three or more	2,044	8.3	10.8
Country			
Colombia	2,043	11.3	4.7
Belgium	986	5.4	4.8
France	1,325	7.3	5.4
Germany	1,287	7.2	4.8
Italy	1,671	9.3	6.0
The Netherlands	1,059	5.6	3.7
Spain	2,008	10.9	10.2
Japan	769	4.3	0.8
Mexico	1,881	10.3	11.9
United States	5,178	28.4	47.8

18 (Table 14.2). Somewhat higher proportions of those with adult obesity – compared to the total sample – met criteria for early-onset depression/anxiety disorders and reported childhood adversities (Table 14.2). Moreover, all mental disorders and all childhood adversities were more common among the adult obesity sample than in the total sample.

14.3.2. Associations between Childhood Adversities and Adult Obesity

After adjustment for age, sex, and country, obese respondents were more likely to report childhood adversities, with an increasing risk depending on the number of adversities experienced (Table 14.3). Univariate ORs were 1.09 ($p > .05$) for one childhood adversity, 1.35 ($p < .01$) for two childhood adversities, and 1.33 ($p < .01$) for three or more childhood adversities. Four specific adversities were significantly associated with adult obesity (Table 14.4): physical abuse (OR = 1.22), parental death (OR = 1.22), other parent loss (OR = 1.38), and family economic adversity (OR = 1.59).

14.3.3. Associations between Early-Onset Anxiety/Depressive Disorders and Adult Obesity

Table 14.4 shows the associations between early-onset anxiety/depressive disorders and adult obesity. In general, specific early-onset anxiety/depressive disorders were not

Table 14.2. Early-onset mood/anxiety disorders and childhood adversities in the total and adult obesity samples

	Weighted %	
	Total cross-national sample ($N = 18{,}207$)	Adult obesity sample ($N = 3{,}126$)
Early-onset (prior to age 21) mental disorders		
Major depressive disorder	4.6	5.3
Generalized anxiety disorder	1.4	1.6
Social phobia	4.9	6.4
Posttraumatic stress disorder	1.7	2.7
Panic/agoraphobia	1.8	2.0
Type of childhood adversity		
Neglect	6.5	6.9
Physical abuse	9.6	10.4
Sexual abuse	2.6	4.0
Parental death	12.9	14.2
Parental divorce	9.9	11.4
Other parent loss	5.2	6.9
Parental mental disorder	7.2	7.4
Parental substance-use disorder	4.9	6.9
Violence in family	9.3	10.7
Criminal behavior in family	3.4	4.6
Family economic adversity	5.8	9.1

Table 14.3. Associations between the number of childhood adversities, early-onset, current anxiety/depressive disorders, and adult obesity

	Odds ratios (95% CI) for obesity (adjusted for age, sex, and country)		
	No adjustment for depressive/anxiety disorders	With adjustment for current depressive/anxiety disorders	With adjustment for early-onset anxiety/depressive disorders
Number of childhood adversities			
None	1.00 (ref)	1.00 (ref)	1.00 (ref)
One	1.09 (0.93–1.27)	1.08 (0.93–1.26)	1.09 (0.93–1.27)
Two	1.35 (1.10–1.66)*	1.34 (1.09–1.65)*	1.36 (1.10–1.67)*
Three or more	1.33 (1.10–1.62)*	1.30 (1.07–1.58)*	1.34 (1.11–1.63)*
Early-onset anxiety/depressive disorders	–	–	0.97 (0.86–1.09)
Current anxiety/depressive disorders	–	1.14 (1.02–1.29)*	–

ref, reference category.
* $p < .05$.

Childhood Adversities and Adult Obesity

Table 14.4. Associations between early-onset anxiety/depressive disorders and childhood adversities with adult obesity

	Odds ratios for obesity (adjusted for age, sex, and country)
Mental disorders	
Any depression/anxiety disorder onset <21 years	1.03 (0.91–1.16), $p = .66$
Major depression episode onset <21 years	1.06 (0.90–1.24), $p = .49$
Generalized anxiety disorder onset <21 years	0.94 (0.71–1.24), $p = .65$
Social phobia onset <21 years	0.99 (0.84–1.17), $p = .91$
Posttraumatic stress disorder onset <21 years	1.36 (1.01–1.84), $p = .04$
Panic/agoraphobia onset <21 years	1.00 (0.78–1.29), $p = .97$
Childhood adversities	
Neglect	1.14 (0.94–1.37), $p = .18$
Physical abuse	1.22 (1.02–1.46), $p = .03$
Family sexual abuse	1.26 (0.96–1.66), $p = .09$
Parental death	1.22 (1.03–1.45), $p = .02$
Parental divorce	1.03 (0.85–1.25), $p = .77$
Other parent loss	1.38 (1.08–1.76), $p = .01$
Parental mental disorder	0.93 (0.78–1.12), $p = .44$
Parental substance-use disorder	1.22 (0.99–1.50), $p = .06$
Family violence	1.05 (0.85–1.29), $p = .66$
Criminal behavior	1.15 (0.94–1.42), $p = .18$
Economic adversity	1.59 (1.23–2.05), $p < .01$

associated with adult obesity (all $p > .49$), except for early-onset posttraumatic stress disorder (OR = 1.36).

14.3.4. Associations between Childhood Adversities, Anxiety/Depressive Disorders, and Adult Obesity

When childhood adversities and early-onset anxiety/depressive disorders were entered into the same statistical model (together with age, sex, and country), only childhood adversities (ORs between 1.34 and 1.36, $p < .01$) yielded a significant association, whereas early-onset anxiety/depressive disorders did not (OR = 0.97, $p = .60$). Conversely, when childhood adversities and current anxiety/depressive disorders were entered into the statistical model (together with age, sex, and country), both childhood adversities (ORs between 1.30 and 1.34, $p < .01$) and current anxiety/depressive disorders (OR = 1.14, $p = .03$) were significantly associated with adult obesity (Table 14.4). Adjusting for current psychological disorder addresses the concern that recall of childhood adversities may be biased by current psychological illness.

Interestingly, after adjusting for either current or early-onset anxiety/depressive disorders, ORs remained significant in the same range for two or more childhood adversities. There was a systematic positive association (ORs in the 1.30–1.36 range) between reporting two or more childhood adversities and obesity in adulthood. Analyses were also undertaken to assess whether there was a statistical interaction between childhood adversities and early-onset anxiety/depressive disorders in their association with adult obesity. We did not observe interaction effects (all p-values > .05). These results are not consistent with early-onset anxiety/depressive disorders mediating the relationship between childhood adversities and adult obesity.

14.4. DISCUSSION

Three main findings stand out from this first cross-national study. First, having experienced multiple childhood adversities is associated with adult obesity. This relationship held after controlling for age, sex, country, prior (i.e., before the age of 21) or current (i.e., in the past 12 months) anxiety/depressive disorders. Second, the presence of a posttraumatic stress disorder prior to the age of 21 was associated with adult obesity. Third, we could not find evidence for an interaction effect between early-onset anxiety/depressive disorders and childhood adversities with regard to their relationship with adult obesity. However, further research on whether early-onset psychological disorder plays a role in the subsequent development of obesity among persons experiencing childhood adversities is needed, given the retrospective nature of the data available in these surveys.

We found a dose–response relationship between the number of childhood adversities and obesity: one experience was not significantly related to an increased risk of obesity in adulthood, whereas multiple adversities had a 1.30- to 1.36-fold increase in adult obesity. This dose–response relationship is consistent with earlier data from the ACE Study. In their study ($N = 9,508$), Felitti et al. (1998) also found that one childhood adversity did not increase the likelihood of meeting the criteria for morbid obesity (defined as a BMI ≥ 35), whereas two or more adversities did.

Post hoc analyses found that specific childhood adversities were associated with obesity. There was a modest increase in risk of obesity among respondents who experienced physical abuse, parental death, other parent loss, or economic adversity before the age of 18. Physical abuse has previously been mentioned as a risk factor for obesity. Huanguang et al. (2004) found that among 239 female gastrointestinal patients, having a history of physical abuse increased the ORs for obesity by 34%. We also found that the loss of one of the parents was a significant early risk factor for adult obesity. Since our study is the first to assess effects of parental loss on obesity, further research is needed to replicate these findings. The effects of economic problems in childhood are in line with prior research (Ziebland et al. 1996). There is substantial evidence supporting a negative association between income and a healthful diet (Apovian 2004; Ludwig, Peterson, & Gortmaker 2001). The relationship between familial sexual abuse and adult obesity was of borderline statistical significance (OR $= 1.26$, $p = .09$). Prior research has reported a 1.3- to 1.6-fold increase in obesity when having experienced childhood sexual abuse (Gustafson & Sarwer 2004). While the association reported here did not reach conventional levels of statistical significance, the OR estimate is similar to that reported in prior research.

Our results thus suggest that there is a significant association between childhood adversities and obesity in adulthood. To the extent that this is the case, why would this be? A possible explanation is that childhood adversities may cause a psychobiological condition that may be linked with obesity. Preclinical and clinical studies have suggested that childhood deprivation may lead to long-lasting dysregulations in hypothalamic–pituitary–adrenocortical axis functioning, manifesting in hypercortisolemia (Heim & Nemeroff 2002). Moreover, high cortisol levels play an important role in the development of body fat (Pasquali et al. 1993; Seematter, Binnert, & Tappy 2005). This hypothesized pathway is consonant with the idea that early adverse experiences may lead to neurobiological conditions that may increase the onset of chronic diseases in adulthood (McEwen 1998).

Our results have implications for both clinical care and prevention. Clinicians should be aware of the significance of the full range of childhood adversities – not just sexual or physical abuse – that may have occurred with increased frequency among adult obese persons. These results are especially relevant to primary or specialty care where obesity is more common than in the general population (Noel et al. 1998; Smith & Haslam 2007) as obesity is a common reason for seeking health care and is associated with chronic diseases that prompt the use of health care (Bertakis & Azari 2005; Raebel et al. 2004). Second, because childhood adversities are associated with adult obesity, increased attention may need to be given to the prevention of these adversities (Felitti et al. 1998). Both universal and selective prevention of childhood adversities are challenging because these require changes in family and social environments (MacMillan et al. 1997). Preventive strategies that identify high-risk families are one possible approach (Felitti et al. 1998). However, there were substantial differences across the 10 countries included in this report in the prevalence of childhood adversities (data not shown), suggesting the possibility that differences in economic, cultural, and/or public policy factors may be capable of changing risks of childhood adversities.

Our observations should be interpreted in light of the following biases that might hamper the interpretation and generalizability of our data. First, the assessment of obesity was limited to the validity of the self-reports of weight and height by respondents. The World Mental Health Surveys were conducted in many population samples and were primarily concerned with assessment of mental health, so it was not feasible to include objective measurement of height and weight. In overweight or obese persons, self-reported height is, on average, greater than measured height and that self-reported weight is, on average, lower than measured weight (Villanueva 2001; Ziebland et al. 1996). This potential bias could have led to an underestimation of the proportion of either overweight or obese persons in the World Mental Health Surveys. Second, the report of childhood adversities was retrospective and could thus have led to a certain recall bias. The possibility of mood-congruent recall bias was addressed by controlling for current mood disorder. The effects of two or more childhood adversities on adult obesity were found to be robust after adjustment for past or current mood disorder. There is also reduced recall due to the time that has elapsed between the childhood experience of adversity and the assessment of it in adulthood. The results reported here support the need for further prospective research concerning the role of multiple childhood adversities occurring in the family context in increasing risks of obesity in adulthood.

REFERENCES

Apovian, C. M. (2004). Sugar-sweetened soft drinks, obesity, and type 2 diabetes. *The Journal of the American Medical Association*, 292, 978–9.

Bertakis, K. D., & Azari, R. (2005). Obesity and the use of health care services. *Obesity Research*, 13, 372–9.

Bruffaerts, R., Demyttenaere, K., Vilagut, G., Martinez, M., Bonnewyn, A., De Graaf, R., Brugha, T. S., Bernert, S., Angermeyer, M. C., Roick, C., & Alonso, J. (2008). The relationship between body mass index, mental health, and functional disability: A European population perspective. *Canadian Journal of Psychiatry*, 53, 37–46.

Comuzzie, A. G., & Allison, D. B. (1998). The search for the human obesity genes. *Science*, 280, 1374–7.

Devlin, M. J., Yanovski, S. Z., & Wilson, G. T. (2000). Obesity: What mental health professionals need to know. *American Journal of Psychiatry*, 157, 854–66.

Felitti, V. J., Anda, R. F., Nordenberg, D., Williamson, D. F., Spitz, A. M., Edwards, V., Koss, M. P., & Marks, J. S. (1998). Relationship of childhood abuse and household dysfunction to many of the leading causes of death in adults: The

Adverse Childhood Experiences (ACE) Study. *American Journal of Preventive Medicine*, **14**, 245–58.

Flegal, K. M., Carroll, M. D., Kuczmarski, R. J., & Johnson, C. L. (1998). Overweight and obesity in the United States: Prevalence and trends, 1960–1994. *International Journal of Obesity and Related Metabolic Disorders*, **22**, 39–47.

Flegal, K. M., Graubard, B. I., Williamson, D. F., & Gail, M. H. (2005). Excess deaths associated with underweight, overweight, and obesity. *The Journal of the American Medical Association*, **20**, 1961–9.

Guallar-Castillón, P., López Garciá, E., Lozano Palacios, L., Gutiérrez-Fisac, J. L., Banegas, J. R., Lafuente Urdinguio, P. J., & Rodriguez Artalejo, F. (2002). The relationship of overweight and obesity with subjective health and use of healthcare services among Spanish women. *International Journal of Obesity and Related Metabolic Disorders*, **26**, 247–52.

Gustafson, T. B., & Sarwer, D. B. (2004). Childhood sexual abuse and obesity. *Obesity Review*, **5**, 129–35.

Heim, C., & Nemeroff, C. B. (2002). Neurobiology of early life stress: Clinical studies. *Seminars in Clinical Neuropsychiatry*, **7**, 147–59.

Hill, J. O., & Peters, J. C. (1998). Environmental contributions to obesity epidemic. *Science*, **280**, 1371–4.

Huanguang, J., Li, J., Leserman, J., Yuming, H., & Drossman, A. (2004). Relationship of abuse history and other risk factors with obesity among female gastrointestinal patients. *Digestive Diseases and Sciences*, **49**, 872–7.

Kessler, R. C., Angermeyer, M., Anthony, J. C., de Graff, R., Demyttenaere, K., Gasquet, I., de Girolamo, G., Gluzman, S., Gureje, O., Haro, J. M., Kawakami, N., Karam, A., Levinson, D., Medina Mora, M. E., Oakley Browne, M. A., Posada-Villa, J., Stein, D. J., Tsang, C. H. A., Aguilar-Gaxiola, S., Alonso, J., Lee, S., Heeringa, S., Pennell, B.-E., Berglund, P. A., Gruber, M., Petukhova, M., Chatterji, S., & Ustun, T. B. (2007). Lifetime prevalence and age-of-onset distributions of mental disorders in the WHO World Mental Health (WMH) Surveys. *World Psychiatry*, **6**, 168–76.

Kress, A. M., Hartzel, M. C., & Peterson, M. R. (2005). Burden of disease associated with overweight and obesity among US military retirees and their dependents, aged 38–64, 2003. *Preventive Medicine*, **41**, 63–9.

Ludwig, D. S., Peterson, K. E., & Gortmaker, S. L. (2001). Relation between consumption of sugar-sweetened drinks and childhood obesity: A prospective, observational analysis. *Lancet*, **17**, 505–8.

MacMillan, H. L., Fleming, J. E., Trocme, N., Boyle, M. H., Wong, M., Racine, Y. A., Beardslee, W. R., & Offord, D. R. (1997). Prevalence of child physical and sexual abuse in the community: Results from the Ontario Health Supplement. *The Journal of the American Medical Association*, **278**, 131–5.

Maillard, G., Charles, M. A., Thibult, N., Vray, M., Borys, J. M., Basdevant, A., Eschwege, E., & Romon, M. (1999). Trends in the prevalence of obesity in the French adult population between 1980 and 1991. *International Journal of Obesity and Related Metabolic Disorders*, **4**, 389–94.

McEwen, B. S. (1998). Protective and damaging effects of stress mediators. *New England Journal of Medicine*, **338**, 171–9.

Neovius, M., Janson, A., & Rössner, S. (2006). Prevalence of obesity in Sweden. *Obesity Review*, **7**, 1–3.

Noel, M., Hickner, J., Ettenhofer, T., & Gauthier, B. (1998). The high prevalence of obesity in Michigan primary care practices. *Journal of Family Practice*, **47**, 39–43.

Pasquali, R., Cantobelli, S., Casimirri, F., Capelli, M., Bortoluzzi, L., Flamia, R., Labate, A. M., & Barbara, L. (1993). The hypothalamic-pituitary-adrenal axis in obese women with different patterns of body fat distribution. *Journal of Clinical Endocrinology and Metabolism*, **77**, 341–6.

Pereira, M. (2006). The possible role of sugar-sweetened beverages in obesity etiology: A review of the evidence. *International Journal of Obesity*, **30**, S28–36.

Pi-Sunyer, F. X. (1993). Medical hazards of obesity. *Annals of Internal Medicine*, **119**, 655–60.

Pi-Sunyer, F. X. (2003). A clinical view of the obesity problem. *Science*, **299**, 859–60.

Raebel, M. A., Mlone, D. C., Conner, D. A., Xu, S., Porter, J. A., & Lanty, F. A. (2004). Health services and health care costs of obese and nonobese individuals. *Archives of Internal Medicine*, **164**, 2135–40.

Salahudeen, A. K., Fleischmann, E. H., Bower, J. D., & Hall, J. E. (2004). Underweight rather than overweight is associated with higher prevalence of hypertension: BP vs BMI in haemodialysis population. *Nephrology, Dialysis, Transplantation*, **19**, 427–32.

Scott, K. M., Bruffaerts, R., Simon, G. E., Alonso, J., Angermeyer, M., de Girolamo, G., Demyttenaere, K., Gasquet, I., Haro, J. M., Karam, E., Kessler, R. C., Levinson, D., Medina Mora, M. E., Oakley Browne, M. A., Ormel, J., Villa, J. P., Uda, H., & Von Korff, M. (2008). Obesity and mental disorders in the general population: Results from the World Mental Health Surveys. *International Journal of Obesity*, **32**, 192–200.

Seematter, G., Binnert, C., & Tappy L. (2005). Stress and metabolism. *Metabolic Syndrome and Related Disorders*, **3**, 8–13.

Seidell, J. C., & Flegal, K. M. (1997). Assessing obesity: Classification and epidemiology. *British Medical Bulletin*, **53**, 238–52.

Simon, G. E., Von Korff, M., Saunders, K., Miglioretti, D. L., Crane, P. K., van Belle, G., & Kessler, R. C. (2006). Association between obesity and psychiatric disorders in the US adult population. *Archives of General Psychiatry*, **63**, 824–30.

Smith, S. C., & Haslam, D. (2007). Abdominal obesity, waist circumference and cardio-metabolic risk: Awareness among primary care physicians, the general population and patients at risk – the Shape of the Nations survey. *Current Medical Research and Opinion*, **23**, 29–47.

Stunkard, A. J., Faith, M. S., & Allison, K. C. (2003). Depression and obesity. *Biological Psychiatry*, **54**, 330–7.

Villanueva, E. (2001). The validity of self-reported weight in US adults: A population based cross-sectional study. *BMC Public Health*, **1**, 11.

World Health Organization. (2004). *Obesity: Preventing and Managing the Global Epidemic. Report of a WHO Consultation.* Geneva: World Health Organization.

Ziebland, S., Thogorood, M., Fuller, A., & Muir, J. (1996). Desire for the body normal: Body image and discrepancies between self-reported and measured height and weight in a British population. *Journal of Epidemiology and Community Health*, **50**, 105–6.

15 Linking Depression–Anxiety Disorders and Headache in a Developmental Perspective: The Role of Childhood Family Adversities

ADLEY TSANG AND SING LEE

15.1. INTRODUCTION

Comorbidity of headache and mental disorders, especially depression and anxiety disorders, is common according to both community and clinical studies (Molgat & Patten 2005; Sheftell & Atlas 2002; Strine, Chapman, & Balluz 2006). A substantial proportion of patients with headache have mental disorders (Radat & Swendsen 2005); many patients with mental disorders also report headache (Bair et al. 2004). Varying patterns of association are likely to exist among different kinds of headaches and mental disorders such as depression, bipolar disorder, phobic anxiety, and substance-use disorder. Regarding migraine and tension headaches that are the most commonly studied types of headaches, different mood and anxiety disorders appear to be similarly frequent (Radat & Swendsen 2005). The specific mechanisms underlying their associations remain to be fully understood. It is possible that there are symmetrical causal links in which one type of disorder is a risk factor for the other or that the disorders share common risk factors (Radat & Swendsen 2005; Sheftell & Atlas 2002). Recent research has begun to demonstrate some specificity in the association between types of headaches and particular mental disorders. For example, migraine increased the risk for the subsequent first onset of depression and vice versa, but preexisting depression did not predict other types of severe headache (Breslau et al. 2003). This specific bidirectional association suggests that migraine and depression may share a common etiology.

Despite a better level of understanding of the association between headache and mental disorder, research has rarely examined how the psychosocial development of an individual may relate to the subsequent unfolding of the association. While headache is common in childhood and is often the presenting symptom of depression–anxiety disorders among children (Fearon & Hotopf 2001; Powers, Gilman, & Hersey 2006), recent research has found that adverse childhood events such as abuse, poverty, and neglect may play a role in the association between headache and mental disorders among adults. For example, Tietjen et al. (2007) found that childhood sexual and physical abuse was more common in women with migraine and concomitant major depression than in those with migraine alone. After accounting for the effects of education, health status, and depression, Sumanen et al. (2007) found that patients with migraine were more likely than control subjects to have a history of long-standing financial difficulty, a family history of chronic illness, serious conflicts, and parental divorce.

Prior research on the topic, nonetheless, has the following limitations: Most of it is based on clinical samples instead of representative community samples. Being characterized by greater severity, chronicity, and/or comorbidity, clinical samples are predisposed to revealing strong associations of the conditions under study. Moreover, most previous studies have focused on depression. This is despite the robust finding that depression and anxiety disorders are usually comorbid with each other (Demyttenaere et al. 2004; Kessler et al. 1996; Scott et al. 2007). Restricting study samples to those having depression would therefore miss a large population of individuals who suffer anxiety disorders. Finally, most studies have been conducted in Western or developed countries, even though headaches, mental disorders, and childhood adversities are prevalent in developing countries as well (Demyttenaere et al. 2004; World Health Organization 2000).

By presenting the results of a large cross-national community survey that includes 10 countries of differing levels of socioeconomic development, this chapter presents the independent and joint effects of significant childhood adversities and depression–anxiety disorders before age 21 (referred to hereafter as early-onset depression–anxiety disorders) on the risk of developing adult-onset (aged 21 years or older) frequent or severe headache.

15.2. APPROACH

Cox proportional hazards models estimated risk of adult-onset headache as a function of number and type of childhood adversities and early-onset depression–anxiety disorder status while adjusting for potential confounders. A chronic physical disorder checklist of the kind commonly used in national health surveys (National Center for Health Studies 1994) examined the occurrence of frequent or severe headache during adulthood, with retrospective self-report of age of onset.

Kaplan–Meier curves were developed for graphical comparison of the age-specific cumulative proportion of respondents reporting onset of headache, comparing three categories of number of childhood adversities: none, one, and two or more adversities. Kaplan–Meier curves were also used to compare onset of headache for persons with and without early-onset depression–anxiety disorder. See Chapter 4 (4.5.5) for further description of the methods that were generic across the physical condition and pain condition outcomes included in this section.

15.3. FINDINGS

Headache in adulthood was common in the countries studied, so were childhood family adversities and early-onset depression–anxiety disorders (Table 15.1). Parental death during childhood was generally the most common form of adversity (Table 15.2).

The hazard ratio for adult-onset headache increased with increasing number of childhood adversities. Those with depression–anxiety disorders before age 21 also had higher risk of adult-onset headache, after the number of childhood family adversities was considered (Table 15.3). Female and younger respondents were found to have higher risk of adult-onset headache.

Sexual abuse, physical abuse, parental mental and substance-use disorders, criminal behavior and violence in family, and other loss of parents during childhood were significantly associated with higher risk of adult-onset headache, whereas parental death, divorce, and economic adversity during childhood were not (Table 15.4). Those who had any of the studied depression–anxiety disorders before age 21, such as panic disorder/agoraphobia, major depression episode,

Table 15.1. Basic demographics of studied countries and their proportion of adult-onset headache, any childhood adversities, and any early-onset mood/anxiety disorders

Country	Sample size (n)	Headache (%)	Any childhood family adversities (%)	Any early-onset depression–anxiety disorders (%)
Belgium	916	9.5	32.9	5.2
Colombia	1,790	17.5	64.5	9.0
France	1,172	11.9	39.8	10.0
Germany	1,150	9.9	31.2	4.6
Italy	1,502	7.5	28.8	4.2
Japan	820	5.9	34.1	2.2
Mexico	1,893	11.0	53.7	5.7
The Netherlands	945	9.9	37.5	7.2
Spain	1,817	8.4	28.5	3.7
United States	4,550	13.1	49.3	17.3
Total	16,555	11.3	43.2	9.1

generalized anxiety disorder, posttraumatic stress disorder and social phobia, had higher risk of adult-onset headache (Table 15.5).

Those with early-onset depression–anxiety disorders, especially those in early adulthood (20–40 years), had higher prevalences of adult-onset headache than those without (Figure 15.1). Similarly, respondents with more childhood family adversities were more likely to have adult onset of headache, compared with those with fewer adversities (Figure 15.2). The risk of onset was greatest in early adulthood, as more than half the adult-onset headache occurred by age 35.

15.4. DISCUSSION

The cross-sectional nature of the data limits our interpretation of the association between childhood family adversities, early-onset depression–anxiety disorders, and adult-onset headache. Given that the lifetime history of these events was ascertained by self-report and recall, the temporal ordering based on such age-of-onset data is an approximation and may be biased. Moreover, we did not assess detailed information about headache, such as its subtypes, chronicity, and frequency of attacks. Because we used a single question to elicit a history of frequent or severe headache, our findings could not be readily compared to research that focused on specific types of headaches and their etiological implications regarding the association between depression and childhood adversities (Breslau et al. 2003; Peterlin et al. 2007; Radat & Swendsen 2005).

In spite of these limitations, our findings provide cross-national support for the comorbidity of adult-onset headache, childhood family adversities, and early-onset depression–anxiety disorders. Although there is variation among participating countries, an overall developmental perspective is warranted: childhood family adversities and early-onset depression–anxiety disorders were independently associated with adult onset of frequent or severe headache. Although some researchers attribute the association between childhood adversities and later headache to depression–anxiety disorders resulting from such adversities, our study showed that these adversities were independently associated with the onset of headache. Thus, depression–anxiety disorder is not

Table 15.2. Distribution of specific family adversities in childhood by country

	Neglect (%)	Physical abuse (%)	Sexual abuse (%)	Parental death (%)	Parental divorce (%)	Other loss of parent (%)	Family economic adversity (%)	Violence in family (%)	Criminal behavior in family (%)	Parental mental disorder (%)	Parental substance-use disorder (%)
Belgium	4.81	2.98	0.90	11.88	6.62	3.35	3.39	1.59	1.99	8.49	3.18
Colombia	11.93	24.02	1.96	20.24	10.71	9.83	5.18	20.41	3.86	8.13	5.25
France	6.80	4.82	1.37	12.38	10.60	5.11	5.74	1.12	1.38	10.20	3.32
Germany	4.72	5.96	1.01	11.69	6.16	2.14	5.11	0.61	0.54	2.80	1.14
Italy	6.05	2.67	0.49	13.90	4.86	1.62	3.89	0.47	0.17	2.42	0.53
Japan	2.14	7.37	0.42	15.25	1.17	5.21	4.23	8.35	0.76	2.56	0.77
Mexico	7.83	20.19	1.60	14.05	5.36	5.47	3.23	20.45	4.23	6.71	9.71
The Netherlands	7.54	5.54	1.38	10.19	9.06	4.07	5.62	2.78	2.24	9.18	1.51
Spain	4.29	3.06	0.14	11.85	7.45	1.73	1.50	0.67	1.03	2.23	1.21
United States	5.21	7.64	5.02	10.21	15.67	6.59	9.85	13.01	6.10	9.24	8.40
Total	6.26	9.24	2.16	12.86	9.48	5.04	5.65	9.09	3.13	6.68	4.82

Table 15.3. Hazard ratios[a] showing the association between adult onset of frequent or severe headache and having one, two, or three or more childhood family adversities, adjusted for gender and age (Model A), with additional predictors: depression–anxiety disorders in previous year (Model B) and early-onset depression–anxiety disorders (Model C)

Risk factor	Model A	Model B	Model C
Number of childhood family adversities			
One	1.43 (1.24–1.64)	1.39 (1.21–1.59)	1.40 (1.22–1.60)
Two	1.47 (1.24–1.75)	1.38 (1.17–1.64)	1.41 (1.19–1.67)
Three or more	1.80 (1.52–2.13)	1.52 (1.28–1.81)	1.63 (1.37–1.95)
Depression–anxiety disorders in previous year		2.16 (1.92–2.44)	
Early-onset depression–anxiety disorder			1.64 (1.42–1.89)
Gender (female)	2.16 (1.91–2.44)	2.07 (1.83–2.44)	2.11 (1.87–2.39)
Age	0.95 (0.94–0.95)	0.95 (0.94–0.96)	0.95 (0.94–0.95)

HR (and 95% CI)

[a] Hazard ratios estimated by Cox regression proportional hazards model based on age of onset of headache. COUNTRY was entered as a stratification variable that permits the hazard functions to differ for each country. Persons with physical disorder onset prior to age 21 are excluded.

universal in adults with frequent or severe headache and a history of childhood adversities.

This association was strongest for persons with three or more adversities. Moreover, in our analysis that decomposed the association of specific childhood family adversities with headache risks, not all the adversities were found to predict increased risks. Sexual and physical abuse, parental mental and

Table 15.4. Hazard ratios[a] for the association of specific childhood adversity as independent predictor of adult-onset frequent or severe headache adjusted for age and gender.

Risk factors	Hazard ratios	95% CI
Sexual abuse	1.73***	1.38–2.17
Physical abuse	1.64***	1.44–1.88
Parental mental disorder	1.52***	1.25–1.83
Family violence	1.51***	1.30–1.76
Criminal behavior in family	1.44**	1.10–1.18
Parental substance-use disorder	1.42***	1.18–1.71
Other loss of parent during childhood	1.29*	1.06–1.58
Neglect	1.21*	1.02–1.43
Economic adversity	1.21 (ns)	0.98–1.48
Parental death	1.10 (ns)	0.93–1.31
Parental divorce	1.01 (ns)	0.84–1.22

[a] Hazard ratios estimated by one Cox regression proportional hazards model per each adversity predictor/each depression–anxiety disorder based on age of onset of headache. COUNTRY was entered as a stratification variable that permits the hazard functions to differ for each country. Persons with physical disorder onset prior to age 21 are excluded.

* $p < 0.05$.
** $p < 0.01$.
*** $p < 0.001$.

Table 15.5. Hazard ratios[a] for the association of specific early-onset depression–anxiety disorders as independent predictors of adult-onset frequent or severe headache, adjusted for age and gender, analyses stratified by country

Risk factors	Hazard ratios	95% CI
Panic/agoraphobia	1.76***	1.37–2.25
Major depressive episode	1.68***	1.40–2.03
Generalized anxiety	1.65***	1.32–2.06
Posttraumatic stress disorder	1.65**	1.19–2.30
Social phobia[b]	1.61***	1.35–1.91

[a] Hazard ratios estimated by one Cox regression proportional hazards model per each adversity predictor/each depression–anxiety disorder based on age of onset of headache. COUNTRY was entered as a stratification variable that permits the hazard functions to differ for each country. Persons with physical disorder onset prior to age 21 are excluded.

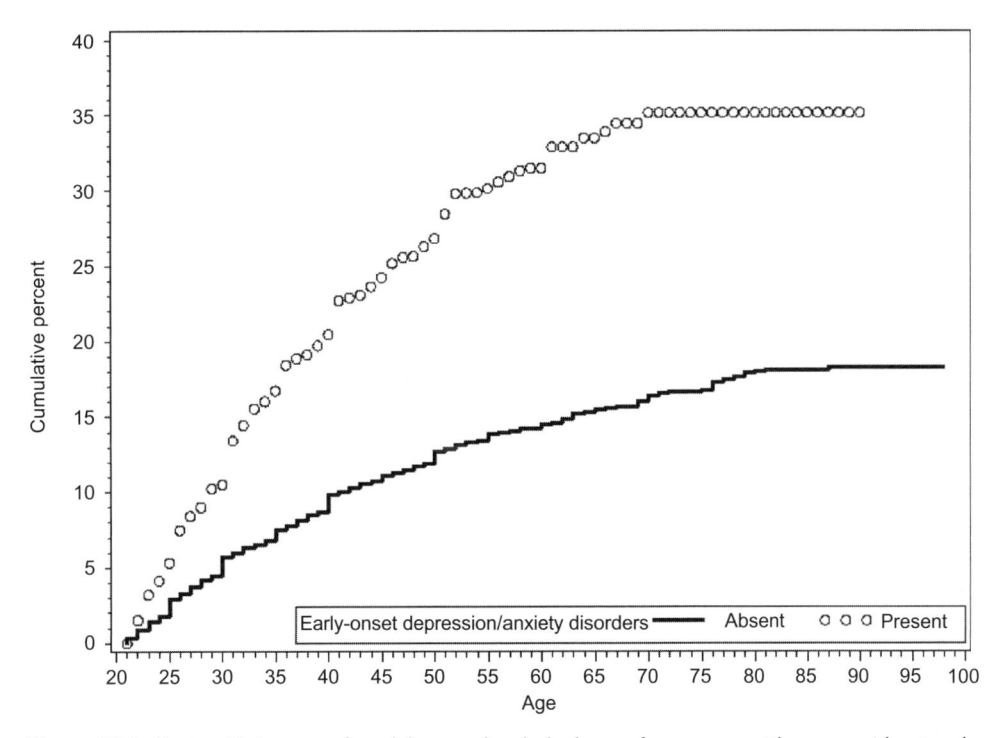

* $p < .05$.
** $p < .01$.
*** $p < .001$.

Figure 15.1. Kaplan–Meier curve for adult-onset headache by age for persons with versus without early-onset depression–anxiety disorders.

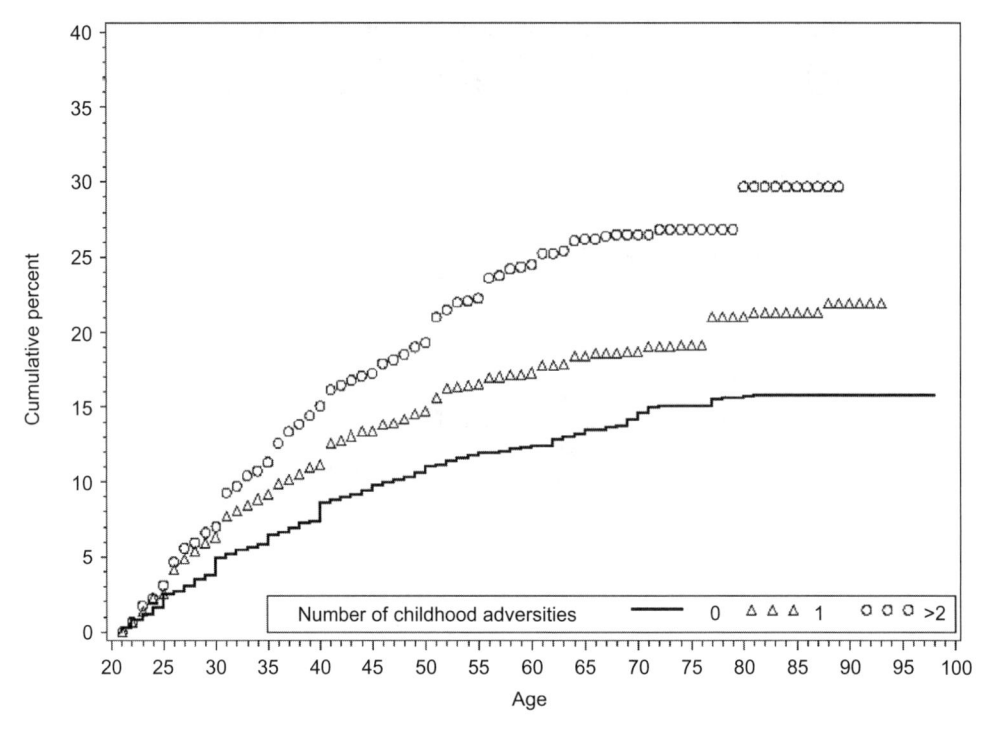

Figure 15.2. Kaplan–Meier curve for the accumulative percent with adult-onset headache by age for persons with none, one, and two or more childhood adversities.

substance-use disorders, and family antisocial behaviors showed the most robust associations with risk of adult-onset headache. Parental death, divorce, and economic adversity were not significantly related. This is different from a previous case-control study that found significant associations between migraine and parental divorce and chronic financial difficulties in the family after adjustment for education, self-reported general physical health, and depression (Sumanen et al. 2007). Differences in methodology, namely, a case-control study versus a community epidemiological study, may contribute to the different findings.

Sexual and physical abuse have been the most frequently studied childhood adversities in relation to adult-onset headache. Our study confirms the association between childhood abuse and headache found in previous research (Golding 1999; Walling et al. 1994), an association that remained significant when early-onset mental disorders were included in our analysis. This is in keeping with studies showing that headache was associated with childhood adversities after controlling for depression (Sumanen et al. 2007) and mental disorders in general (Goodwin et al. 2003).

While our analyses did not identify interaction or synergistic effects between the number of childhood adversities and the presence of early-onset depression–anxiety disorder, our results suggest that childhood adversities may predispose individuals to adult-onset headache via mechanisms in addition to DSM-IV Axis I Disorders. For example, some studies have shown that inadequate coping style and maladaptive personality factors were present among people who had experienced childhood adversities (Passchier et al. 1991; Romans et al. 2002). These difficulties in coping and personality factors may produce distress that manifests as headache. Indeed, neuroimaging studies have indicated that the brain areas activated during the distress caused by social adversities such as exclusion were also activated during physical pain (Eisenberger, Lieberman, & Willams 2003). Future studies that examine personality and brain functioning may clarify the complex mechanisms that mediate the associations we found.

In summary, we have shown in a large cross-national sample that the risk of developing frequent and/or severe headache during adulthood is independently associated with both the number of childhood adversities and the presence of early-onset depression–anxiety disorder. Although the etiology of headache remains poorly understood, a broad developmental perspective taking account of early-life risk factors for developing severe or frequent headache is needed to work out how life stressors influence risks in combination with depression–anxiety disorders. This perspective has clinical implications, in that childhood adversities should be considered in the psychosocial assessment of patients who present with frequent headache in primary health care services. Similarly, mental health professionals should be prepared to address comorbid chronic pain conditions, especially headache, when treating patients with depression–anxiety disorders and childhood adversities.

ACKNOWLEDGMENT

Some material in this chapter appeared in Lee et al. (2009). This material is reprinted with the permission of the *British Journal of Psychiatry*.

REFERENCES

Bair, M. J., Robinson, R. L., Eckert, G. J., Stang, P. E., Groghan, T. W., & Kroenke, K. (2004). Impact of pain on depression treatment response in primary care. *Psychosomatic Medicine*, **66**, 17–22.

Breslau, N., Lipton, R. B., Steward, W. F., Schultz, L. R., & Welch, K. M. (2003). Comorbidity of migraine and depression: Investigating potential etiology and prognosis. *Neurology*, **60**, 1308–12.

Demyttenaere, K., Bruffaerts, R., Posada-Villa, J., Gasquet, I., Kovess, V., Lepine, J. P., Angermeyer, M. C., Bernert, S., Girolamo, G., Morosini, P., Polidori, G., Kikkawa, T., Kawakami, N., Ono, Y., Takeshima, T., Uda, H., Karam, E. G., Fayyad, J. A., Karam, A. N., Mneimneh, Z. N., Medina-Mora, M. E., Borges, G., Lara, G., Graaf, R., Ormel, J., Gureje, O., Shen, Y., Huang, Y., Zhang, M., Alonso, J., Haro, J. M., Vilagut, G., Bromet, E. J., Gluzman, S., Webb, C., Kessler, R. C., Merikangas, K. R., Anthony, J. C., Korff, M. R. V., Wang, P. S., Alonso, J., Brugha, T. S., Aguilar-Gaxiola, S., Lee, S., Heeringa, S., Pennell, B. E., Zaslavsky, A. M., Ustun, T. B., & Chatterji, S. (2004). Prevalence, severity, and unmet need for treatment of mental disorders in the World Health Organization World Mental Health Surveys. *The Journal of the American Medical Association*, **291**, 2581–90.

Eisenberger, N. I., Lieberman, M. D., & Williams, K. D. (2003). Does rejection hurt? An FMRI study of social exclusion. *Science*, **302**, 290–2.

Fearon, P., & Hotopf, M. (2001). Relation between headache in childhood and physical and psychiatric symptoms in adulthood: National birth cohort study. *British Medical Journal*, **322**, 1–5.

Golding, J. M. (1999). Sexual assault history and headache: Five general population studies. *The Journal of Nervous and Mental Disease*, **187**, 624–9.

Goodwin, R. D., Hoven, C. W., Murison, R., & Hotopf, M. (2003). Association between childhood physical abuse and gastrointestinal disorders and migraine in adulthood. *American Journal of Public Health*, **93**, 1065–7.

Kessler, R. C., Nelson, C. B., McGonagle, K. A., Liu, J., Swartz, M., & Blazer, D. G. (1996). Comorbidity of DSM-III-R major depression disorder in the general population: Results from the US National Comorbidity Survey. *British Journal of Psychiatry*, **168**, 17–30.

Lee, S., Tsang, A., Von Korff, M., de Graaf, R., Benjet, C., Haro, J. M., Angermeyer, M., Demyttenaere, K., de Girolamo, G., Gasquet, I., Merikangas, K., Posada-Villa, J., Takeshima, T., & Kessler, R. C. (2009). Association of headache with childhood adversity and mental disorder: Cross-national study. *British Journal of Psychiatry*, **194**, 111–16.

Molgat, C. V., & Patten, S. B. (2005). Comorbidity of major depression and migraine – A Canadian population-based study. *Canadian Journal of Psychiatry*, **50**, 832–7.

National Center for Health Studies. (1994). Evaluation of National Health Interview Survey diagnostic reporting. *Vital and health statistics 2*, **120**, 1–116.

Passchier, J., Schouten, J., Van Der Donk, J., & van Romunde, L. K. (1991). The association of frequent headaches with personality and life events. *Headache*, **31**, 116–21.

Peterlin, B. L., Ward, T., Lidicker, J., & Levin, M. (2007). A retrospective, comparative study on the frequency of abuse in migraine and chronic daily headache. *Headache*, **47**, 397–401.

Powers, S. W., Gilman, D. K., & Hershey, A. D. (2006). Headache and psychological functioning in children and adolescents. *Headache: The Journal of Head and Face Pain*, **46**, 1404–15.

Radat, F., & Swendsen, J. (2005). Psychiatric comorbidity in migraine: A review. *Cephalalgia*, **25**, 165–78.

Romans, S., Belaise, C., Martin, J., Morris, E., & Raffi, A. (2002). Childhood abuse and later medical disorders in women: An epidemiological study. *Psychotherapy and Psychosomatics*, **71**, 141–50.

Scott, K. M., Bruffaerts, R., Tsang, A., Ormel, J., Alonso, J., Angermeyer, M. C., Benjet, C., Bromet, E., de Girolamo, G., de Graaf, R., Gasquet, I., Gureje, O., Haro, J. M., He, Y., Kessler, R. C., Levinson, D., Mneimneh, Z. N., Oakley Browne, M. A., Posada-Villa, J., Stein, D. J., Takeshima, T., & Von Korff, M. (2007). Depression-anxiety relationships with chronic physical conditions: Results from the World Mental Health surveys. *Journal of Affective Disorders*, **103**, 113–20.

Sheftell, F. D., & Atlas, S. J. (2002). Migraine and psychiatric comorbidity: From theory and hypothesis to clinical application. *Headache*, **42**, 934–44.

Strine, T. W., Chapman, D. P., & Balluz, L. S. (2006). Population-based U.S. study of severe headaches in adults: Psychological distress and comorbidities. *Headache*, **46**, 223–32.

Sumanen, M., Rantala, A., Sillanmaki, L. H., & Mattila, K. J. (2007). Childhood adversities experienced by working-age migraine patients. *Journal of Psychosomatic Research*, **62**, 139–43.

Tietjen, G. E., Brandes, J. L., Digre, K. B., Baggaley, S., Martin, V. T., Recober, A., Geweke, L. O., Hafeez, F., Aurora, S. K., Herial, N. A., Utley, C., & Khuder, S. A. (2007). History of childhood maltreatment is associated with comorbid depression in women with migraine. *Neurology*, **69**, 959–68.

Walling, M. K., O'Hara, M. W., Reiter, R. C., Milburn, A. K., Lily, G., & Vincent, S. D. (1994). Abuse history and chronic pain in woman. A multivariate analysis of abuse and psychological morbidity. *Obstetrics and Gynecology*, **84**, 200–6.

World Health Organization. (2000). *Headache Disorders and Public Health: Education and Management Implication*. Geneva: World Health Organization.

16 Women, Depression, and Mental–Physical Comorbidity: Chronic Pain as a Mediating Factor

OYE GUREJE AND BIBILOLA OLADEJI

16.1. INTRODUCTION

Evidence for the higher prevalence of depression in women is provided by the results of several studies (Kessler et al. 1993; Maier et al. 1999). The replication of this observation across different cultures (Weissman et al. 1996) makes it a robust epidemiological phenomenon for which different explanatory hypotheses have been suggested. Such hypotheses include those averring developmental, social, biological, or social origins (Hankin & Abramson 1999; Kessler et al. 1993; Steiner, Dunn, & Born 2003). However, since females are also at elevated risk for chronic pain as well as several chronic medical conditions (Blyth et al. 2001; Fillingim 2000; Gureje et al. 2008; Rustoen et al. 2004), which are themselves risk factors for depression (Gureje et al. 2008), it is plausible to ask whether the increased female vulnerability to depression is not mediated by their higher likelihood to experience chronic physical conditions.

Even though it is less consistently studied, there is evidence that females are also at elevated risk for anxiety disorders (Kessler, Keller, & Wittchen 2001). The association of anxiety disorders with chronic pain conditions, also much less studied, is now known to be about as strong as that between depression and chronic pain (Gureje 2007; Gureje et al. 2008). It is therefore plausible to ask the same question for anxiety disorders: Are women more likely to have these disorders because of their greater vulnerability to experience chronic physical conditions? This chapter examines these questions. Specifically, it seeks to address the following questions: (1) Can the observation of a higher prevalence of depression in women be replicated across different countries with varying socioeconomic status? (2) Can the often reported higher occurrence of chronic physical conditions in women be replicated across these countries? (3) If the higher prevalence of both depression and chronic physical conditions is consistent across countries, is there evidence that the former observation is mediated by the latter? (4) Is such a mediating role consistent across developed and developing countries?

16.2. APPROACH

This chapter reports 12-month prevalence rates of any depressive disorder (major depressive disorder or dysthymia) and any anxiety disorder (generalized anxiety disorders, panic/agoraphobia, social phobia, or posttraumatic stress disorder) among males and females in each country, in developing and developed countries, and in the total sample pooled across all countries. It also reports the 12-month rates of chronic pain and chronic medical conditions. Four chronic pain conditions as well as fifteen chronic medical conditions were inquired about. Included, among others, were questions about chronic back and neck pains, arthritis, chronic headaches,

Table 16.1. Prevalence (95% CI) of 12-month depression and any anxiety disorders among males and females

Country	Depression Females	Depression Males	Any anxiety disorder Females	Any anxiety disorder Males
Colombia	7.7 (6.7, 8.9)	4.4 (3.4, 5.7)	7.2 (5.8, 8.9)	4.5 (3.2, 6.4)
Mexico	5.4 (4.5, 6.5)	2.9 (2.0, 4.0)	5.2 (4.3, 6.3)	2.5 (1.7, 3.7)
United States	10.4 (9.5, 11.4)	6.3 (5.5, 7.3)	16.6 (15.3, 18.0)	10.3 (9.2, 11.5)
Japan	2.5 (1.7, 3.6)	2.1 (1.3, 3.5)	2.6 (1.7, 3.9)	2.7 (1.6, 4.5)
Beijing	1.7 (1.1, 2.6)	3.1 (1.8, 5.2)	2.2 (1.3, 3.7)	1.5 (0.8, 3.0)
Shanghai	2.4 (0.8, 6.4)	1.2 (0.6, 2.6)	1.8 (0.4, 7.3)	0.3 (0.1, 1.0)
New Zealand	8.3 (7.4, 9.3)	5.0 (4.1, 6.1)	12.7 (11.5, 13.9)	7.9 (6.9, 8.9)
Belgium	7.4 (5.1, 10.7)	4.7 (3.1, 7.2)	4.3 (2.8, 6.7)	3.7 (1.9, 7.0)
France	8.5 (6.7, 10.7)	4.8 (3.4, 6.9)	9.8 (7.4, 12.8)	4.2 (3.0, 5.7)
Germany	4.1 (3.1, 5.5)	2.6 (1.7, 4.1)	4.5 (3.4, 5.9)	2.1 (1.2, 3.5)
Italy	5.0 (4.1, 6.1)	2.1 (1.5, 2.9)	4.4 (3.4, 5.6)	1.8 (1.1, 2.7)
The Netherlands	7.5 (5.9, 9.6)	3.4 (2.1, 5.6)	8.2 (5.7, 11.7)	2.9 (1.7, 4.7)
Spain	6.2 (5.1, 7.6)	2.5 (1.9, 3.4)	3.5 (2.7, 4.5)	1.7 (1.0, 2.7)
Ukraine	12.7 (10.6, 15.2)	6.7 (5.2, 8.6)	9.5 (7.8, 11.6)	4.5 (2.9, 7.2)
Lebanon	7.5 (5.3, 10.5)	3.8 (2.4, 5.8)	7.3 (5.0, 10.6)	1.6 (1.0, 2.4)
Nigeria	1.0 (0.7, 1.5)	1.2 (0.8, 2.0)	0.4 (0.1, 1.1)	0.7 (0.2, 2.5)
Israel	7.4 (6.4, 8.6)	4.7 (3.9, 5.7)	5.4 (4.5, 6.4)	3.2 (2.6, 4.0)
South Africa	6.4 (5.2, 7.9)	3.0 (2.2, 4.2)	11.0 (9.5, 12.7)	5.5 (4.3, 7.0)

diabetes, heart disease, asthma, and hypertension. Logistic regression was used to assess the association of gender with the presence of mood and anxiety disorders. Unadjusted odds ratios as well as odds ratios adjusted for the presence of comorbid chronic pain and chronic medical conditions are presented.

16.3. FINDINGS

Other than Beijing and Nigeria, depression was more common among females than males in all the surveys (Table 16.1). The same was true for anxiety disorders, with Japan and Nigeria being the only 2 of the 18 sites where rates were higher in males than females. Pooled across the surveys, the data show that both depression and anxiety disorders were much more common among females than males (Table 16.2). This pattern was similar in both developed and developing countries.

We next examined the occurrence of any chronic medical disorder and any chronic

Table 16.2. Prevalence (95% CI) of 12-month depression and any anxiety disorders among males and females – developing, developed, and all countries combined

	Depression Females	Depression Males	Any anxiety disorder Females	Any anxiety disorder Males
Developing	6.1 (5.6, 6.7)	3.3 (2.9, 3.7)	6.9 (6.3, 7.5)	3.3 (2.8, 3.9)
Developed	7.8 (7.4, 8.2)	4.6 (4.2, 4.9)	9.6 (9.1, 10.2)	5.7 (5.2, 6.1)
All countries	7.2 (6.9, 7.5)	4.1 (3.8, 4.4)	8.6 (8.2, 9.0)	4.8 (4.5, 5.2)

Table 16.3. Prevalence (standard error) of any chronic medical condition and any chronic pain in the prior 12 months

Country	Any chronic medical condition Females	Any chronic medical condition Males	Any chronic pain Females	Any chronic pain Males
Developing				
Colombia	23.4 (1.7)	15.1 (1.8)	35.3 (2.2)	17.7 (1.6)
Mexico	13.4 (1.0)	9.4 (1.2)	29.2 (2.2)	18.5 (1.9)
Beijing	18.3 (2.2)	16.9 (1.5)	41.8 (3.8)	32.6 (3.2)
Shanghai	25.9 (3.3)	27.4 (3.0)	44.1 (3.9)	25.6 (3.2)
Ukraine	40.3 (2.2)	27.1 (2.4)	71.9 (2.0)	46.1 (2.5)
Lebanon	13.2 (2.3)	9.8 (1.7)	34.0 (3.4)	19.4 (3.0)
Nigeria	7.6 (1.0)	7.6 (0.9)	33.3 (2.3)	27.5 (1.7)
South Africa	25.6 (1.2)	18.9 (0.9)	56.0 (1.4)	39.4 (2.1)
Developed				
United States	32.6 (1.0)	32.4 (1.2)	49.7 (1.6)	37.3 (1.4)
Japan	25.3 (3.1)	34.4 (3.9)	30.9 (2.3)	24.7 (2.4)
New Zealand	32.3 (1.1)	30.6 (1.3)	44.2 (1.2)	33.5 (1.3)
Belgium	22.5 (2.4)	26.7 (2.5)	46.3 (3.4)	34.2 (3.2)
France	22.2 (2.1)	25.3 (2.1)	54.4 (2.7)	44.3 (3.2)
Germany	23.0 (2.4)	24.2 (2.1)	39.1 (1.8)	25.3 (2.1)
Italy	14.7 (1.6)	19.2 (1.9)	52.4 (2.3)	38.1 (2.0)
The Netherlands	23.7 (2.3)	26.7 (2.7)	40.2 (4.1)	26.0 (3.1)
Spain	17.9 (1.4)	23.1 (2.1)	44.5 (1.8)	24.8 (2.2)
Israel	27.9 (0.9)	30.5 (0.9)	39.1 (1.0)	27.4 (0.9)

pain across the surveys (Table 16.3). In all of the countries, without exception, the 12-month prevalence of chronic pain was higher among women than men. The picture was very different for the presence of chronic medical conditions. In all of the surveys conducted in developing countries, except those in Shanghai and Nigeria, women reported higher prevalence of chronic medical condition. In Shanghai, the prevalence among men was higher while in Nigeria the prevalence was the same for both sexes. On the other hand, men had higher rates of chronic medical condition in 8 of the 10 surveys in developed countries, while in the remaining two, the United States and the Netherlands, women had marginally higher rates than men. Pooled across the surveys, the data show that chronic pain was more common among females than males in both developing and developed countries. On the other hand, while chronic medical conditions were more common among females than males in developing countries, the reverse was marginally the case in developed countries (Table 16.4).

The effect of gender on the likelihood of having depression in the prior 12 months was examined next. The results are presented in the form of odds ratios for the difference between males and females in Table 16.5. In all the surveys, except those in Japan and Nigeria where no gender effect was observed, there was an almost consistent doubling of risk for depression for females compared to males. The pattern was not affected when the presence of chronic pains alone or both

Table 16.4. Prevalence (standard error) of any chronic medical condition and any chronic pain in the prior 12 months among males and females – developing, developed, and all countries combined

	Any chronic medical condition		Any chronic pain	
	Females	Males	Females	Males
Developing	21.7 (0.61)	15.9 (0.56)	45.0 (0.86)	29.6 (0.86)
Developed	27.4 (0.47)	28.8 (0.55)	44.8 (0.61)	32.4 (0.60)
All countries	25.4 (0.37)	24.2 (0.41)	44.9 (0.50)	31.4 (0.50)

chronic pains and chronic medical conditions were entered in the regression model: females were at elevated risk for depression in every instance. There was a striking similarity in the strength of this observation, as shown by the values of the odds ratios, between developing and developed countries (Table 16.6).

Even though there was some variability in the association, females also showed elevated risk for anxiety disorders in almost all the sites, the exception being Nigeria (Table 16.7). The pattern was statistically significant in 13 of the 18 surveys. Controlling for the presence of chronic pains alone or the joint effect of chronic pains and physical disorders reduced the strength of association between female gender and anxiety disorders in a few surveys, but only in

Table 16.5. Odds ratios (95% CI) for effect of female gender on presence of 12-month depression

Country	[1]Adjusted OR	[2]Adjusted OR	[3]Adjusted OR
Colombia	1.8 (1.3, 2.5)*	1.5 (1.1, 2.0)*	1.4 (1.0, 1.9)*
Mexico	1.9 (1.3, 2.7)*	1.6 (1.1, 2.3)*	1.6 (1.1, 2.3)*
United States	1.8 (1.5, 2.1)*	1.6 (1.3, 1.9)*	1.6 (1.3, 1.9)*
Japan	1.3 (0.6, 2.6)	1.4 (0.6, 2.8)	1.5 (0.7, 3.2)
Beijing	0.5 (0.3, 1.0)*	0.5 (0.2, 0.9)*	0.5 (0.2, 0.9)*
Shanghai	2.0 (0.5, 7.4)	1.2 (0.4, 3.5)	1.3 (0.4, 3.7)
New Zealand	1.7 (1.4, 2.2)*	1.6 (1.3, 2.0)*	1.6 (1.3, 2.0)*
Belgium	1.7 (0.9, 3.2)	1.5 (0.8, 3.0)	1.6 (0.8, 3.2)
France	1.9 (1.2, 2.9)*	1.8 (1.1, 2.8)*	1.8 (1.1, 2.9)*
Germany	1.7 (0.9, 3.1)	1.5 (0.9, 2.7)	1.6 (0.9, 2.8)
Italy	2.3 (1.5, 3.4)*	2.0 (1.4, 3.0)*	2.3 (1.5, 3.5)*
The Netherlands	2.4 (1.5, 3.8)*	2.1 (1.4, 3.2)*	2.2 (1.4, 3.5)*
Spain	2.6 (1.7, 3.9)*	2.1 (1.4, 3.2)*	2.3 (1.5, 3.4)*
Ukraine	1.8 (1.4, 2.5)*	1.3 (1.0, 1.9)	1.4 (1.0, 1.9)
Lebanon	2.1 (1.2, 3.4)*	1.9 (0.7, 5.5)	2.0 (0.7, 5.6)
Nigeria	0.8 (0.5, 1.6)	0.8 (0.4, 1.4)	0.8 (0.4, 1.5)
Israel	1.6 (1.3, 2.1)*	1.4 (1.1, 1.8)*	1.4 (1.1, 1.9)*
South Africa	2.1 (1.4, 3.1)*	1.8 (1.2, 2.8)*	1.8 (1.2, 2.8)*
Pooled odds ratio	1.8 (1.7, 1.9)*	1.6 (1.4, 1.7)*	1.6 (1.4, 1.7)*

Note: [1]Adjusted for age and education; [2]Adjusted for age, education, and number of pain conditions; [3]Adjusted for age, education, number of pain conditions, and number of physical conditions.
* $p < .05$.

Table 16.6. Odds ratios (95% CI) for effect of female gender on presence of 12-month depression – developing, developed, and all countries

	[1]Adjusted OR		[2]Adjusted OR		[3]Adjusted OR	
	OR	p-value	OR	p-value	OR	p-value
Developing	1.9 (1.6, 2.2)*	.0000	1.6 (1.3, 1.8)*	.0000	1.5 (1.3, 1.8)*	.0000
Developed	1.8 (1.6, 2.0)*	.0000	1.6 (1.5, 1.8)*	.0000	1.6 (1.5, 1.8)*	.0000
All countries	1.8 (1.7, 2.0)*	.0000	1.6 (1.5, 1.7)*	.0000	1.6 (1.5, 1.8)*	.0000

Note: [1]Adjusted for age and education; [2]Adjusted for age, education, and number of pain conditions; [3]Adjusted for age, education, number of pain conditions, and number of physical conditions.
* $p < .05$.

Colombia did the association thereby lose its statistical significance. In 12 of the 13 surveys, controlling for chronic pains alone or for both chronic pains and chronic medical conditions did not substantially alter the overall pattern of higher risk among females than males. The pattern of association between female gender and anxiety disorders was similar between developed and developing countries (Table 16.8).

Table 16.7. Odds ratios (95% CI) for effect of female gender on presence of 12-month anxiety disorder

Country	[1]Adjusted OR	[2]Adjusted OR	[3]Adjusted OR
Colombia	1.6 (1.1, 2.5)*	1.5 (0.9, 2.3)	1.4 (0.9, 2.2)
Mexico	2.1 (1.4, 3.3)*	1.8 (1.1, 2.8)*	1.7 (1.1, 2.7)*
United States	1.8 (1.6, 2.1)*	1.6 (1.4, 1.9)*	1.6 (1.4, 1.9)*
Japan	1.0 (0.5, 2.1)	1.0 (0.5, 2.2)	1.2 (0.5, 2.8)
Beijing	1.4 (0.5, 3.7)	1.3 (0.5, 3.6)	1.3 (0.5, 3.5)
Shanghai	6.2 (0.6, 68.1)	3.7 (0.3, 50.3)	3.4 (0.3, 41.9)
New Zealand	1.7 (1.4, 2.0)*	1.6 (1.3, 1.9)*	1.6 (1.3, 1.9)*
Belgium	1.3 (0.6, 2.8)	1.1 (0.5, 2.3)	1.1 (0.5, 2.3)
France	2.6 (1.6, 4.2)*	2.5 (1.6, 4.0)*	2.6 (1.6, 4.3)*
Germany	2.4 (1.4, 4.3)*	2.1 (1.1, 3.8)*	2.1 (1.1, 3.9)*
Italy	2.6 (1.6, 4.1)*	2.3 (1.4, 3.7)*	2.4 (1.5, 3.9)*
The Netherlands	3.1 (1.5, 6.4)*	2.7 (1.3, 5.5)*	3.3 (1.5, 6.9)*
Spain	2.2 (1.3, 3.6)*	1.8 (1.1, 2.9)*	2.0 (1.2, 3.2)*
Ukraine	2.1 (1.2, 3.7)*	1.5 (0.9, 2.6)	1.5 (0.9, 2.7)
Lebanon	5.0 (3.1, 8.0)*	10.9 (2.6, 45.2)*	10.8 (2.6, 44.5)*
Nigeria	0.5 (0.1, 2.6)	0.4 (0.1, 2.1)	0.3 (0.1, 1.9)
Israel	1.7 (1.3, 2.3)*	1.4 (1.0, 1.9)*	1.4 (1.0, 1.9)*
South Africa	2.1 (1.5, 2.8)*	1.8 (1.3, 2.4)*	1.8 (1.3, 2.4)*
Pooled odds ratio	1.9 (1.8, 2.1)*	1.7 (1.5, 1.8)*	1.7 (1.5, 1.8)*

Note: [1]Adjusted for age and education; [2]Adjusted for age, education, and number of pain conditions; [3]Adjusted for age, education, number of pain conditions, and number of physical conditions.
* $p < .05$.

Table 16.8. Odds ratios (95% CI) for effect of female gender on pressure of 12-month anxiety disorders – developing, developed, and all countries

	[1]Adjusted OR		[2]Adjusted OR		[3]Adjusted OR	
	OR	p-value	OR	p-value	OR	p-value
Developing	2.1 (1.8, 2.5)*	.0000	1.7 (1.4, 2.1)*	.0000	1.7 (1.4, 2.1)*	.0000
Developed	1.8 (1.7, 2.0)*	.0000	1.6 (1.5, 1.8)*	.0000	1.7 (1.5, 1.8)*	.0000
All countries	1.9 (1.7, 2.1)*	.0000	1.6 (1.5, 1.8)*	.0000	1.7 (1.5, 1.8)*	.0000

Note: [1]Adjusted for age and education; [2]Adjusted for age, education, and number of pain conditions; [3]Adjusted for age, education, number of pain conditions, and number of physical conditions.
* $p < .05$.

16.4. DISCUSSION

The results of the analyses presented in this chapter can be summarized thus: (1) the higher prevalence of depression and anxiety disorders among women than men is similar in developed as well as developing countries; (2) females are more likely to experience chronic pains and chronic medical conditions than are males; and (3) the higher occurrence of depression, and to a lesser extent anxiety disorders, among women was not attributable to their greater tendency to experience chronic pains or chronic medical conditions than that among men.

The observation of a higher prevalence of depression, and to a lesser extent of anxiety disorder, among women than men compliments what has been commonly reported in the literature (Demyttenaere et al. 2004; Kessler et al. 1993, 2001, 2007). The use of an identical ascertainment procedure allows us to extend this observation to developing countries where such a relationship has not been widely examined. The almost consistent pattern of the association between the disorders and female gender would suggest that the nature of the risk for women transcends cultural boundaries and probably reflects a biological vulnerability. A higher prevalence of chronic pain among females than males was also found in all the surveys, with no exception. The consistency of these observations provides a rationale for the question, "Is the higher occurrence of depression (and anxiety disorders) among women a reflection of their higher likelihood to suffer from chronic physical conditions?" Also, given that chronic pain is often comorbid with chronic medical conditions, a further consideration of the effect of chronic medical condition on the association between mood and anxiety disorders and female sex seems plausible. Previous research suggests that chronic pain is as likely to precede the occurrence of depression as depression is to precede chronic pain (Gureje, Simon, & Von Korff 2001). This bidirectional relationship makes the question about the direction of causality between pain and depression an open one. Nevertheless, the joint occurrence of chronic pain and depression more commonly among women than men could be plausibly assumed to suggest that the higher occurrence of one might be mediated by the higher vulnerability to the other. Our findings suggest that the answer to the question is negative. That is, the elevated risk of women to have depression and anxiety disorders is independent of their higher vulnerability to suffer from chronic pain and medical conditions.

The design of the World Mental Health Surveys does not permit an examination of whether chronic pains are antecedents or consequences of depression and anxiety disorders (Fishbain et al. 1997). What the findings of their higher prevalence in women suggest is that they may be more likely to co-occur in females, irrespective of the direction of causality. If depression and anxiety disorders are consequences of chronic pain, it could be that females are more likely to develop emotional disorders in reaction to pain. Some studies have found gender differences in emotional states that are associated with the experience of pain, but the findings for depression have not commonly been in the same direction as those of anxiety disorders (Bolton 1994; Edwards, Augustson, & Fillingim 2000; Keogh, McCracken, & Eccleston 2006). If pain mediates the association of depression and anxiety disorders with female gender, however, then the strength of that association should be reduced when the presence of chronic pain is controlled for. Clearly, our findings did not support such a relationship.

Could a shared mechanism or origin underlie the emergence of both mental disorders and chronic physical illness? Such a mechanism may relate to social, psychological, or biological factors. For example, the suggestion that perhaps women are at elevated risk for depression as a result of their social roles and demands may also apply to their greater tendency to experience chronic pain (Hankin & Abramson 1999; Myers, Riley, & Robinson 2003; Wiesenfeld-Hallin 2005). Likewise, if their vulnerability to depression has its origin in their unique hormonal status (Steiner et al. 2003), the same could be true of the higher prevalence of chronic physical conditions among them (Blackburn-Munro & Blackburn-Munro 2003; Wiesenfeld-Hallin 2005). In this respect, the occurrence of one is independent of the occurrence of the other, even though a shared mechanism may be at play. This possibility is supported, but not proved, by the results presented in this chapter. It is of course also possible that the mechanism by which women become more vulnerable to developing depression and anxiety disorders is independent of that which makes them to be at an elevated risk for chronic pain.

In conclusion, this chapter has presented evidence to show that the common observation of higher prevalence of depression and anxiety disorders among women is applicable across countries with diverse socioeconomic status. This risk is not mediated by their equally consistent vulnerability to experience chronic pains across these diverse settings. The possibility that these conditions have a shared origin is a plausible one. Only further research, however, can confirm or refute this.

REFERENCES

Blackburn-Munro, G., & Blackburn-Munro, R. (2003). Pain in the brain: Are hormones to blame? *Trends in Endocrinology and Metabolism*, **14**, 20–7.

Blyth, F. M., March, L. M., Nicholas, M. K., & Cousins, M. J. (2001). Chronic pain in Australia: A prevalence study. *Pain*, **89**, 127–34.

Bolton, J. E. (1994). Psychological distress and disability in back pain patients: Evidence of sex differences. *Journal of Psychosomatic Research*, **38**, 849–58.

Demyttenaere, K., Bruffaerts, R., Lee, S., Posada-Villa, J., Gasquet, I., Kovess, V., Lepine, J. P., Angermeyer, M. C., Bernet, S., de Girolamo, G., Morosini, P., Polidori, G., Kikkawa, T., Kawakami, N., Ono, Y., Takeshima, T., Uda, H., Karam, E. G., Fayyad, J. A., Karam, A. N., Mneimneh, Z. N., Medina-Mora, M. E., Borges, G., Lara, C., de Graaf, R., Ormel, J., Gureje, O., Shen, Y., Huang, Y., Zhang, M., Alonso, J., Haro, J. M., Vilagut, G., Bromet, E. J., Gluzman, S., Webb, C., Kessler, R. C., Merikangas, K. R., Anthony, J. C., Von Korff, M. R., Wang, P. S., Brugha, T. S., Aguilar-Gaxiola, S., Lee, S., Heeringa, S., Pennell, B. E., Zaslavsky, A. M., Ustun, T. B., Chatterji, S., & WHO World Mental Health Survey Consortium. (2004). Prevalence, severity, and unmet need for treatment of mental disorders in the World Health Organization

World Mental Health Surveys. *The Journal of the American Medical Association*, 291, 2581–90.

Edwards, R., Augustson, E. M., & Fillingim, R. B. (2000). Sex-specific effects of pain-related anxiety on adjustment to chronic pain. *Clinical Journal of Pain*, 16, 46–53.

Fillingim, R. B. (2000). Sex, gender, and pain: Women and men really are different. *Current Reviews of Pain*, 4, 24–30.

Fishbain, D. A., Cutler, R., Rosomoff, H. L., & Rosomoff, R. S. (1997). Chronic pain-associated depression: Antecedent or consequence of chronic pain? A review. *The Clinical Journal of Pain*, 13, 116–37.

Gureje, O. (2007). Psychiatric aspects of pain. *Current Opinion in Psychiatry*, 20, 42–6.

Gureje, O., Simon, G. E., & Von Korff, M. (2001). A cross-national study of the course of persistent pain in primary care. *Pain*, 92, 195–200.

Gureje, O., Von Korff, M., Kola, L., Demyttenaere, K., He, Y., Posada-Villa, J., Lepine, J. P., Angermeyer, M. C., Levinson, D., de Girolamo, G., Iwata, N., Karam, A., Guimaraes Borges, G. L., de Graaf, R., Browne, M. O., Stein, D. J., Haro, J. M., Bromet, E. J., Kessler, R. C., & Alonso, J. (2008). The relation between multiple pains and mental disorders: Results from the World Mental Health Surveys. *Pain*, 135, 82–91.

Hankin, B. L., & Abramson, L. Y. (1999). Development of gender differences in depression: Description and possible explanation. *Annals of Medicine*, 31, 372–9.

Keogh, E., McCracken, L. M., & Eccleston, C. (2006). Gender moderates the association between depression and disability in chronic pain patients. *European Journal of Pain*, 10, 413–22.

Kessler, R. C., Angermeyer, M., Anthony, J. C., D. E. Graaf, R., Demyttenaere, K., Gasquet, I., D. E. Girolamo, G., Gluzman, S., Gureje, O., Haro, J. M., Kawakami, N., Karam, A., Levinson, D., Medina Mora, M. E., Oakley Browne, M. A., Posada-Villa, J., Stein, D. J., Adley Tsang, C. H., Aguilar-Gaxiola, S., Alonso, J., Lee, S., Heeringa, S., Pennell, B. E., Berglund, P., Gruber, M. J., Petukhova, M., Chatterji, S., & Üstün T. B. (2007). Lifetime prevalence and age-of-onset distributions of mental disorders in the World Health Organization's World Mental Health Survey Initiative. *World Psychiatry*, 6, 168–76.

Kessler, R. C., Keller, M. B., & Wittchen, H. U. (2001). The epidemiology of generalized anxiety disorder. *Psychiatric Clinics of North America*, 24, 19–39.

Kessler, R. C., McGonagle, K. A., Swartz, M., Blazer, D. G., & Nelson, C. B. (1993). Sex and depression in the National Comorbidity Survey I. Lifetime prevalence, chronicity and recurrence. *Journal of Affective Disorders*, 2, 85–96.

Maier, W., Gansike, M., Gater, R., Rezaki, M., Tiemens, B., & Urzúa, R. F. (1999). Gender differences in the prevalence of depression: A survey in primary care. *Journal of Affective Disorders*, 53, 241–52.

Myers, C. D., Riley, J. L., & Robinson, M. E. (2003). Psychosocial contributions to sex-correlated differences in pain. *Clinical Journal of Pain*, 19, 225–32.

Rustoen, T., Wahl, A. K., Hanestad, B. R., Lerdal, A., Paul, S., & Miaskowski, C. (2004). Gender differences in chronic pain – Findings from a population-based study of Norwegian adults. *Pain Management Nursing*, 5, 105–17.

Steiner, M., Dunn, E., & Born, L. (2003). Hormones and mood: From menarche to menopause and beyond. *Journal of Affective Disorders*, 74, 67–83.

Weissman, M. M., Bland, R. C., Canino, G. J., Faravelli, C., Greenwald, S., Hwu, H. G., Joyce, P. R., Karam, E. G., Lee, C. K., Lellouch, J., Lépine, J. P., Newman, S. C., Rubio-Stipec, M., Wells, J. E., Wickramaratne, P. J., Wittchen, H., & Yeh, E. K. (1996). Cross-national epidemiology of major depression and bipolar disorder. *The Journal of the American Medical Association*, 276, 293–9.

Wiesenfeld-Hallin, Z. (2005). Sex differences in pain perception. *Gender Medicine*, 2, 137–45.

PART THREE

Consequences of Mental–Physical Comorbidity

17 Understanding Consequences of Mental–Physical Comorbidity

MICHAEL R. VON KORFF

17.1. INTRODUCTION

For chronic disease, there is greater continuity between factors that cause disease and those that influence outcomes than often acknowledged. For example, behavioral risk factors such as tobacco use, sedentary lifestyle, and obesity not only increase risks of developing diverse chronic diseases, but influence outcomes as well. Similarly, the presence of multiple indicators of the metabolic syndrome – such as high triglycerides, high low-density lipoprotein levels, elevated blood pressure, and elevated fasting glucose levels – not only affect risks of developing cardiovascular disease and diabetes, but also influence disease outcomes subsequent to onset. The preceding chapters presented results showing that early-onset depression and anxiety disorders may influence risks of onset of chronic physical conditions. The following chapters present compelling data showing that depression and anxiety disorders, also referred to as internalizing psychological disorders (Goldberg & Goodyer 2005) or as emotional disorders, also influence disease outcomes after onset, particularly in the case of functional disability.

Broad-spectrum risk factors refer to common causes of multiple disorders whose effects are realized across the developmental stages of those disorders, including onset, duration, recurrence, and adaptation to disease. Depression and anxiety disorders appear to meet this definition of a broad-spectrum risk factor for chronic physical disease. They are associated with increased risks of onset of diverse chronic physical conditions and with increased risks of adverse outcomes subsequent to onset.

Early-onset emotional disorders may increase risks of physical disease through their influence on health risk behaviors including tobacco use, sedentary lifestyle, unhealthful dietary patterns, and abuse of alcohol and drugs. Subsequent to disease onset, internalizing psychological disorders may impair abilities to change these harmful health behaviors, thereby increasing risks of a poor outcome. A second pathway through which early-onset emotional disorders may increase risks of onset of physical disease is through dysregulation of homeostatic processes in cardiovascular, metabolic, neuroendocrine, immune, and autonomic nervous systems (McEwen 1998). Subsequent to onset, the role of depression and anxiety disorders in dysregulation of homeostatic processes complicates achieving adequate disease control. A third pathway through which emotional disorders influence chronic disease outcomes is through their deleterious effects on chronic disease self-management, increasing risks of unfavorable physiologic and functional outcomes.

Living with a chronic disease taxes an individual's adaptive capacities. Key tasks in managing chronic illness include the following: (1) engaging in activities that promote health, sustain and build physiologic reserve, and prevent adverse sequelae; (2) adhering to medical regimens and changing health behaviors; (3) working with health care providers to develop and modify treatment plans; (4) monitoring health status and adapting to observed changes; and (5) managing the impacts of illness on one's ability to function in key life roles in work, family, and social life (Clark et al. 1991; Lorig 1993; Von Korff et al. 1997; Wagner, Austin, & Von Korff 1996). Depression and anxiety make each of these tasks in managing chronic illness more difficult and less likely to be carried out successfully. People who are depressed or anxious are less able to engage fully in life activities in work, family, and social and self-care spheres. Emotional disorders rob people of their motivation, energy, and self-confidence. Depression and anxiety undermine the ability to work effectively with others and sustain effort in the face of adversities. Pain and other physical symptoms tend to be more severe and debilitating among persons who are psychologically distressed, whether the physical symptoms are "medically explained" or not. For these reasons, when depression and anxiety co-occur with a chronic physical condition, the negative effects of both physical and psychological illness are magnified. Despite the central importance of emotional disorders in undermining self-management of chronic physical disease, many patients and physicians believe that functional disability is largely explained by physical impairments due to disease or injury. The results presented in this section provide compelling evidence that psychological and physical impairments influence disability outcomes in tandem.

This chapter reviews prior research concerning mechanisms through which psychological impairments influence disease outcomes including effects on symptom burden, self-regulation of illness, functional disability, health care use, and physiological outcomes of disease, including mortality. A key idea is that depression and anxiety have deleterious effects on the physiologic, emotional, cognitive, and behavioral functioning of persons with well-defined chronic physical diseases such as diabetes and heart disease, not only outcomes of persons with symptomatic conditions such as back pain and headache. This chapter provides context for understanding how it is possible for depression and anxiety to influence the symptom burden, self-regulation of illness, functional disability, health care use, and physiological outcomes of chronic physical conditions.

17.2. SYMPTOM BURDEN

The association of psychological distress with physical symptoms has been explained by three related but conceptually distinct phenomena: (1) patients whose physical symptoms are due to excessive bodily preoccupation and illness worry; (2) patients with medically unexplained symptoms and functional somatic syndromes (e.g., irritable bowel, chronic fatigue, and chronic idiopathic pain); and (3) patients with physical symptoms that are secondary to an underlying mood or anxiety disorder (Kirmayer & Sartorius 2007). Some hold that medically unexplained symptoms due to illness worry, psychosomatic syndromes, and underlying psychological disorder are strongly influenced by culture-specific ways of understanding the body, interpreting symptoms, and expressing distress (Kirmayer & Young 1998). A contrasting view is that the association of depression and anxiety disorders with nonspecific physical symptoms is universal across cultures, but that cultural differences in norms regarding presentation of physical versus psychological illness influence what kinds of symptoms patients bring to the attention of physicians (Escobar & Gureje 2007; Simon et al. 1999). There is now a large body of epidemiological, clinical, and experimental research that sheds light on these relationships.

Although it has been known for decades that pain and depression are associated in clinical populations (Bair et al. 2003; Romano & Turner 1985), extensive data from representative population samples now show that chronic pain is more common among persons with both depression and anxiety disorders and that this phenomenon is observed across diverse countries and cultures (Gureje 2007; Verhaak et al. 1998). In the past, the relationship of psychological impairment and chronic pain was explained in terms of diverse forms of psychosomatic illness such as a pain-prone disorder (Blumer & Heilbronn 1982), psychogenic pain (Haber, Kuczmierczyk, & Adams 1985), masked depression (Lesse 1983), and a chronic pain syndrome (Addison 1984). However, the association of pain and other unpleasant physical symptoms with depression and anxiety is not limited to psychosomatic illness. Kisely and Simon (2006), reporting data from a cross-national study of primary care patients, found that medically explained and medically unexplained physical symptoms were both associated with psychiatric morbidity and functional disability. They found little difference in disability outcomes at follow-up between persons with medically explained versus medically unexplained symptoms. Ludman et al. (2004) found, in a large sample of persons with clinically confirmed diabetes, that depression was a stronger predictor of number of diabetes symptoms than glycemic control or diabetes complications. Similarly, Richardson et al. (2006) found that among young persons with asthma, those with a depression or anxiety disorder reported more asthma symptoms than those without psychological impairment after controlling for objective measures of asthma severity and medical comorbidity. In a study of burn patients, Loncar, Bras, and Mickovic (2006) found that higher levels of anxiety and depression were associated with higher pain ratings and that percent of body surface burned was associated with both psychological distress and pain ratings. Thus, psychological distress appears to be associated with dysphoric physical symptoms in general, not only "medically unexplained" physical symptoms.

Experimental research has shown that cognitive–behavioral therapy and (possibly) antidepressant medications are effective in reducing physical symptoms among persons with diffuse, ill-defined physical symptoms (Kroenke 2007; Sumathilpala 2007). However, experimental research has also shown that depression treatment can reduce physical pain and other somatic symptoms among persons with well-defined medical disorders. Lin et al. (2003) found that enhanced depression treatment among depressed elders with arthritis reduced arthritis pain relative to control patients who did not receive enhanced depression treatment. Similarly, Mohr, Hart, and Vella (2007) reported that cognitive–behavioral treatment of depression among persons with multiple sclerosis reduced fatigue and improved functional outcomes relative to a control treatment.

These results are supported by longitudinal and prospective observational studies. Several systematic reviews have concluded that depression and anxiety predict increased risks of pain running a chronic course (Hasenbring, Hallner, & Klasen 2001; Mallen et al. 2007b). Prospective studies have also found that psychological distress is associated with increased risks of onset of physical pain problems (Linton 2000). Three recent randomized controlled trials of depression treatment have yielded findings with provocative implications for the role of severe pain in influencing depression outcomes. Thielke et al. (2007),

Kroenke et al. (2008), and Mavandadi et al. (2007) each found that the presence of moderate-to-severe pain interference blunted the effectiveness of evidence-based depression treatment for improving depression outcomes. In each of these three randomized trials, intervention versus control differences in depression outcomes were significantly less for persons with severe pain at baseline than for persons with lower levels of pain dysfunction at baseline. These results suggest that chronic pain is a risk factor for treatment-resistant depression, which is entirely consistent with research finding that depression is a risk factor for pain running a chronic course. Thus, the relationships between pain and internalizing psychological disorders are likely reciprocal, each having a negative influence on the other.

Taken together, these findings support Barsky's concept of somatosensory amplification (Barsky 1979; Barsky et al. 1988) in which psychological distress amplifies physical symptoms in general, whether medically explained or not. The idea that ill-defined physical symptoms are typically a manifestation of an underlying masked psychological illness needs to be reconsidered. In its stead, an integrated understanding of the dynamic interplay between symptoms attributed to physical origins (e.g., bodily pain) and those attributed to psychological origins (e.g., depression and anxiety) is needed. Both physical and psychological symptoms have an underlying physical substrate and both are amplified or reduced by central neurophysiologic and psychological processes modulating symptom perception. Unpleasant physical symptoms and psychological distress appear to have reciprocating effects that increase risks of both physical and psychological symptoms being amplified and becoming chronic. A shift in focus is needed to understand underlying mechanisms modulating both physical and psychological symptoms (Von Korff & Simon 1996a), rather than identifying specific physical or psychological causes of symptoms.

Positing mechanisms that modulate "physical" and "psychological" symptoms alike is consistent with the observation that patients who are depressed or anxious often present to medical care with chronic pain or multisymptom somatic syndromes (e.g., chronic fatigue syndrome). Such mechanisms are also consistent with the prevalence of depression and anxiety disorders being high among patients with multisymptom somatic syndromes. It should not be surprising that there is considerable overlap between mood and anxiety disorders on the one hand, defined by the presence of multiple psychological and somatic symptoms, and somatic syndromes on the other, defined by the presence of multiple physical and psychological symptoms.

17.3. CHRONIC ILLNESS SELF-REGULATION

From the perspective of many physicians, the central task in managing a chronic disease, such as diabetes, is to carry out treatment regimens to control key disease parameters (e.g., maintaining glycemic control and blood pressure at optimal levels). From the patients' perspective, managing symptoms and engagement in valued life activities may seem more important than disease management per se. The self-regulatory model (Leventhal, Meyer, & Nerenz 1980) holds that cognitive representations of illness influence how patients cope with illness experiences (e.g., symptom burden and functional limitations). Self-regulation of illness is goal oriented, problem-solving behavior directed at return to health or minimizing adverse consequences of illness (Carver & Scheier 1998). Cognitive representations of illness concern its identify (e.g., diagnosis), what is causing the illness, potential consequences of the illness, the timeline or course the illness is expected to take, and how the illness can be managed or cured. Kleinman's (1988) cross-cultural explanatory model of illness identifies similar categories for the commonsense understanding of illness by patients. The self-regulatory model posits three stages in managing chronic illness: *interpretation* of symptoms to arrive at an understanding of the problem; *coping*, in which an ameliorative plan of action is developed and executed; and *appraisal*, in which the success of the coping strategy is considered and revisions made based on experience gained.

The role of symptom interpretation and appraisal in chronic illness has been studied most extensively for chronic pain. For chronic pain, two coping styles have been extensively studied and found to be associated with adverse outcomes: catastrophizing (Keefe et al. 2004) and fear-avoidance (Vlaeyen & Linton 2000). Catastrophizing is a constellation of cognitive and emotional responses characterized by feelings of helplessness, magnification of the severity of pain symptoms, and a pessimistic orientation to the likely consequences of pain (Edwards et al. 2006). Catastrophizing has been observed in idiopathic chronic pain conditions (Proctor, Gatchel, & Robinson 2000), in rheumatologic disorders, including arthritis and fibromyalgia (Edwards et al. 2006), and in cancer pain (Zaza & Baine 2002). Catastrophizing is associated with affective distress and depression, but associations with disability and pain severity are not fully explained by depression (Edwards et al. 2006). A systematic review found evidence that psychological distress, depression, and somatization predict risks of transition from acute to chronic back pain, with weaker support for the prognostic significance of catastrophizing after controlling for depression (Pincus et al. 2002).

Research concerning the fear-avoidance model yields a similar picture. Fear-avoidance is characterized by avoidance of behaviors that might increase pain and by attribution of pain to an underlying condition that could be harmed by movement, lifting, or exercise (Vlaeyen & Linton 2000). Fear-avoidance is correlated with pain severity, pain-related disability, and affective distress (Leeuw et al. 2007). Prospective studies of patients with acute back pain suggest that affective distress is a better predictor of risks of transition to chronic pain than are measures of fear-avoidance beliefs, although fear-avoidance may be associated with less favorable prognosis among persons with persistent back pain (Pincus et al. 2006). While catastrophizing and fear-avoidance have been most extensively studied for chronic pain conditions, these coping styles have also been identified in patients with other chronic diseases including asthma, diabetes, and heart disease (Olson et al. 1993; van Ittersum et al. 2003; Zvolensky et al. 2003).

Catastrophizing and fear-avoidance are conceptually related to important features of internalizing psychological disorders (e.g., helplessness, pessimistic outlook, avoidance, and symptom amplification). There is considerable evidence that catastrophizing and fear-avoidance are associated with psychological distress. Despite these links, there is confusion about how to integrate research concerning the role of catastrophizing and fear-avoidance with that concerning the role of depression and anxiety in determining illness outcomes. Catastrophizing and fear-avoidance define specific psychological mechanisms through which depressed mood and anxiety symptoms may influence coping with chronic illness. In clarifying the extent to which depression and anxiety influence chronic disease outcomes versus specific modes of interpreting and responding to symptoms, it would be helpful if specific effects of catastrophizing and fear-avoidance above and beyond those attributable to general effects of psychological distress were evaluated.

While the self-regulatory model has been applied most frequently to symptom interpretation and response, it is also relevant to broader aspects of chronic illness self-management. As noted earlier, goal-directed behaviors that are part of chronic illness self-management include engaging in activities that promote health, sustain and build physiologic reserve, and prevent adverse sequelae; adhering to medical regimens and changing health behaviors; working with health care providers to develop and modify treatment plans; monitoring health status and adapting to observed changes; and managing the impact of illness on one's ability to function in key life roles in work, family, and social life (Clark et al. 1991; Lorig 1993; Von Korff et al. 1997; Wagner et al. 1996). Psychological distress has deleterious effects on each of these broader domains of chronic illness self-management. DiMatteo, Lepper, and Croghan (2000), in a meta-analysis of noncompliance with medical treatments, found that depressed patients were three times as likely to be noncompliant with treatment recommendations compared to nondepressed patients. In a systematic review of medication adherence among persons with diabetes, Odegard and Capoccia (2007) found that depression predicted increased noncompliance with medical regimens. The self-regulatory model is also relevant to understanding the effects of depression and anxiety on functional disability outcomes among persons with chronic physical conditions.

17.4. FUNCTIONAL DISABILITY

The triad of impairment, disability, and participation articulated in the International Classification of Functioning, Disability and Health (ICF) (World Health Organization 2001) provides a framework for understanding how psychological impairments influence functional disability. "Impairment" is defined as a health-related loss or abnormality of psychological, physiological, or anatomical structure or function, including psychological illness and pain. "Disability" is defined as a health-related restriction or lack of ability to perform an activity, within the range considered normal. "Participation" is the extent of involvement in meaningful and rewarding life activities.

Early research on disability, largely in geriatric populations, focused on activities of daily living, such as self-care and mobility inside the home, and instrumental activities of daily living, such as household maintenance and mobility outside the home (Katz & Akpom 1976; Pope & Tarlov 1991). Subsequently, as researchers began to consider the nature and determinants of disability in nongeriatric populations, disability concepts expanded to encompass broader domains of functioning. Wiersma, DeJong, and Ormel (1988) advanced the idea that disability should be defined in terms of performance of key social roles including self-care, occupational, partner, and household maintenance roles. Disability measures that assessed both activities of daily living and broader aspects of social role functioning were developed, including the Medical Outcomes Survey SF-36 (Ware et al. 1995), the Sickness Impact Profile (Bergner et al. 1981), the Arthritis Impact Measurement Scale (Mason, Anderson, & Meenan 1988), the Dartmouth Co-op Charts (Nelson et al., 1987), the Groningen Social Disabilities Schedule (Wiersma et al. 1988), and others. Research using such measures found consistent relationships between internalizing psychological impairments and disability (Berkman et al. 1986; Broadhead et al. 1990; Dohrenwend et al. 1983; Turner & Noh 1988; Wohlfarth et al. 1993), both for activities of daily living and for broader domains of social role function. The association of psychological illness with functional disability was subsequently shown to be present among medical patients in many different cultures in both developed and developing countries (Ormel et al. 1994; Von Korff et al. 1996b).

Physical disease impairs physical abilities including respiratory capacity, muscle strength, fine and gross motor coordination, vision, and hearing. But resilience in social role performance in the face of severe physical impairments is not unusual. In contrast, psychological illness impairs the highest-order human capacities central to social role performance. Impairments resulting from psychological illness include loss of motivation and energy, reduced ability to engage in planned action, loss of self-confidence, avoidance of important activities due to unfounded fears, greater difficulties in working harmoniously with others, and reduced abilities to sustain effort toward achieving goals when difficulties and frustrations arise. Thus, it is understandable that psychological impairments are at least as disabling as physical impairments (Von Korff 1999; Von Korff et al. 1992), because depression and anxiety undermine problem-solving abilities that are central to chronic illness self-regulation.

In seminal work on psychological disorders and disability, Wells, Golding, and Burnman (1988) reported that persons with psychological disorder reported more physical limitations and activity restrictions than persons without psychological illness, after controlling for chronic disease status (Wells et al. 1988), and that depressed persons showed poorer functioning than patients with major chronic physical diseases (Wells et al. 1989). Subsequent prospective studies found that internalizing psychological disorders are a risk factor for the onset of functional disability (Armenian et al. 1998; Bruce et al. 1994; Manninen et al. 1997; Ormel et al. 1999; Pennix et al. 1998). Longitudinal studies among persons with significant medical conditions have also shown that disability is reduced over time among patients whose psychological illness improves, whereas disability does not improve among persons whose depression runs a chronic course (Ormel et al. 1993; Von Korff et al. 1992). These cross-sectional, prospective, and longitudinal studies support the hypothesis that psychological impairments amplify functional disability among persons with chronic physical disease.

A second line of research also supports the hypothesis that psychological impairments play a causal role in functional disability. There is now substantial evidence that psychological disorder has a substantial influence on disability among persons with specific chronic physical diseases after accounting for condition-specific objective measures of physical impairment. Sullivan et al. (1997) found that depression and anxiety were important prognostic factors for disability outcomes among persons with coronary artery disease, whereas the number of vessels with stenosis, as assessed by angiography, did not predict functional outcomes at 1 year. These findings were subsequently found to hold over a 5-year follow-up (Sullivan et al. 2000). Mallen et al. (2007a) reported that among older adults with knee pain, anxiety predicted poor functional outcomes at 18 months after controlling for radiographic findings. Creamer, Lethbridge-Cejku, and Hochberg (2000) found that anxiety was associated with functional disability among patients with knee osteoarthritis, while radiographic findings were not. In a study of persons with chronic obstructive pulmonary disease (COPD), Peruzza et al. (2003) found that reduced respiratory capacity was the strongest predictor of deterioration in functional status, but that depression was an independent predictor of quality of life after controlling for respiratory capacity. Ng et al. (2007) found that depressive symptoms among COPD patients were associated with less favorable functional outcomes at 1 year after controlling for measures of disease severity at baseline. Von Korff et al. (2005b) found that depression was a stronger predictor of functional disability among persons with diabetes than was the number of diabetes complications, glycemic control, or the extent of chronic disease comorbidity. Among working-age adults, it was also found that depression was the strongest predictor of being unable to work, missing more than 5 days from work in the prior month, and reporting severe difficulties with work tasks after accounting for measures of glycemic control, complications, and chronic disease comorbidity (Von Korff et al. 2005a). Simon, Von Korff, and Lin (2005) reported that depressed patients with diabetes, COPD, and ischemic heart disease showed significant improvements in depressive symptoms and functional disability subsequent to initiation of depression treatment, suggesting that disability is influenced by depression among persons with progressive chronic physical diseases.

Experimental research also supports the hypothesis that psychological impairments play a causal role in determining functional disability, although results have been inconsistent, depending on the population, intervention, and disability measure. Coulehan et al. (1997) found that patients who received active treatment for depression experienced more favorable disability outcomes than did control patients who received care as usual. In contrast, Simon et al. (1998) in a less severely depressed population in which usual care patients were often adequately treated found that a collaborative care program for depression produced more favorable outcomes than did usual care for depression and somatic distress, but not for disability outcomes. Lin et al. (2000) found that patients whose depression was treated with a collaborative care program reported that illness interfered less with work, family, and social activities, and a trend toward greater improvement in social functioning, but no difference in the SF-36 role function subscale. Among patients at high risk of depression relapse who received maintenance pharmacotherapy, intervention patients had greater improvement in SF-36 social functioning at 1 year and a nonsignificant trend toward greater improvement in ratings of interference in work, family, and social functioning (Von Korff et al. 2003).

Telephone case management for depressive illness improved both symptom and disability outcomes over a 1-year follow-up period (Katzelnick et al. 2000). Wells et al. (2000) found that employed depressed patients who were cared for at clinics randomly assigned to participate in a depression quality improvement program were more likely to sustain employment at 1 year than were control patients from usual care clinics. Among depressed patients with arthritis, intervention patients reported more favorable outcomes for arthritis pain and reduced interference with activities due to pain than did control patients with arthritis who received care as usual (Lin et al. 2003). Depressed employees who received enhanced depression treatment showed significantly greater job retention and significantly more hours worked over a 1-year follow-up period relative to control patients who did not receive the case management program (Wang et al. 2007).

In a trial of telephone-administered cognitive–behavioral therapy for depressed persons with multiple sclerosis, Mohr et al. (2007) found that depression treatment relative to a control treatment resulted in significantly greater reductions in functional disability and fatigue. Endicott et al. (2007) reported results from three independent randomized controlled trials of pharmacotherapy for generalized anxiety disorder that showed that intervention patients achieved greater improvements in social role functioning than did control patients. Roy-Bryne et al. (2005) found, in a multicenter trial, that a combined pharmacotherapy and cognitive–behavioral intervention for panic disorder increased panic disorder remission rates and also yielded significantly greater improvements on multiple disability outcome measures relative to patients receiving usual care. Although the results vary across trials, taken together, there is now considerable evidence that enhanced treatment of depressive and anxiety disorders improves disability outcomes and that psychological impairments amplify functional disability. In light of the self-regulatory model, this makes sense because reducing depression and anxiety enhances the abilities of patients to solve problems and carry out goal-directed behaviors required to effectively manage the deleterious effects of chronic illness.

17.5. HEALTH CARE USE

Research over the last two decades has conclusively established that depression and anxiety disorders are associated with health care utilization and costs that are at least 50% higher than those for persons without psychological illness, after adjusting for the effects of comorbid physical conditions on health care use (Katon et al. 2003; Koopmans & Lamars 2006; Simon et al. 1995a; Simon, Von Korff, & Barlow 1995a; Unutzer et al. 1997). These studies have also established that increased health care utilization and costs among persons with depression and anxiety disorders are not explained by treatment of psychological disorder. Studies of health care use by patients with symptomatic conditions have shed light on the nature of health care use by persons who are psychologically distressed. Many studies have shown that most of the health care utilization and costs utilized by persons with symptomatic conditions are not explained by their index condition and that increased utilization is sustained over extended time periods (Engel, Von Korff, & Katon 2004; Levy et al. 2001; Turner et al. 2004; Von Korff et al. 2007). Von Korff et al. (2007) found that the increased utilization of health care among patients with back pain, headache, and orofacial pain was due to increased use of health care for a broad range of conditions including well-defined and ill-defined medical conditions and mental health problems, whereas no differences in preventive care were observed. Engel et al. (2004) reported that back pain patients with elevated depression had higher health care costs overall, but did not have higher costs for back pain care specifically. Thus, it is likely that increased health care use by persons with psychological illness is at least partially explained by their more severe and diffuse health problems, including both symptomatic conditions and chronic physical diseases.

Randomized trials of depression treatment have generally not found significant reductions in health care utilization or costs (Araya et al. 2006; Simon et al. 2001a, 2001b; Von Korff et al. 1998). It remains unclear why depression treatment does not reduce health care utilization and costs given the strong association of depression with health care use. Even so, since increased costs of depression treatment are typically modest and time limited, economic evaluations have generally concluded that improved depression treatment is cost-effective. Two recent cost-effectiveness studies of depression treatment among persons with diabetes have noted nonsignificant trends toward reduced health care costs in the year after the intervention program was completed (Katon et al. 2006; Simon et al. 2007). In a structured review of randomized trials assessing effects of interventions for somatoform disorders on health care utilization or costs, Kroenke (2007) observed that 10 of 11 trials reporting relevant results found reductions in either health care use or costs. Since the interventions tested and study populations were very heterogeneous, however, it is not clear what specific mechanisms accounted for reductions in health care utilization and costs. Interventions that resulted in reduced use of services included (1) a letter sent from a consulting psychiatrist to the primary care physician, suggesting more conservative care; (2) physician training in managing somatoform disorders; and (3) multisession cognitive–behavioral therapy.

These results suggest that altering health care utilization may be more responsive to behavioral interventions that target health care use specifically than to psychological interventions that reduce psychological symptoms. Given the substantial health care utilization and costs among persons who are psychologically distressed, and the questionable medical value of some of the services rendered, there is a need for further research to shed light on what kinds of services, and for what conditions, depressed and anxious patients seek care and how the frequency of providing services of low medical value to these patients might be reduced.

17.6. PHYSIOLOGICAL OUTCOMES AND MORTALITY

There is a large body of evidence that internalizing psychological disorders are associated with less favorable physiological outcomes of diverse chronic diseases. Depression is associated with poor glycemic control among persons with diabetes (Katon et al. 2004a; Lustman & Clouse 2005; Selby et al. 2007). Inadequate blood pressure control (Scalco et al. 2005) and increased rates of cardiovascular events (Smoller et al. 2007) are also associated with depression and anxiety among persons with cardiovascular disease. Reasons offered for poor chronic disease control among psychologically distressed patients include poor treatment adherence and physiologic mechanisms that undermine disease control. Research also shows that depression and anxiety disorders are associated with increased mortality among persons with diverse chronic physical diseases after controlling for behavioral risk factors, chronic disease severity, and chronic disease comorbidity (Ang et al. 2005; Everson et al. 1998; Gallo et al. 2005; Katon et al. 2005; Kinder et al. 2008; Szekely et al. 2007; Unutzer et al. 2002).

Unfortunately, the most recent large-scale trials of depression treatment among persons with diabetes and heart disease have not shown beneficial effects on disease control or events (Berkman et al. 2003; Glassman et al. 2002; Katon et al. 2004b; Williams et al. 2004). A recent randomized controlled trial of enhanced depression treatment did find reduced mortality among depressed persons with diabetes who received enhanced care relative to that among control patients (Bogner et al. 2007). This result is difficult to explain, however, in light of modest treatment effects on depressive symptoms and the absence of evidence that depression treatment improved disease control. Given that effects of depression and anxiety on key physiologic parameters such as blood pressure and glycemic control are likely to be accrued over extended periods of time, it may be unrealistic to expect that short-term treatment of a depressive or anxiety disorder will, by itself, produce significant improvements in disease control, reduced rates of cardiovascular disease events, or reduced mortality. It is possible that improved disease outcomes may require reductions in depression and anxiety that are sustained over longer periods of time, accompanied by changes in health risk behaviors and adherence to treatment regimens that are also sustained over time. In light of substantial evidence that depression and anxiety disorders are associated with less favorable disease outcomes, including mortality, we need to better understand the complex mechanisms through which these adverse effects are realized and how they might be reversed.

17.7. SYNTHESIS

There is now compelling evidence that depression and anxiety play an important role in influencing important outcomes of diverse chronic physical conditions including symptom burden; effectiveness of chronic illness self-management and adherence to medical treatments; severity and duration of functional disability; and key disease outcomes (e.g., glycemic control and blood pressure), rates of cardiovascular disease events, and mortality. There is strong evidence that treatment of depression and anxiety disorders can have significant benefits in reducing functional disability among persons with comorbid chronic physical disorders. There is also evidence that psychological treatments can have beneficial effects on symptom burden for well-defined physical diseases as well as for ill-defined symptom disorders. The traditional emphasis on the role of depression and anxiety in the experience and reporting of medically unexplained, psychosomatic symptoms appears to be too narrow. Rather, the evidence suggests that depression and anxiety play a central role in determining physiologic, symptomatic, and behavioral outcomes of all chronic conditions, including conditions that are medically well defined as well as conditions that are medically ill defined.

Early-onset depression and anxiety disorders may increase risks of developing diverse chronic physical conditions. The evidence reviewed here shows that depression and anxiety disorders also influence diverse features of adaptation to and management of chronic disease. This supports viewing these psychological disorders as broad-spectrum risk factors. The evidence is consistent with a reciprocal causation model, similar to those posited by Evans et al. (2005) and by Piette, Richardson, and Valenstein (2004), in which psychological illness influences physical disease status and vice versa. However, a reciprocal causation model should not be reified to mean only that psychological disease causes physical illness and that physical illness, in turn, causes psychological disorder. Rather, a systems perspective in which physiological, symptomatic, psychological, and behavioral processes are inherently integrated provides a more compelling framework for understanding how internalizing psychological disorders influence outcomes of chronic physical disorders. While evidence to date suggests that enhanced management of depression and anxiety improves functional and symptomatic outcomes of diverse chronic physical conditions, we should not lose sight of the broader role that depression and anxiety appear to play in the pathogenesis of physical disease and in the management of and adaptation to chronic physical conditions subsequent to onset.

REFERENCES

Addison, R. (1984). Chronic pain syndrome. *American Journal of Medicine*, 77, 54–8.

Ang, D. C., Choi, H., Kroenke, K., & Wolfe, F. (2005). Comorbid depression is an independent risk factor for mortality in patients with rheumatoid arthritis. *Journal of Rheumatology*, 32, 1013–19.

Araya, R., Flynn, T., Rojas, G., Fritsch, R., & Simon, G. (2006). Cost-effectiveness of a primary care treatment program for depression in low-income women in Santiago, Chile. *American Journal of Psychiatry*, 163, 1379–87.

Armenian, H. K., Pratt, L. A., Gallo, J., & Eaton, W. W. (1998). Psychopathology as a predictor of disability: A population-based follow-up study in Baltimore, Maryland. *American Journal of Epidemiology*, 148, 269–75.

Bair, M. J., Robinson, R. L., Katon, W., & Kroenke, K. (2003). Depression and pain comorbidity: A literature review. *Archives of Internal Medicine*, 163, 2433–45.

Barsky, A. J. (1979). Patients who amplify bodily sensations. *Annals of Internal Medicine*, **91**, 63–70.

Barsky, A. J., Goodson, J. D., Lane, R. S., & Cleary, P. D. (1988). The amplification of somatic symptoms. *Psychosomatic Medicine*, **5**, 510–19.

Bergner, M., Bobbitt, R. A., Carter, W. B., & Gilson, B. S. (1981). The sickness impact profile: Development and final revision of a health status measure. *Medical Care*, **19**, 787–805.

Berkman, L. F., Blumenthal, J., Burg, M., Carney, R. M., Catellier, D., Cowan, M. J., Czajkowski, S. M., DeBusk, R., Hosking, J., Jaffe, A., Kaufmann, P. G., Mitchell, P., Norman, J., Powell, L. H., Raczynski, J. M., & Schneiderman, N. (2003). Effects of treating depression and low perceived social support on clinical events after myocardial infarction. The Enhancing Recovery in Coronary Heart Disease (ENRICHD) Randomized Trial. *The Journal of the American Medical Association*, **289**, 3106–16.

Berkman, L. L. S., Berkman, C. S., Kasl, S., Freeman, D. M., Leo, L., Ostfeld, A. M., Coroni-Huntley, J., & Brody, J. A. (1986). Depressive symptoms in relation to physical health and functioning in the elderly. *American Journal of Epidemiology*, **115**, 684–94.

Blumer, D., & Heilbronn, M. (1982). Chronic pain as a variant of depressive disease: The pain-prone disorder. *The Journal of Nervous and Mental Disease*, **170**, 381–406.

Bogner, H. R., Morales, K. H., Post, E. P., & Bruce, M. L. (2007). Diabetes, depression and death: A randomized controlled trials of a depression treatment program for older adults based in primary care (PROSPECT). *Diabetes Care*, **30**, 3005–10.

Broadhead, W. E., Blazer, D. G., George, L. K., & Tse, C. K. (1990). Depression, disability days and days lost from work in a prospective epidemiologic study. *The Journal of the American Medical Association*, **264**, 2524–8.

Bruce, M. L., Seeman, T. E., Merrill, S. S., & Blazer, D. G. (1994). The impact of depressive symptomatology on physical disability: MacArthur Studies of Successful Aging. *American Journal of Public Health*, **84**, 1796–9.

Carver, C. S., & Scheier, M. F. (1998). *On the Self-Regulation of Behavior*. New York: Cambridge University Press.

Clark, N. M., Becker, M. H., Janz, N. K., Lorig, K., Rakowski, W., & Anderson, L. (1991). Self-management of chronic disease by older adults: A review and questions for research. *Journal of Aging and Health*, **3**, 3–27.

Coulehan, J. L., Schulberg, H. C., Block, M. R., Madonia, M. J., & Rodriguez, E. (1997). Treating depressed primary care patients improves their physical, mental, and social functioning. *Archives of Internal Medicine*, **157**, 1113–20.

Creamer, P., Lethbridge-Cejku, M., & Hochberg, M. C. (2000). Factors associated with functional impairment in symptomatic knee osteoarthritis. *Rheumatology (Oxford)*, **39**, 490–6.

DiMatteo, M. R., Lepper, H. S., & Croghan, T. W. (2000). Depression is a risk factor for noncompliance with medical treatment: meta-analysis of the effects of anxiety and depression on patient adherence. *Archives of Internal Medicine*, **160**, 2101–7.

Dohrenwend, B. S., Dohrenwend, B. P., Link, B., & Levav, I. (1983). Social functioning of psychiatric patients in contrast with community cases in the general population. *Archives of General Psychiatry*, **40**, 1174–82.

Edwards, R. R., Bingham, C. O., III, Bathon, J., & Haythornwaite, J. (2006). Catastrophizing and pain in arthritis, fibromyalgia and other rheumatic diseases. *Arthritis and Rheumatism*, **55**, 325–32.

Endicott, J., Russell, J. M., Raskin, J., Detke, M. J., Erickson, J., Ball, S. G., Marciniak, M., & Swindle, R. W. (2007). Duloxetine treatment for role functioning improvement in generalized anxiety disorder: Three independent studies. *Journal of Clinical Psychiatry*, **68**, 518–24.

Engel, C. C., Von Korff, M., & Katon, W. J. (2004). Back pain in primary care: Predictors of high health care costs. *Pain*, **65**, 197–204.

Escobar, J. I., & Gureje, O. (2007). Influence of cultural and social factors on the epidemiology of idiopathic somatic complaints and syndromes. *Psychosomatic Medicine*, **69**, 841–5.

Evans, D. L., Charney, D. S., Lewis, L., Golden, R. N., Gorman, J. M., Krishnan, K. R., Nemeroff, C. B., Bremner, J. D., Carney, R. M., Coyne, J. C., Delong, M. R., Frasure-Smith, N., Glassman, A. H., Gold, P. W., Grant, I., Gwyther, L., Ironson, G., Johnson, R. L., Kanner, A. M., Katon, W. J., Kaufmann, P. G., Keefe, F. J., Ketter, T., Laughren, T. P., Leserman, J., Lyketsos, C. G., McDonald, W. M., McEwen, B. S., Miller, A. H., Musselman, D., O'Connor, C., Petitto, J. M., Pollock, B. G., Robinson, R. G., Roose, S. P., Rowland, J., Sheline, Y., Sheps, D. S., Simon,

G., Spiegel, D., Stunkard, A., Sunderland, T., Tibbits, P., Jr., & Valvo, W. J. (2005). Mood disorders in the medically ill: Scientific review and recommendations. *Biological Psychiatry*, **58**, 175–89.

Everson, S. A., Roberts, R. E., Golderbg, D. E., & Kaplan, G. A. (1998). Depressive symptoms and increased risk of stroke mortality over a 29 year period. *Archives of Internal Medicine*, **158**, 1133–8.

Gallo, J. J., Bogner, H. R., Morales, K. H., Post, E. P., Ten Have, T., & Bruce, M. L. (2005). Depression, cardiovascular disease, diabetes and two-year mortality among older, primary care patients. *American Journal of Geriatric Psychiatry*, **13**, 748–55.

Glassman, A. H., O'Connor, C. M., Califf, R. M., Swedberg, K., Schwartz, P., Bigger, J. T., Jr., Krishnan, K. R., van Zyl, L. T., Swenson, J. R., Finkel, M. S., Landau, C., Shapiro, P. A., Pepine, C. J., Mardekian, J., Harrison, W. M., Barton, D., & McLvor, M. (2002). Sertraline treatment of major depression in patients with acute MI or unstable angina. *The Journal of the American Medical Association*, **288**, 701–9.

Goldberg, D., & Goodyer, I. (2005). *The Origins and Course of Common Mental Disorders*. London: Routledge.

Gureje O. (2007). Psychiatric aspects of pain. *Current Opinion in Psychiatry*, **20**, 42–6.

Haber, J., Kuczmierczyk, A., & Adams, H. (1985). Tension headaches: Muscle overactivity or psychogenic pain. *Headache*, **25**, 23–9.

Hasenbring, M., Hallner, D., & Klasen, B. (2001). Psychological mechanisms in the transition from acute to chronic pain: over- or underrated? *Schmerz*, **15**, 442–7.

Katon, W., Unutzer, J., Fan, M. Y., Williams, J. W., Jr., Schoenbaum, M., Lin, E. H., & Hunkeler, E. M. (2006). Cost-effectiveness and net benefit of enhanced treatment of depression for older adults with diabetes and depression. *Diabetes Care*, **29**, 265–70.

Katon, W., Von Korff, M., Ciechanowski, P., Russo, J., Lin, E., Simon, G., Ludman, E., Walker, E., Bush, T., & Young, B. (2004a). Behavioral and clinical factors associated with depression among individuals with diabetes. *Diabetes Care*, **27**, 914–20.

Katon, W., Von Korff, M., Lin, E. H. B., Simon, G., Ludman, E., Russo, J., Ciechanowski, P., Walker, E., & Bush, T. (2004b). The Pathways Study: A randomized trial of collaborative care in patients with diabetes and depression. *Archives of General Psychiatry*, **61**, 1042–9.

Katon, W. J., Lin, E., Russo, J., & Unutzer, J. (2003). Increased medical costs of a population-based sample of depressed elderly patients. *Archives of General Psychiatry*, **60**, 897–903.

Katon, W. J., Rutter, C., Simon, G., Lin, E. H., Ludman, E., Ciechanowski, P., Kinder, L., Young, B., & Von Korff, M. (2005). The association of comorbid depression with mortality in patients with type 2 diabetes. *Diabetes Care*, **28**, 2668–72.

Katz, S., & Akpom, C. A. (1976). Index of ADL. *Medical Care*, **14**, 116–18.

Katzelnick, D. J., Simon, G. E., Pearson, S. D., Manning, W. G., Helstad, C. P., Henk, H. J., Cole, S. M., Lin, E. H., Taylor, L. H., & Kobak, K. A. (2000). Randomized trial of a depression management program in high utilizers of medical care. *Archives of Family Medicine*, **9**, 345–51.

Keefe, F., Rumble, M. E., Scipio, C. D., Giordano, L. A., & Perri, L. M. (2004). Psychological aspects of persistent pain: Current state of the science. *Journal of Pain*, **5**, 195–211.

Kinder, L. S., Bradley, K. A., Katon, W. J., Ludman, E., McDonnell, M. B., & Bryson, C. L. (2008). Depression, posttraumatic stress disorder, and mortality. *Psychosomatic Medicine*, **70**, 20–6.

Kirmayer, L. J., & Sartorius, N. (2007). Cultural models and somatic symptoms. *Psychosomatic Medicine*, **69**, 832–40.

Kirmayer, L. J., & Young, A. (1998). Culture and somatization: Clinical, epidemiological, and ethnographic perspectives. *Psychosomatic Medicine*, **60**, 420–30.

Kisely, S., & Simon, G. (2006). An international study comparing the effect of medically explained and unexplained somatic symptoms on psychosocial outcomes. *Journal of Psychosomatic Research*, **60**, 125–30.

Kleinman, A. (1998). *The Illness Narratives: Suffering, Healing and the Human Condition*. New York: Basic Books.

Koopmans, G. T., & Lamers, L. M. (2006). Is the impact of depressive complaints on the use of general health care services dependent on severity of somatic morbidity? *Journal of Psychosomatic Research*, **61**, 41–50.

Kroenke, K. (2007). Efficacy of treatment for somatoform disorders: A review of randomized controlled trials. *Psychosomatic Medicine*, **69**, 881–8.

Kroenke, K., Shen, J., Oxman, T. E., Williams, J. W., Jr., & Dietrich, A. J. (2008). Impact of pain on the outcomes of depression treatment: Results for the RESPECT trial. *Pain*, **134**, 209–15.

Leeuw, M., Goosens, M. E., Linton, S. J., Crombez, G., Boersma, K., & Vlaeyen, J. W. (2007). The fear-avoidance model of musculoskeletal pain: Current status of scientific evidence. *Journal of Behavioral Medicine*, **30**, 77–94.

Lesse, S. (1983). The masked depression syndrome – Results of a seventeen year clinical study. *American Journal of Psychotherapy*, **37**, 456–75.

Leventhal, H., Meyer, D., & Nerenz, D. (1980). The common sense representation of illness danger. In *Medical Psychology*, vol. **2**, ed. S. Rachman, pp. 7–30. New York: Permagon Press.

Levy, R. L., Von Korff, M., Whitehead, W. E., Stang, P., Saunders, K., Jhingran, P., Barghout, V., & Feld, A. D. (2001). Costs of care for irritable bowel syndrome patients in a health maintenance organization. *American Journal of Gastroenterology*, **96**, 3122–9.

Lin, E. H., Katon, W., Von Korff, M., Tang, L., Williams, J. W., Jr., Kroenke, K., Hunkeler, E., Harpole, L., Hegel, M., Arean, P., Hoffing, M., Della Penna, R., Langston, C., Unutzer, J., & IMPACT Investigators. (2003). Effect of improving depression care on pain and functional outcomes among older adults with arthritis: A randomized controlled trial. *The Journal of the American Medical Association*, **290**, 2428–34.

Lin, E. H., Von Korff, M., Russo, J., Katon, W., Simon, G. E., Unutzer, J., Bush, T., Walker, E., & Ludman, E. (2000). Can depression treatment in primary care reduce disability? A stepped care approach. *Archives of Family Medicine*, **9**, 1052–8.

Linton, S. J. (2000). A review of psychological risk factors in back and neck pain. *Spine*, **25**, 1148–56.

Loncar, Z., Bras, M., & Mickovic, V. (2006). The relationships between burn pain, anxiety and depression. *Collegium antropologicum*, **30**, 319–25.

Lorig, K. (1993). Self-management of chronic illness: A model for the future. *Generations*, 11–14.

Ludman, E. J., Katon, W., Russo, J., Von Korff, M., Simon, G., Ciechanowski, P., Lin, E., Bush, T., Walker, E., & Young, B. (2004). Depression and diabetes symptom burden. *General Hospital Psychiatry*, **26**, 430–6.

Lustman, P. J., & Clouse, R. E. (2005). Depression in diabetic patients: The relationship between mood and glycemic control. *Journal of Diabetes and Its Complications*, **19**, 113–22.

Mallen, C. D., Peat, G., Thomas, E., Dunn, K. M., & Croft, P. R. (2007a). Prognostic factors for musculoskeletal pain in primary care: A systematic review. *British Journal of General Practice*, **57**, 655–61.

Mallen, C. D., Peat, G., Thomas, E., Lacey, R., & Croft, P. (2007b). Predicting poor functional outcome in community-dwelling older adults with knee pain: Prognostic value of generic indicators. *Annals of the Rheumatic Diseases*, **66**, 1456–61.

Manninen, P., Heliovaara, M., Riihimaki, H., & Makela, P. (1997). Does psychological distress predict disability? *International Journal of Epidemiology*, **26**, 1063–70.

Mason, J. H., Anderson, J. J., & Meenan, R. F. (1988). A model of health status for rheumatoid arthritis. A factor analysis of the Arthritis Impact Measurement Scales. *Arthritis and Rheumatism*, **31**, 714–20.

Mavandadi, S., Ten Have, T. R., Katz, I. R., Durai, U. N., Krahn, D. D., Llorente, M. D., Kirchner, J. E., Olsen, E. J., Van Stone, W. W., Cooley, S. L., & Oslin, D. W. (2007). Effect of depression treatment on depressive symptoms in older adulthood: The moderating role of pain. *Journal of the American Geriatric Society*, **55**, 202–11.

McEwen, B. S. (1998). Protective and damaging effects of stress mediators. *New England Journal of Medicine*, **338**, 171–7.

Mohr, D. C., Hart, S., & Vella, L. (2007). Reduction in disability in a randomized controlled trial of telephone-administered cognitive-behavioral therapy. *Health Psychology*, **26**, 554–63.

Nelson, E., Wasson, J., Kirk, J., Keller, A., Clark, D., Dietrich, A., Stewart, A., & Zubkoff, M. (1987). Assessment of function in routine clinical practice: Description of the COOP Chart method and preliminary findings. *Journal of Chronic Disease*, **40**, S55–69.

Ng, T. P., Niti, M., Tan, W. C., Cao, Z., Ong, K. C., & Eng, P. (2007). Depressive symptoms and chronic obstructive pulmonary disease: Effect on mortality, hospital readmission, symptom burden, functional status and quality of life. *Archives of Internal Medicine*, **8**, 60–7.

Odegard, P. S., & Capoccia, K. (2007). Medication taking and diabetes: A systematic review of the literature. *Diabetes Education*, **33**, 1014–29.

Olson, A. L., Johansen, S. G., Powers, L. E., Pope, J. B., & Klein, R. B. (1993). Cognitive coping strategies of children with chronic illness.

Journal of Developmental and Behavioral Pediatrics, **14**, 217–23.
Ormel, J., Von Korff, M., Oldehinkel, A. J., Simon, G., Tiemens, T. G., & Ustun, T. B. (1999). Onset of disability in depressed and non-depressed primary care patients. *Psychological Medicine*, **29**, 847–53.
Ormel, J., Von Korff, M., Ustun, T. B., Pini, S., Korten, A., & Oldehinkel, T. (1994). Common mental disorders and disability: A strong and cross-culturally consistent relationship. Results from the WHO Collaborative Study. *The Journal of the American Medical Association*, **272**, 1741–8.
Ormel, J., Von Korff, M., Van Den Brink, W., Katon, W., Brilman, E., & Oldehinkel, T. (1993). Depression, anxiety and disability show synchrony of change: A 3 1/2 year longitudinal study in primary care. *American Journal of Public Health*, **83**, 385–90.
Penninx, B. W., Guralnik, J. M., Ferrucci, L., Simonsick, E. M., Deeg, D. J., & Wallace, R. B. (1998). Depressive symptoms and physical decline in community-dwelling older persons. *The Journal of the American Medical Association*, **279**, 1720–6.
Peruzza, S., Sergi, G., Vianello, A., Pisent, C., Tiozzo, F., Manzan, A., Coin, A., Inelmen, E. M., & Enzi, G. (2003). Chronic obstructive pulmonary disease (COPD) in elderly subjects: Impact on functional status and quality of life. *Respiratory Medicine*, **97**, 612–17.
Piette, J., Richardson, C., & Valenstein, M. (2004). Addressing the needs of patients with multiple chronic illnesses: the case of diabetes and depression. *The American Journal of Managed Care*, **10**, 152–62.
Pincus, T., Burton, A. K., Vogel, S., & Field, A. P. (2002). A systematic review of psychological factors as predictors of chronicity/disability in prospective cohorts of low back pain. *Spine*, **27**, E109–20.
Pincus, T., Vogel, S., Burton, A. K., Santos, R., & Field, A. P. (2006). Fear avoidance and prognosis in back pain: A systematic review and synthesis of current evidence. *Arthritis and Rheumatism*, **54**, 3999–4010.
Pope, A. M., & Tarlov, A. R., eds. (1991). *Disability in America: Toward a National Agenda for Prevention of Disabilities*. Washington, DC: National Academy Press.
Proctor, T., Gatchel, R. J., & Robinson, R. C. (2000). Psychosocial factors and risk of pain and disability. *Occupational Medicine*, **15**, 803–12.
Richardson, L. P., Lozano, P., Russo, J., McCauley, E., Bush, T., & Katon, W. (2006). Asthma symptom burden: Relationship to asthma severity and anxiety and depression symptoms. *Pediatrics*, **118**, 1042–51.
Romano, J., & Turner, J. (1985). Chronic pain and depression: Does the evidence support a relationship? *Psychological Bulletin*, **97**, 18–34.
Roy-Bryne, P. P., Craske, M. G., Stein, M. B., Sullivan, G., Bystritsky, A., Katon, W., Golinelli, D., & Sherbourne, C. D. (2005). A randomized trial of cognitive-behavioral and medication for primary care panic disorder. *Archives of General Psychiatry*, **62**, 290–8.
Scalco, A. Z., Scalco, M. Z., Azul, J. B., & Lotufo Neto, F. (2005). Hypertension and depression. *Clinics*, **60**, 241–50.
Selby, J. V., Swain, B. E., Geroff, R. B., Karter, A. J., Waitzfelder, B. E., Brown, A. F., Ackermann, R. T., Duru, O. K., Ferrara, A., Herman, W., Marrero, D. G., Caputo, D., & Narayan, K. M. for the TRIAD Study Group. (2007). Understanding the gap between good processes of diabetes care and poor intermediate outcomes: Translating Research into Action for Diabetes (TRIAD). *Medical Care*, **45**, 1144–53.
Simon, G., Katon, W., Von Korff, M., Lin, E., Robinson, P., Bush, T., Walker, E., Ludman, E., Russo, J., & Rutter, C. (1998). Impact of improved depression treatment in primary care on daily functioning and disability. *Psychological Medicine*, **28**, 693–701.
Simon, G., Ormel, J., Von Korff, M., & Barlow, W. (1995a). Health care costs associated with depressive and anxiety disorders in primary care. *American Journal of Psychiatry*, **152**, 352–7.
Simon, G. E., Katon, W. J., Von Korff, M., Unutzer, J., Lin, E. H., Walker, E. A., Bush, T., Rutter, C., & Ludman, E. (2001a). Cost-effectiveness of a collaborative care program for primary care patients with persistent depression. *American Journal of Psychiatry*, **158**, 1638–44.
Simon, G. E., Manning, W. G., Katzelnick, D. J., Pearson, S. D., Henk, H. J., & Helstad, C. S. (2001b). Cost-effectiveness of systematic depression treatment for high utilizers of general medical care. *Archives of General Psychiatry*, **58**, 181–7.
Simon, G. E., Von Korff, M., & Barlow, W. (1995b). Health care costs of primary care patients with

recognized depression. *Archives of General Psychiatry*, **52**, 850–6.

Simon, G. E., Von Korff, M., Piccinelli, M., Fullerton, C., & Ormel, J. (1999). An international study of the relation between somatic symptoms and depression. *New England Journal of Medicine*, **341**, 1329–35.

Simon, G. E., Katon, W. J., Lin, E. H., Rutter, C., Manning, W. G., Von Korff, M., Ciechanowski, P., Ludman, E. J., & Young B. (2007). Cost-effectiveness of systematic depression treatment among people with diabetes mellitus. *Archives of General Psychiatry*, **64**, 65–72.

Simon, G. E., Von Korff, M., & Lin, E. (2005). Clinical and functional outcomes of depression treatment in patients with and without chronic medical conditions. *Psychological Medicine*, **35**, 271–9.

Smoller, J. W., Pollack, M. H., Wassertheil-Smoller, S., Jackson, R. D., Oberman, A., Wong, N. D., & Sheps, D. (2007). Panic attacks and risk of incident cardiovascular events among postmenopausal women in the Women's Health Initiative Study. *Archives of General Psychiatry*, **64**, 1153–60.

Sullivan, M. D., LaCroix, A. Z., Baum, C., Grothaus, L. C., & Katon, W. J. (1997). Functional status in coronary artery disease: A one-year prospective study of the role of anxiety and depression. *American Journal of Medicine*, **103**, 348–56.

Sullivan, M. D., LaCroix, A. Z., Spertus, J. A., & Hecht, J. (2000). Five-year prospective study of the effects of anxiety and depression in patients with coronary artery disease. *American Journal of Cardiology*, **86**, 1135–8.

Sumathilpala, A. (2007). What is the evidence for the efficacy of treatments for somatoform disorders? A critical review of previous intervention studies. *Psychosomatic Medicine*, **69**, 889–900.

Szekely, A., Balog, P., Benko, E., Breuer, T., Szekely, J., Kertai, M. D., Horkay, F., Kopp, M. S., & Thayer, J. F. (2007). Anxiety predicts mortality and morbidity after coronary artery and valve surgery – A 4 year follow-up study. *Psychosomatic Medicine*, **69**, 625–31.

Thielke, S. M., Fan, M. Y., Sullivan, M., & Unutzer, J. (2007). Pain limits the effectiveness of collaborative care for depression. *American Journal of Geriatric Psychiatry*, **15**, 699–707.

Turner, J. A., Ciol, M. A., Von Korff, M., Rothman, I., & Berger, R. E. (2004). Healthcare use and costs of primary care secondary care patients with prostatitis. *Urology*, **63**, 1031–5.

Turner, R. J., & Noh, S. (1988). Physical disability and depression: A longitudinal analysis. *Journal of Health and Social Behavior*, **29**, 23–37.

Unutzer, J., Patrick, D. L., Marmon, T., Simon, G. E., & Katon, W. J. (2002). Depressive symptoms and mortality in a prospective study of 2,588 older adults. *American Journal of Geriatric Psychiatry*, **10**, 521–30.

Unutzer, J., Patrick, D. L., Simon, G., Grembowski, D., Walker, E., Rutter, C., & Katon, W. (1997). Depressive symptoms and the cost of health services in HMO patients aged 65 years and older. A 4 year prospective study. *The Journal of the American Medical Association*, **277**, 1618–23.

Van Ittersum, M., de Greef, M., van Gelder, I., Coster, J., Brugemaan, J., & van der Schans, C. (2003). Fear of exercise and health-related quality of life in patients with an implantable cardioconverter defibrillator. *Journal of Rehabilitation Research*, **26**, 117–22.

Verhaak, P. F. M., Kerssens, J. J., Dekker, J., Sorbi, M. J., & Bensing, J. M. (1998). Prevalence of chronic benign pain disorder among adults: A review of the literature. *Pain*, **77**, 231–9.

Vlaeyen, J. W., & Linton, S. J. (2000). Fear-avoidance and its consequences in chronic musculoskeletal pain: A state of the art. *Pain*, **85**, 317–32.

Von Korff, M. (1999). Disability and psychological illness in primary care. In *Common Mental Disorders in Primary Care: Essays in Honour of Professor Sir David Goldberg*, ed. M. Tansella & G. Thornicroft, pp. 52–63. London: Routledge Press.

Von Korff, M., Gruman, J., Schaefer, J., Curry, S., & Wagner, E. H. (1997). Collaborative management of chronic illness. *Annals of Internal Medicine*, **127**, 1097–102.

Von Korff, M., Katon, W., Bush, T., Lin, E., Simon, G. E., Saunders, K., Ludman, E., Walker, E., & Unutzer, J. (1998). Treatment costs, cost offset and cost-effectiveness of collaborative management of depression. *Psychosomatic Medicine*, **60**, 143–9.

Von Korff, M., Katon, W., Lin, E. H., Simon, G., Ciechanowski, P., Ludman, E., Oliver, M., Rutter, C., & Young, B. (2005a). Work disability among individuals with diabetes. *Diabetes Care*, **28**, 1326–32.

Von Korff, M., Katon, W., Lin, E. H., Simon, G., Ludman, E., Oliver, M., Ciechanowski, P., Rutter, C., & Young, B. (2005b). Potentially modifiable factors associated with disability among people with diabetes. *Psychosomatic Medicine*, **67**, 233–40.

Von Korff, M., Katon, W., Rutter, C., Ludman, E., Simon, G., Lin, E., & Bush T. (2003). Effect on disability outcomes of a depression relapse prevention program. *Psychosomatic Medicine*, **65**, 938–43.

Von Korff, M., Lin, E. H., Fenton, J. J., & Saunders, K. (2007). Frequency and priority of pain patients' health care use. *Clinical Journal of Pain*, **23**, 400–8.

Von Korff, M., Ormel, J., Katon, W., & Lin, E. H. B. (1992). Disability and depression in medical patients: A longitudinal analysis. *Archives of General Psychiatry*, **49**, 91–100.

Von Korff, M., & Simon, G. (1996a). The relationship between pain and depression. *British Journal of Psychiatry*, **168**, 101–8.

Von Korff, M., Ustun, T. B., Ormel, J., Kaplan, I., & Simon, G. (1996b). Self-report disability in an international primary care study of psychological illness. *Journal of Clinical Epidemiology*, **49**, 297–303.

Wagner, E. H., Austin, B. T., & VonKorff, M. (1996). Organizing care for patients with chronic illness. *The Milbank Quarterly*, **74**, 511–44.

Wang, P. S., Simon, G. E., Avorn, J., Azocar, F., Ludman, E. J., McCulloch, J., Petukhova, M. Z., & Kessler, R. C. (2007). Telephone screening, outreach, and care management for depressed workers and impact on clinical and work productivity outcomes: A randomized controlled trial. *The Journal of the American Medical Association*, **298**, 1401–11.

Ware, J. E., Jr., Kosinski, M., Bayliss, M. S., McHorney, C. A., Rogers, W. H., & Raczek, A. (1995). Comparison of methods for the scoring and statistical analysis of SF-36 health profile and summary measures: Summary of results from the Medical Outcomes Study. *Medical Care*, **33**, AS264–79.

Wells, K. B., Golding, J. M., & Burnham, M. A. (1988). Psychiatric disorder and limitations in physical functioning in a sample of the Los Angeles general population. *American Journal of Psychiatry*, **145**, 712–17.

Wells, K. B., Scherbourne, C., Schoenbaum, M., Duan, N., Meredith, L., Unutzer, J., Miranda, J., Carney, M. F., & Rubenstein, L. V. (2000). Impact of disseminating quality improvement programs for depression in managed primary care: A randomized control trial. *The Journal of the American Medical Association*, **283**, 212–20.

Wells, K. B., Stewart, A., Hays, R. D., Burnham, A., Rogers, W., Daniels, M., Berry, S., Greenfield, S., & Ware, J. (1989). The functioning and well-being of depressed patients. *The Journal of the American Medical Association*, **262**, 914–19.

Wiersma, D., DeJong, A., & Ormel, J. (1988). The Groningen Social Disabilities Schedule: Development, relationship with I.C.I.D.H., and psychometric properties. *International Journal of Rehabilitation Research*, **11**, 213–24.

Williams, J. W., Jr., Katon, W., Lin, E. H., Noel, P. H., Worchel, J., Cornell, J., Harpole, L., Fultz, B. A., Hunkeler, E., Mika, V. S., & Unutzer, J. (2004). The effectiveness of depression care management on depression and diabetes-related outcomes in older patients with both conditions. *Annals of Internal Medicine*, **140**, 1015–24.

Wohlfarth, T. D., Van Den Brink, W., Ormel, J., Koeter, M. W., & Oldehinkel, A. J. (1993). The relationship between social dysfunctioning and psychopathology among primary care attenders. *British Journal of Psychiatry*, **163**, 37–44.

World Health Organization. (2001). *International Classification of Functioning, Disability and Health: ICF*. Geneva: World Health Organization.

Zaza, C., & Baine, N. (2002). Cancer pain and psychosocial factor: A critical review of the literature. *Journal of Pain and Symptom Management*, **24**, 526–542.

Zvolensky, M. J., Eifert, G. H., Feldner, M. T., & Leen-Feldner, E. (2003). Heart-focused anxiety and chest pain in post angiography medical patient. *Journal of Behavioral Medicine*, **26**, 197–209.

18 Disability and Treatment of Specific Mental and Physical Disorders

JOHAN ORMEL, MARIA V. PETUKHOVA, MICHAEL R. VON KORFF, AND RONALD C. KESSLER

18.1. INTRODUCTION

As health care costs continue to rise, health care resource allocation decisions will need to be based on information about prevalence, severity, and chronicity of disorders, including associated disability, and on cost-effectiveness of interventions, not only on mortality (Goetzel et al. 2003; Katschnig, Freeman, & Sartorius 1997; Murray & Lopez 1996; Spitzer et al. 1995; Sprangers et al. 2000; Verbrugge & Patrick 1995; Ware et al. 1986, 1989). Studies from developed countries have documented significant impairment and loss of quality of life among patients treated in specialty mental health settings, among patients with mental disorders treated in primary care settings, as well as among persons with untreated mental disorders in the community (Andrews, Henderson, & Hall 2001; Bijl & Ravelli 2000; Kessler & Frank 1997; Ormel et al. 1994). Consistently, people with one or more mental disorders reported higher levels of disability compared to people without mental illness. The burden of mental disorders in the population at large is substantial. The World Bank's Burden of Disease estimates suggest that common mental disorders account for at least a fifth of all disability-adjusted life-years (DALYs) in individuals aged 15–44 years worldwide (Murray & Lopez 1996). The burden of common mental disorders is due to the combination of a significant impact at the individual level, their high prevalence, early age of onset compared to most chronic physical conditions, and the recurrent chronic course of many mental disorders.

Existing data used for cross-national comparison of disability burden have significant limitations. Most studies have used country-specific methods or, if cross-national, targeted only one or a few common mental disorders (Tylee et al. 1999). One exception, the World Health Organization (WHO) study on Psychological Problems in Primary Health Care (PPGHC) (Ustun & Sartorius 1995) used identical methods in each participating country. In this study, patients with one or more mental disorders (irrespective of whether the general practitioner had diagnosed a mental disorder) showed higher levels of disability compared to patients attending for other ailments without mental health problems (Ormel et al. 1994). These findings were consistent across the 15 participating countries, despite large cross-national differences in prevalence of mental disorders and disability. However, this study was limited to patients presenting in primary care settings, not to a population-based sample.

A second major limitation is that few studies assessed condition-specific disability for a broad range of mental and physical disorders. In a condition-specific approach, respondents are asked to rate the interference in role functioning caused by a particular disorder rather than the interference caused by all their health problems. Most studies have assessed overall disability, which makes it difficult to compare condition-specific disabilities, particularly when comorbidity is present. Furthermore, nearly all studies that used condition-specific approaches to estimate the effects of specific disorders on disability were performed in developed countries (Berto et al. 2000; Maetzel & Li 2002; Reed, Lee, & McCrory 2004). Comparable studies are rare in developing countries (Moussavi et al. 2007). Therefore, international data on the burden of mental disorders are incomplete and have limited comparability. A third limitation is that few studies have assessed both mental and physical disorders (Buist-Bouwman et al. 2005; Kessler et al. 2003).

The aim of this chapter is to examine, in a cross-national, population-based study that used condition-specific disability assessments for both mental and physical disorders, whether common mental disorders are as seriously disabling as common physical disorders according to respondent self-reports.

18.2. APPROACH

The World Mental Health (WMH) Surveys were carried out in six countries classified by the World Bank (World Bank 2003) as developing (Colombia, Lebanon, Mexico, People's Republic of China, South Africa, and Ukraine) and nine as developed (Belgium, France, Germany, Italy, Japan, the Netherlands, New Zealand, Spain, and the United States of America). The total sample size was 73,441, with individual country samples from 2,372 (the Netherlands) to 12,992 (New Zealand).

18.2.1. Measures

Physical disorders were assessed with a standard chronic disorders checklist (Centers for Disease Control and Prevention 2004; Schoenborn, Adams, & Schiller 2003) containing ten conditions that included asthma, cancer, cardiovascular disease (hypertension and other heart disease), diabetes, musculoskeletal diseases (arthritis and chronic back/neck pain), chronic headaches, other chronic pain disorders, and ulcers. Respondents were asked to report whether they had each of the symptom-based conditions (e.g., chronic headaches) in the past 12 months and to say whether a doctor ever told them they had each of the medically diagnosed chronic conditions (e.g., diabetes, heart disease, and hypertension).

Checklists of this sort yield more complete and accurate reports about chronic conditions than do open-ended questions (Knight, Stewart-Brown, & Fletcher 2001). Methodological studies have documented moderate to good concordance between checklist reports and medical records in developed countries (Baker, Stabile, & Deri 2001; Bergmann et al. 1998; Kriegsman et al. 1996; National Center for Health Statistics 1994). Self-reports are obviously less accurate than assessments based on biological tests. Caution is consequently needed in interpreting the results of studies, like this one, that use self-report to assess physical conditions. The implications of this imperfect assessment were evaluated by replicating analyses only for treated cases of physical disorders. Treated cases are both more likely to meet full diagnostic criteria and more disabling than self-reported untreated cases. A remaining bias is that the conditions included in the checklist did not include infectious diseases prevalent in developing countries.

Mental disorders were assessed with version 3.0 of the WHO Composite International Diagnostic Interview (CIDI) (Kessler & Ustun 2004), a fully structured lay-administered interview that generates research diagnoses of commonly occurring Diagnostic and Statistical Manual of Mental Disorders, Fourth Edition (DSM-IV) mental disorders (American

Psychiatric Association 1994). The 10 disorders considered here include anxiety disorders (panic disorder, generalized anxiety disorder, specific phobia, social phobia, and posttraumatic stress disorder (PTSD)), mood disorders (major depressive disorder or dysthymia and bipolar disorder), and impulse-control disorders (intermittent explosive disorder, adult attention-deficit/hyperactivity disorder (ADHD), and oppositional-defiant disorder). Only disorders present in the past 12 months are considered.

Treatment was assessed for physical disorders by asking respondents if they saw a medical doctor or other health professional in the past 12 months for the disorder. For mental disorders, disorder-specific treatment was assessed by asking each respondent if "you ever in your life talk(ed) to a medical doctor or other professional about (the disorder)," and if so, if "you receive(d) professional treatment for (the disorder) at any time in the past 12 months." Treatment of mental disorders was also assessed in a series of more general questions that asked respondents if they in the past 12 months went to each of a long list of types of professionals (the list varying across countries depending on the types of professionals available in the country) "for problems with your emotions, nerves, or your use of alcohol or drugs." Self-reports about treatment have been shown in previous methodological studies to have generally good concordance with archival health care utilization records (Reijneveld & Stronks 2001), although this research has been carried out exclusively in developed countries.

Disability was assessed with the Sheehan Disability Scales (SDS), a widely used self-report measure of condition-specific disability that, although heretofore used only in the assessment of mental disorders, can just as well be used to assess disability caused by physical disorders. The SDS consists of four questions, each asking the respondent to rate on a 0–10 scale the extent to which a particular disorder "interfered with" activities in one of four role domains during the month in the past year when the disorder was most severe. The four domains include (1) "your home management, like cleaning, shopping, and taking care of the (house/apartment)" (home); (2) "your ability to work" (work); (3) "your social life" (social); and (4) "your ability to form and maintain close relationships with other people" (close relationships). The 0–10 response options were presented in a visual analog format with labels for the response options of none (0), mild (1–3), moderate (4–6), severe (7–9), and very severe (10). A global SDS score was also created by assigning each respondent the highest SDS domain score reported across the four domains.

Previous methodological studies have documented good internal consistency reliability across the SDS domains (Hambrick et al. 2004; Leon et al. 1997), a result that we replicated in the WMH data by finding that Cronbach's alpha (a measure of internal consistency reliability) was 0.82–0.92 across countries. Reliability was high in both developed countries (median .86; interquartile range .84–.88) and developing countries (median .90; interquartile range .88–.90). Previous methodological studies have also documented good discrimination between role functioning of cases and controls based on SDS scores in studies of social phobia (Hambrick et al. 2004), PTSD (Connor & Davidson 2001), panic disorder (Leon et al. 1997), and substance abuse (Pallanti, Bernardi, & Quercioli 2006). Similar results were found in the WMH Surveys–based responses to a question asked after the SDS about "how many days out of 365 in the past year were you totally unable to work or carry out you normal activities because of (the illness)?" We examined the strength of SDS scores predicting variation in this relatively objective measure of disability. If the SDS measures disability accurately, we would expect correlations to be significant and comparable for physical and mental disorders. This was confirmed. In developed countries, the multiple correlations of the four SDS domain scores predicting days out of role were .55 for mental disorders and .50 for physical disorders, while the comparable correlations in less developed countries were .39 for mental disorders and .36 for physical disorders.

It is important to recognize that the SDS scales are *condition specific*. Respondents were asked to rate the interference in role functioning caused by a particular disorder rather than the interference caused by all their health problems. This focused approach to questioning allows SDS scores to be compared across disorders without adjusting for comorbidity. However, this requires respondents with multiple health problems to sort out the relative effects of their various conditions on their overall functioning. An indication that respondents are able to do this comes from controlled treatment studies that have documented significant improvements in SDS measures of condition-specific role functioning with treatment for generalized anxiety disorder (Davidson et al. 2004), panic disorder (Bertani et al. 2004), and major depression (Hudson et al. 2007).

Because they are condition specific, the SDS scales were administered separately for each of the 10 mental disorders considered in this report. In the case of the physical disorders, for which assessments were necessarily more limited in the WMH Surveys, the SDS scales were administered only for one physical disorder per respondent. This one disorder was selected randomly from among all the physical disorders reported by the respondent as being in existence during the 12 months before interview. This method of selection underrepresents comorbid physical disorders, which may be more severe than pure disorders, as a function of number of such disorders. In order to correct this bias, a weight was applied to each case equal to the number of physical conditions reported by the respondent.

18.2.2. Statistical Analysis

Since respondents could report multiple physical and psychological disorders, the unit of analysis is the disorder. However, among respondents who reported multiple physical disorders, one was selected at random for asking questions about disability.

Significance tests were used to test the statistical significance of pairwise differences in SDS scores across all pairs of conditions. Within-disorder comparisons were also made to determine whether disability ratings differ in developing and developed countries. Between-disorder comparisons were made to determine whether disability ratings are systematically different for physical disorders than mental disorders within countries. All these analyses were then replicated using only the subsample of respondents with treated physical disorders. Finally, all pairwise comparisons were repeated on a within-person basis: that is, by comparing SDS scores for specific pairs of conditions for the same individual (e.g., a single person who had both depression and cancer and who provided separate SDS ratings for these conditions). All these significance tests adjusted for the clustering and weighting of observations using the jackknife repeated replications pseudo-replication simulation method (Kish & Frankel 1974). Significance was consistently evaluated at the .05 level with two-sided tests.

18.3. FINDINGS

18.3.1. Self-Reported Disorder Prevalence and Treatment

The broad pattern of prevalence estimates for physical and mental disorders was similar for developed and developing countries (Table 18.1), albeit there were often significant differences in these rates. However, the percent of respondents that reported being in treatment for the focal disorders at the time of interview was generally considerably higher in developed than developing countries. The difference in rates of treatment among prevalent cases between developed and developing countries was particularly large for mental disorders.

The broad rank-ordering of mental disorder prevalence estimates was also fairly similar across developed and developing countries despite the fact that, unlike physical disorders, most mental disorders were significantly more prevalent in developed than developing countries. Specific phobia, depression, and social phobia were most prevalent disorders, while oppositional-defiant disorder and ADHD were the least common. As with physical disorders, the percent of respondents that reported being in treatment for the focal disorder at the time of interview was consistently higher in developed than developing countries.

The physical disorders were more likely to be treated than the mental disorders. In developed countries, 64.4% ($n = 6,746$) of all the physical disorders were treated versus 23.7% ($n = 2,642$) of all the mental disorders. In developing countries, only 7.7% ($n = 319$) of the mental disorders were treated versus 51.9% ($n = 2,908$) of the physical disorders. This pattern also held for severely disabling disorders, with 35.3% ($n = 1,380$) of severe mental disorders treated in developed countries and 11.9% ($n = 145$) treated in developing countries compared to 77.6% ($n = 2,172$) of severe physical disorders treated in developed countries and 63.6% ($n = 763$) treated in developing countries. It is noteworthy that these results show the mental–physical treatment gap to be considerably higher in developing than developed countries.

18.3.2. Individual-Level Disability

The physical disorders with the highest mean SDS global disability ratings in both subsamples were chronic pain disorders, although between-disorder variation in disability ratings was much greater in developed than developing countries. Three physical disorders – back/neck pain, headaches, and other chronic pain disorders – had significantly higher mean SDS global disability ratings in developed countries. Three others – asthma, diabetes, and hypertension – had significantly higher ratings in developing countries. A similar pattern of relative disability was found for the proportion of cases rated severely disabled in the total sample (Table 18.2) as well as among treated cases (Table 18.3).

The mental disorders with the highest mean SDS global disability ratings in both subsamples were bipolar disorder and depression. The lowest SDS ratings were for specific phobia. Four mental disorders – bipolar disorder, depression, generalized anxiety disorder, and PTSD – had significantly higher mean global disability ratings in developed countries. None had a significantly higher rating in developing countries. A similar pattern of relative disability was found for the proportion of cases rated severely disabled in the total sample (Table 18.2) as well as among treated cases (Table 18.3).

The SDS disability ratings for mental disorders were generally higher than for physical disorders. This was true, as evaluated by Mann–Whitney tests, both for mean disability ratings ($z = 3.0$, $p = .002$ developing; $z = 3.0$, $p = .002$ developed) and for the proportions rated severely disabled ($z = 2.5$, $p = .011$ developing; $z = 2.7$, $p = .007$ developed). Of the 100 possible pairwise disorder-specific mental–physical comparisons (Table 18.4), mean ratings were higher for the mental disorder in 91 comparisons in developed and 91 in developing countries.

Table 18.1. Twelve-month prevalence of disorders and treatment in developed and developing WMH countries

	Disorder prevalence								Treatment prevalence among cases							
	Developed		Developing						Developed		Developing					
	N^a	%	SE	N^a	%	SE	c^2	p	N^b	%	SE	N^b	%	SE	c^2	p
I. Physical disorders																
Arthritis	4,434	18.1	0.4	1,627	10.0	0.3	73.6	<.001	1,127	50.9	1.8	229	46.6	4.1	1.0	.31
Asthma	2,524	10.0	0.3	542	3.5	0.2	305.2	<.001	494	51.0	3.7	122	61.4	5.4	0.1	.74
Back/neck pain	5,150	19.3	0.4	3,375	22.0	0.5	51.7	<.001	1,632	64.8*	1.6	548	43.7	2.3	56.6	<.001
Cancer	903	4.0	0.2	112	0.6	0.1	107.1	<.001	165	51.8	5.2	26	59.6	10.2	0.2	.64
Chronic pain	1,791	6.0	0.2	1,240	8.0	0.3	32.4	<.001	472	71.5*	3.2	217	52.4	4.4	12.4	<.001
Diabetes	1,108	4.6	0.2	564	3.9	0.2	1.4	.237	373	94.4*	1.2	168	76.6	5.7	10.0	.002
Headaches	3,363	10.9	0.3	3,260	20.8	0.6	221.6	<.001	833	49.7	1.8	677	49.7	2.2	0.0	.96
Heart disease	1,168	4.7	0.2	1,063	5.9	0.2	87.2	<.001	310	77.7*	2.9	171	50.9	5.3	13.1	<.001
High blood pressure	3,382	14.0	0.4	2,033	13.1	0.4	30.1	<.001	1,194	90.2*	1.4	553	69.8	2.7	42.7	<.001
Ulcer	529	1.9	0.1	786	5.2	0.3	156.5	<.001	120	67.7	5.4	173	60.6	4.8	1.7	.19
II. Mental disorders																
ADHD	249	0.7	0.1	59	0.2	0.0	45.7	<.001	81	29.9*	3.7	9	12.8	4.2	10.8	.001
Bipolar disorder	612	1.4	0.1	174	0.7	0.1	78.6	<.001	165	29.1*	2.0	23	13.4	3.4	9.4	.002
Depression	2,509	5.7	0.2	1,360	5.2	0.2	8.8	.003	737	29.3*	1.1	107	8.1	1.1	79.0	<.001
GAD	1,064	2.4	0.1	360	1.4	0.1	36.2	<.001	327	31.6*	1.8	22	7.2	1.9	33.1	<.001
IED	391	1.1	0.1	357	1.8	0.1	4.4	.037	71	16.7*	2.2	25	5.2	1.1	25.9	<.001
ODD	76	0.2	0.0	34	0.2	0.0	5.0	.025	24	33.4	7.5	2	13.5	10.8	2.7	.10
Panic disorder	685	1.6	0.1	211	0.7	0.1	72.0	<.001	212	33.1*	2.2	24	9.4	2.4	19.6	<.001
PTSD	962	2.3	0.1	211	0.9	0.1	59.4	<.001	284	29.5*	1.9	11	8.1	3.2	10.3	.001
Social phobia	1,621	4.1	0.1	419	1.9	0.1	133.2	<.001	342	20.8*	1.1	37	9.3	2.0	14.4	<.001
Specific phobia	2,643	6.9	0.2	829	3.4	0.2	142.1	<.001	394	13.2*	0.8	59	5.5	0.9	29.1	<.001

Note: Data obtained from administrative databases and registries estimate that the highest prevalence of cancer is in North America, with 1.5% of the population aged 15 years and older affected and diagnosed within the past 5 years, followed by Western Europe (1.2%), Australia and New Zealand (1.1%), Japan (1.0%), Eastern Europe (0.7%), Latin America and the Caribbean (0.4%), and the rest of the world (0.2%) (Pisani P et al. 2002). Although cancer survivors who were diagnosed and treated more than 5 years ago have the same survival as the general population, it is likely that the higher prevalence of self-reported cancer in the WMH Surveys than in these administrative databases reflects the fact that some long-term cancer survivors consider themselves still to have cancer.

[a] Number of respondents with the disorder.
[b] Number of cases in treatment.

ADHD, attention-deficit hyperactivity disorder; GAD, generalized anxiety disorder; IED, intermittent explosive disorder; ODD, oppositional-defiant disorder; PTSD, posttraumatic stress disorder.

* Significant difference between developed and developing at the .05 level, two-sided test.

Table 18.2. Disorder-specific global SDS ratings in developed and developing WMH countries (total sample)

	Mean disability ratings								Proportion rated severely disabled							
	Developed			Developing					Developed			Developing				
	N^a	Mean	SE	N^a	Mean	SE	c^2	p	N^b	%	SE	N^b	%	SE	c^2	p
I. Physical disorders
Arthritis	2,140	3.5	0.1	580	3.8	0.2	0.5	49	526	23.3	1.5	127	22.8	3.0	0.1	73
Asthma	1,040	1.9*	0.2	228	3.7	0.4	7.4	007	119	8.2*	1.4	44	26.9	5.4	9.0	003
Back/neck pain	2,602	4.8*	0.1	1,379	3.9	0.1	30.6	<.0001	912	34.6*	1.5	305	22.7	1.8	27.0	<.0001
Cancer	285	2.0	0.3	42	3.5	0.7	1.9	16	60	16.6	3.2	8	23.9	10.3	0.0	87
Chronic pain	685	5.2*	0.2	418	3.8	0.3	18.2	<.0001	296	40.9*	3.6	109	24.8	3.8	12.9	<.0001
Diabetes	408	2.1*	0.4	215	3.5	0.5	3.9	050	49	13.6	3.4	39	23.7	6.1	1.4	23
Headaches	1,709	5.4*	0.1	1,440	4.3	0.2	18.4	<.0001	751	42.1*	1.9	401	28.1	2.1	15.7	<.0001
Heart disease	396	3.3	0.3	319	3.8	0.4	0.3	59	83	26.5	3.9	63	27.8	5.2	0.3	56
High blood pressure	1,365	1.2*	0.1	797	3.5	0.2	74.9	<.0001	91	5.3*	0.9	144	23.8	2.6	50.0	<.0001
Ulcer	170	2.9	0.4	312	3.3	0.4	0.8	385	31	15.3	3.9	59	18.3	3.6	0.1	79
II. Mental disorders
ADHD	228	5.4	0.2	45	5.1	0.5	0.1	78	87	37.6	3.6	14	24.3	7.4	0.8	36
Bipolar disorder	588	7.4*	0.1	158	6.4	0.3	9.5	002	419	68.3*	2.6	87	52.1	4.9	7.9	005
Depression	1,536	7.1*	0.1	1,241	6.3	0.1	35.0	<.0001	1,028	65.8*	1.6	622	52.0	1.8	30.4	<.0001
GAD	1,002	6.6*	0.1	328	5.5	0.3	11.9	001	576	56.3*	1.9	127	42.0	4.2	7.9	005
IED	387	4.9	0.2	345	4.4	0.3	2.4	12	136	36.3	2.8	106	27.8	3.6	2.0	15
ODD	67	5.3	0.5	32	5.4	0.6	0.0	98	29	34.2	6.0	12	41.3	10.3	1.2	27
Panic disorder	641	5.8	0.2	189	5.2	0.4	2.9	09	317	48.4*	2.6	67	38.8	4.7	4.3	040
PTSD	571	6.5*	0.2	112	5.6	0.4	5.3	020	329	54.8*	2.8	53	41.2	7.3	4.2	040
Social phobia	1,621	5.0	0.1	419	5.4	0.2	2.1	15	593	35.1	1.4	164	41.4	3.6	2.6	11
Specific phobia	2,643	3.4	0.1	829	3.3	0.1	0.5	49	537	18.6	1.1	144	16.2	1.6	1.9	17

[a] Number of respondents with valid SDS scores for the randomly selected physical disorder or the mental disorder. Note that the numbers for physical disorder are substantially lower than those in Table 18.2 because the prevalence estimates in Table 18.2 were based on all respondents who reported the disorder, while the SDS scores were obtained only for the subsample of randomly selected physical disorders. The numbers for mental disorders in Table 18.3 are slightly lower than those in Table 18.2 because cases with missing values on SDS scores were omitted from Table 18.3, but not Table 18.2. Skip errors in the Western European surveys led to the number of cases with missing SDS scores being higher than would normally be expected based on t, respondent refusals, and interviewer recording errors.

[b] Number of cases rated severely disabled.

ADHD, attention-deficit hyperactivity disorder; GAD, generalized anxiety disorder; IED, intermittent explosive disorder; ODD, oppositional-defiant disorder; PTSD, posttraumatic stress disorder.

* Significant difference between developed and developing at the .05 level, two-sided test.

Table 18.3. Disorder-specific global SDS ratings for disorders in treatment in developed and developing WMH countries (treated cases only)

| | Mean disability ratings ||||||||| Proportion rated severely disabled |||||||||
| | Developed ||| Developing ||||| Developed |||| Developing ||||
	N^a	Mean	SE	N^a	Mean	SE	c^2	p	N^b	%	SE	N^b	%	SE	c^2	p
							I. Physical disorders								
Arthritis	1,127	4.8	0.2	229	4.5	0.2	1.1	.29	404	36.1	2.3	70	28.9	4.5	2.1	.15
Asthma	494	2.9	0.3	122	4.5	0.6	1.5	.22	94	13.6	2.8	32	35.5	7.6	2.5	.12
Back/neck pain	1,632	5.5*	0.1	548	4.5*	0.2	18.1	<.0001	707	42.5*	2.0	148	27.8*	2.9	20.0	<.0001
Cancer	165	3.0	0.5	26	4.7	0.8	2.1	.15	48	27.1	5.7	5	27.7	15.0	0.3	.60
Chronic pain	472	5.8*	0.2	217	4.3*	0.4	12.4	<.0001	242	47.2*	4.5	72	29.5	4.8	7.7	.006
Diabetes	373	2.2*	0.4	168	3.9*	0.6	6.8	.009	47	14.2	3.6	36	30.2	7.1	3.6	.06
Headaches	833	6.4*	0.2	677	4.9*	0.2	22.2	<.0001	449	53.5*	2.6	211	31.4*	3.0	17.6	<.0001
Heart disease	310	3.5*	0.3	171	5.0*	0.4	6.2	.01	73	27.3	4.2	48	41.1	6.9	1.4	.24
High blood pressure	1,194	1.2*	0.1	553	3.8*	0.2	62.6	<.0001	82	5.2*	1.0	102	27.4*	3.1	46.8	<.0001
Ulcer	120	3.0	0.5	173	3.7	0.6	0.2	.61	26	17.8	5.2	39	20.1	5.3	0.0	.93
							II. Mental disorders								
ADHD	78	6.2	0.4	6	6.0	0.6	1.2	.26	39	48.4	7.3	2	30.9	20.1	0.1	.75
Bipolar disorder	163	8.2	0.2	23	7.2	0.8	1.9	.17	133	80.6	4.1	15	72.7	11.3	0.6	.42
Depression	451	7.8	0.1	96	7.5	0.2	1.8	.19	346	76.8	2.5	59	73.6	4.8	1.4	.23
GAD	313	7.5	0.2	17	7.2	0.8	0.5	.47	223	71.7	2.9	12	71.1	12.8	0.1	.75
IED	69	5.5	0.4	25	6.8	0.8	0.5	.47	29	40.6	5.8	12	52.9	11.3	0.6	.44
ODD	22	5.4*	0.9	2	9.1*	0.2	16.4	<.0001	12	36.0	11.4	2	100.0	0.0	1.6	.20
Panic disorder	201	7.4	0.2	21	6.4	0.8	2.7	.10	147	73.9	3.4	12	65.1	12.1	1.2	.27
PTSD	209	7.2	0.2	5	4.3	2.6	1.4	.23	139	65.1	4.1	2	43.8	27.0	0.5	.47
Social phobia	342	6.0	0.2	37	6.5	0.7	0.0	.97	188	54.7	2.8	19	59.9	11.0	0.1	.74
Specific phobia	394	4.3*	0.2	59	3.0*	0.4	7.1	.008	122	31.4*	2.8	10	13.5*	4.5	4.3	.04

[a] Numbers of respondents with the disorder.
[b] Number of cases rated severely disabled.
ADHD, attention-deficit hyperactivity disorder; GAD, generalized anxiety disorder; IED, intermittent explosive disorder; ODD, oppositional-defiant disorder; PTSD, post-traumatic stress disorder.
* Significant difference between developed and developing countries at the .05 level, two-sided test.

Nearly all the comparisons in which disability was higher for psychological disorder than for physical disorder were statistically significant at the .05 level. Comparable results were obtained for severe disability ratings and also for both mean and severe disability ratings when respondent age, sex, and education were controlled. Similar results were obtained when analyses were limited to cases in treatment (data not shown).

Consistently higher mental than physical disability ratings were found in both developed and developing countries when individual SDS domains were considered rather than global ratings (Table 18.5). These differences were much more pronounced for disability in social life and personal relationships than for work or household management. For example, the proportions of severe disability in work functioning associated with mental disorders in developing and developed countries (19.4–21.7%, $n = 673$–2,135) were only slightly higher than the proportions associated with physical disorders (17.9–18.1%, $n = 874$–2,028). The proportions of severe disability in social functioning associated with mental disorders (21.8–28.0%, $n = 775$–2,758), in comparison, were dramatically higher than those associated with physical disorders (10.3–8.9%, $n = 513$–1,168). Similar patterns were found when mean disability ratings were compared. In addition, an attenuated version of the same general pattern holds when treated physical disorders were compared to all (i.e., treated or not) mental disorders to address the concern about the more superficial assessment of physical than mental disorders, possibly leading to inclusion of subthreshold cases of physical disorders that might have low disability (results not reported).

18.4. DISCUSSION

Four key findings emerged. First, respondents generally attributed more disability to mental than physical disorders. Second, the higher disability of the mental than physical disorders held equally in developing and developed countries. Third, the higher aggregate disability of mental than physical disorder was more pronounced for disability in social and personal relationships than in productive (work and housework) roles. Fourth, the proportion of cases in treatment at the time of interview was much lower for mental than physical disorders in developed countries and even more so in developing countries. This was true both overall and among cases rated severely disabled. These findings substantially extend results of prior research, none of which documented comparability in the disabilities associated with such a varied a set of physical and mental disorders or disaggregated disability into the domains considered here to detect the greater relative impact of mental than physical disorders in social–personal domains than productive role domains (Berto et al. 2000; Goetzel et al. 2003; Hays et al. 1995; Katschnig et al. 1997; Maetzel & Li 2002; Moussavi et al. 2007; Ormel et al. 1994, 1998; Reed et al. 2004; Spitzer et al. 1995; Sprangers et al. 2000; Verbrugge & Patrick 1995; Ware et al. 1986; Wells et al. 1989; Wells & Sherbourne 1999).

These results need to be interpreted with sampling and measurement limitations in mind. With regard to sampling, results could be influenced by a truncation of the severity spectrum of physical disorders. For example, people facing the end stage of chronic physical disease might be institutionalized or not willing or able to participate in an interview to a greater extent than people with severe mental disorders, leading to underestimation of the relative disability of physical compared to mental disorders. Whether such a difference in sample bias actually exists, though, is unknown. The physical conditions checklist did not include infectious diseases that are more prevalent in developing

Table 18.4. Pairwise differences in mean global SDS disability ratings for all mental–physical disorder pairs in developed and developing countries[a]

	ADHD	Bipolar disorder	Depression	GAD	IED	ODD	Panic disorder	PTSD	Social Phobia	Specific phobia
			I. Developed countries							
Arthritis	1.9*	3.9*	3.6*	3.1*	1.4*	1.8*	2.3*	3.0*	1.5*	−0.1
Asthma	3.5*	5.5*	5.2*	4.7*	3.0*	3.4*	3.9*	4.6*	3.1*	1.5*
Back/neck pain	0.6	2.6*	2.3*	1.8*	0.1	0.5	1.0*	1.7*	0.2	−1.4*
Cancer	3.4*	5.4*	5.1*	4.6*	2.9*	3.3*	3.8*	4.5*	3.0*	1.4*
Chronic pain	0.2	2.2*	1.9*	1.4*	−0.3*	0.1	0.6	1.3*	−0.2	−1.8*
Diabetes	3.3*	5.3*	5.0*	4.5*	2.8*	3.2*	3.7*	4.4*	2.9*	1.3*
Headaches	0.0	2.0*	1.7*	1.2*	−0.5*	−0.1	0.4	1.1*	−0.4*	−2.0*
Heart disease	2.1*	4.1*	3.8*	3.3*	1.6*	2.0*	2.5*	3.2*	1.7*	0.1
High blood pressure	4.2*	6.2*	5.9*	5.4*	3.7*	4.1*	4.6*	5.3*	3.8*	2.2*
Ulcer	2.5*	4.5*	4.2*	3.7*	2.0*	2.4*	2.9*	3.6*	2.1*	0.5
			II. Developing countries							
Arthritis	1.3*	2.6*	2.5*	1.7*	0.6	1.6*	1.4*	1.8*	1.6*	−0.5
Asthma	1.4*	2.7*	2.6*	1.8*	0.7*	1.7*	1.5*	1.9*	1.7*	0.4
Back/neck	1.2*	2.5*	2.4*	1.6*	0.5	1.5*	1.3*	1.7*	1.5*	0.6
Cancer	1.6*	2.9*	2.8*	2.0*	0.9	1.9*	1.7	2.1	1.9*	0.2
Chronic pain	1.3*	2.6*	2.5*	1.7*	0.6	1.6*	1.4*	1.8*	1.6*	0.5
Diabetes	1.6*	2.9*	2.8*	2.0*	0.9	1.9*	1.7*	2.1*	1.9*	0.2
Headaches	0.8*	2.1*	2.0*	1.2*	0.1	1.1*	0.9	1.3	1.1*	−1.0*
Heart disease	1.3*	2.6*	2.5*	1.7*	0.6	1.6*	1.4*	1.8*	1.6*	0.5
High blood pressure	1.6*	2.9*	2.8*	2.0*	0.9*	1.9*	1.7*	2.1*	1.9*	0.2
Ulcer	1.8*	3.1*	3.0*	2.2*	1.1*	2.1*	1.9*	2.3*	2.1*	0.0

[a] Each coefficient represents the difference in the mean global disability rating between the mental disorder in the column and the physical disorder in the row. A positive coefficient means that the mental disorder has a higher mean than the physical disorder.

ADHD, attention-deficit hyperactivity disorder; GAD, generalized anxiety disorder; IED, intermittent explosive disorder; ODD, oppositional-defiant disorder; PTSD, post-traumatic stress disorder.

* Significant physical–mental difference at the .05 level, two-sided test.

Table 18.5. SDS global and domain-specific ratings (proportion rated severely disabled) aggregated across physical (total and treated) and mental (total) disorders in developed and developing WMH countries

	Physical disorders			Treated physical disorders			Mental disorders			Physical vs. mental		Treated physical vs. mental	
	N^a	%	SE	N^a	%	SE	N^a	%	SE	χ^{2b}	p	χ^{2b}	p
					Global disability								
Developed	2918	23.8	0.7	2172	28.6	1.0	4051	41.3*	0.8	178.8	<.001	33.9	<.0001
Developing	1299	24.5	1.2	763	29.4	1.6	1396	37.6*	1.3	46.6	<.001	12.0	0005
χ^2		0.4			1.5			12.1					
p		55			22			001					
					Work disability								
Developed	2028	18.1	0.7	1546	22.4	1.0	2135	21.7*	0.7	0.8	38	14.4	0001
Developing	874	17.9	1.0	517	21.7	1.4	673	19.4*	0.9	1.4	24	0.7	41
χ^2		0.7			3.2			8.8					
p		40			07			003					
					Home disability								
Developed	2,146	17.8	0.6	1,608	21.3^{c,*}	0.9	2,011	19.9	0.7	0.6	44	10.7	001
Developing	881	16.7^c	1.0	517	19.8*	1.4	795	20.5^c	1.0	8.5	004	1.1	30
χ^2		2.0			5.0			0.1					
p		16			025			72					
					Social disability								
Developed	1,168	8.9^c	0.4	887	10.7^c	0.6	2,758	28.0*	0.8	393.6	<.001	187.2	<.0001
Developing	513	10.3^c	0.7	324	13.7^c	1.1	775	21.8*	1.0	67.9	<.001	17.4	<.0001
χ^2		0.0			0.1			27.5					
p		92			76			<.001					
					Close relations								
Developed	850	6.5^c	0.4	630	7.8^c	0.6	2,375	24.3*	0.7	428.0	<.001	213.2	<.0001
Developing	495	9.0^c	0.7	305	11.7^c	1.0	785	21.3*	1.1	105.3	<.001	34.2	<.0001
χ^2		2.8			2.2			7.9					
p		10			14			005					

^{a} Number of cases rated severely disabled.
^{b} Significant difference between physical and mental disorders at the .05 level, two-sided test.
^{c} The χ^2 and p values were calculated based on a multivariate model that controlled for sociodemographics. These significance tests are sometimes different from those based on bivariate associations.
* Significant difference between developed and developing at the .05 level, two-sided test.

than developed countries. Our results consequently can be generalized only to chronic cardiovascular, digestive, metabolic, musculoskeletal, pain, and respiratory conditions. Despite this limitation, the physical conditions considered are important sources of morbidity in developing as well as developed countries.

Another measurement problem was that the physical disorders were assessed by self-report rather than by abstracting medical records or administering medical examinations. Mental disorders were assessed more comprehensively with a fully structured lay-administered diagnostic interview. The more superficial assessment of physical disorders could have led to the inclusion of more sub-threshold cases than mental disorders, introducing an artificial lowering of the estimated disability of physical disorders, although this was addressed in the analysis of treated physical conditions. In addition, the use of a self-report checklist likely led to underestimation of undiagnosed silent physical conditions. As the latter are likely to be less disabling than symptom-based conditions or diagnosed silent conditions, though, this bias presumably increased the estimated disability of physical disorders.

Some of the WMH physical disorder prevalence estimates were lower than those based on gold-standard assessments. For example, the population prevalence of diabetes has been assessed in a number of community surveys using glucose tolerance tests from blood samples (e.g., King & Rewers 1993; Roglic et al. 2005). A meta-analysis of these studies suggests that the prevalence of diabetes is highest in North America (9.2%) and Europe (8.4%), lower in India and most of Latin America (5–8%), and lowest in most of Africa and China (2–5%) (International Diabetes Federation 2005). The WMH prevalence estimates, 4.6% in developed countries and 3.9% in developing countries, are lower than these gold-standard estimates, presumably reflecting the fact that the latter include undiagnosed cases.

In other cases, the WMH prevalence estimates were higher than those in gold-standard assessments. For example, cancer prevalence data have been assembled from various administrative databases and registries in a number of countries (Pisani, Bray, & Parkin 2002). Meta-analysis of these data suggest that cancer is much more common in developed than developing countries, with the highest prevalence in North America (1.5% of the population aged 15 years and older diagnosed within the past 5 years), followed by Western Europe (1.2%), Australia and New Zealand (1.1%), Japan (1.0%), Eastern Europe (0.7%), Latin America, and the Caribbean (0.4%), with a much lower estimated prevalence in the rest of the world (0.2%). The much higher cancer prevalence estimates in the WMH data, 4.0% in developed countries and 0.6% in developing countries, presumably reflect the fact that cancer survivors who were diagnosed and treated more than 5 years ago, although not counted in cancer prevalence estimates because they have the same survival rates as the general population, would have reported that they had been diagnosed by a doctor as having cancer.

Based on comparisons such as these with gold-standard assessments, caution is needed in interpreting the WMH prevalence estimates of physical disorders. However, the fact that the same general pattern of higher disability among mental than physical disorders held in comparisons of treated physical disorders argues strongly that the finding of higher SDS disability associated with mental rather than physical disorders is not due to imprecision in the measurement of physical disorders.

Another measurement problem involves the fact that disability was assessed with brief self-report scales rather than clinical evaluations. This might have introduced upward bias in the reported disability caused by mental disorders compared to physical disorders to the extent that people with mental disorders gave overly pessimistic appraisals of their functioning. This would seem to be an unlikely interpretation, though, in that the associations of SDS ratings with reported numbers of days out of role – a more objective indicator of disability than the SDS ratings – were found to be equivalent for mental and physical disorders. Furthermore, within-person comparison, which controlled for individual differences in perceptions, found similar results.

Another possibility is that the SDS questions might have been biased in the direction of assessing the disabilities associated with mental more than physical disorders. This would seem unlikely, though, as the SDS questions are quite broad and cover all the main areas of adult role functioning. Another possible limitation is that the SDS focused on the "worst month" in the past year, introducing recall error that possibly was more extreme for physical than mental disorders. In addition, between-disorder differences in persistence were not taken into consideration, which means that particular disorders might have been more dominant in severity ratings than suggested here if they were more persistently severe than others. The aggregate disability estimates should be interpreted cautiously due to these limitations regarding the recall period.

A final measurement problem concerning the assessment of disability relates to our use of a "condition-specific" measurement approach. This is an attractive approach from a statistical perspective in comparison to an unconditional measurement approach (i.e., an approach that simply assesses overall disability without asking the respondent to make inferences about the conditions that caused the disability). This approach produces condition-specific estimates directly, avoiding the need to rely on multivariate equations that adjust for the effects of comorbidity in predicting overall disability. This advantage in analytic simplicity, however, is achieved by requiring respondents with comorbid conditions to perform the potentially difficult task of making judgments about the effects of individual conditions on their functioning. Because of likely imprecision in these assessments, it would be useful to replicate the results reported here in multivariate analyses that evaluated the separate and joint effects of comorbid conditions in predicting an unconditional measure of disability. Unfortunately, the statistical methods needed to estimate models of this sort are complex (Merikangas et al. 2007).

Within the context of these limitations, the results reported here are consistent with previous comparative burden-of-illness studies in suggesting that musculoskeletal disorders and major depression are the disorders with the largest contribution to disability at the individual level both in developed and developing countries. Previous studies have documented this pattern only for the United States (Druss, Rosenheck, & Sledge 2000; Goetzel et al. 2003; Manuel, Schultz, & Kopec 2002; Wang et al. 2003), although the importance of depression has also been documented throughout the world in the World Health Surveys (WHS; Moussavi et al. 2007). The current report replicates the WHS results regarding depression and documents for the first time the cross-national importance of musculoskeletal disorders. As noted previously, the WMH results also suggest that mental disorders are especially disabling to personal relationships and social life, which implies that they are more disabling because they create psychological barriers than physical barriers to functioning. Among these barriers are limitations in cognitive and motivational capacities, affect regulation, embarrassment and stigma (Buist-Bouwman et al. 2005), and a tendency to amplify physical symptoms (Barsky et al. 1988) and associated disability (Kessler et al. 2003).

18.4.1. Mediators and Modifiers of the Disorder–Disability Relationship

Considerable progress has been made in understanding the relationship between psychopathology and disability, since the introduction of the International Classification of Impairments, Disabilities and Handicaps (ICIDH) in 1980 (World Health Organization 1980). The triad of impairment, disability, and handicap provided the framework for expanding disease concepts to include their impact on physical and psychosocial functioning. The ICIDH has recently been replaced by the International Classification of Functioning, Disability, and Health (ICF) in 2001 (World Health Organization 2001). Both classifications provide a common language that was issued by the WHO to study the consequences of disease. Their underlying principles as a classification of health-related functioning and disability are its (a) universality; that is, it is applicable to all people irrespective of country of origin; (b) parity; that is, there should not be a distinction between mental and physical health conditions; (c) neutrality; that is, classification can express both positive and negative aspects of functioning; and (d) the inclusion of contextual factors. Three levels of functioning are identified: (1) body and structures, for example, speech function, musculoskeletal function, and structure and functioning of the nervous system; (2) activities, for example, communication and mobility; and (3) participation, for example, work and social life. Disability as assessed by the SDS – which ask the respondent to indicate on a 1–100 scale to what extent a particular disorder "interfered with" activities in one of four role domains – refers largely to limitations in participation as defined by the ICF. Within the ICF model, body function, activities, and participation are viewed as a complex process in which pathology, personal characteristics, and context characteristics interact.

A better understanding of the pathways between psychopathology and participation could provide cues for reducing the burden of disease. The ICF asserts that a disorder may lead to activity limitations that, in turn, lead to participation restrictions. The activity limitations via which mental and physical disorders cause limitations in participation are likely to differ. Physical disorders may produce participation restrictions because of limitations in physical capacities such as mobility, vision, aerobic capacity, lower and upper body strength, manual dexterity, and incontinence, whereas mental disorders may produce participation restrictions via cognitive and motivational capacities, affect regulation, social perception, and a tendency to amplify physical symptoms such as fatigue and pain. Treatment may benefit from insight into which activity limitations mediate effects on participation of which disorders.

The association between mental disorder and disability is strong but there is considerable heterogeneity in the functional status of persons with the same mental disorder. Many people with a mental disorder function at a high level, whereas others are significantly impaired. This raises the question of what environmental factors and person characteristics dampen or enhance the impact of psychopathology on disability. Such knowledge may help enhance the effectiveness of treatments for mental illness itself, in addition to possible benefits for disability outcomes.

18.4.2. Treatment Implications

Given this greater disability of mental than physical disorders, it is disturbing to find that only a minority of even severe cases of mental disorder receive treatment and that treatment was substantially more common among comparably severe physical disorders. In developed countries, seriously disabling mental disorders were only about half as likely to be treated as seriously disabling physical disorders (35.3% vs. 77.6%), while they were about only 20% as likely to be treated as comparably severe physical disorders in developing countries (11.9% vs. 63.6%). This low treatment rate is consistent with the low rate of recognition and treatment of mental disorders in primary care, especially if comorbid with physical disorders (Thompson et al. 2000; Tiemens et al. 1999; Ustun & Sartorius 1995). In combination with the burden of disability that mental disorders produce, the low treatment rates call for more attention to mental disorders.

Implications of the WMH findings for treatment are not clear because, even though treatment effectiveness trials document that common anxiety and mood disorders can often be successfully treated (Hyman et al. 2006; Nathan & Gorman 1998), uncertainties exist regarding long-term outcomes. In particular, long-term functional outcomes are important to track because residual disability and recurrence are major problems with chronic mental disorders (Ormel et al. 2004). Another limitation of existing trials is that they typically focused on symptoms and did little to assess the effects of treatment on reduced disability (Hyman et al. 2006; Nathan & Gorman 1998), notwithstanding some notable exceptions that suggest that effective treatment of depression improves functional outcomes (Coulehan et al. 1997; Katzelnick, Simon, & Pearson 2000; Mintz et al. 1992; Mynors-Wallis et al. 1995). Despite this uncertainty about long-term outcomes, though, the results reported here strongly argue that, on the basis of population disease burden associated with disorder-specific disability, more attention should be given to the treatment of mental disorders and that this is especially so in developing countries.

18.4.3. Future Directions

A promising direction for further research rests on conceptualizing disability in terms of social role performance. We lack insight into the development and course of the behavioral effects of mental disorders on social roles. Is there a hierarchical structure in the impairment of social roles? Work on severe mental illness suggests that social activities and family roles are the first to become impaired, followed by work role, and finally the self-care role (Wiersma, DeJong, & Ormel 1988). Does loss and recovery of social role performance follow the reverse pattern? We also know little about the lag times between onset and remission of mental disorders and associated social role disabilities.

The evidence that disability due to physical conditions is a risk factor for the onset of anxiety and depression raises intriguing questions regarding bidirectional effects between mental disorders and disability. To what extent does disability, triggered by physical conditions, propel the onset and maintenance of depression? Recently, we examined the reciprocal effects between depressive symptoms and functional disability and their temporal character in a multiwave community-based cohort of 753 older people with physical limitations (Ormel et al. 2002). We compared structural equation models that differed in terms of direction and speed of effects between patient-reported disability in activities of daily living (ADLs) and depressive symptoms. The association between disability and depression could be separated into three components: (1) a strong contemporaneous effect of change in disability on depressive symptoms, (2) a weaker 1-year lagged effect of change in depressive symptoms on disability (probably indirect via physical health), and (3) a weak correlation between the trait (or stable) components of depression and disability. These results were remarkably similar to the findings of Aneshensel et al. (1984) in a younger but unselected sample. Further research on the complex, possibly multidirectional, effects among physical disease, mental disorder, and social role functioning is needed.

Another aspect of the association between mental disorders and functional limitations that remains ambiguous is the amount of residual disability after remission of the disorder. Some authors reported that mean disability levels returned to normal levels among patients who had recovered from a major depressive episode (e.g., Ormel et al. 1993; Von Korff et al. 1992), while others found evidence of scarring, that is, persistent disability after remission of the mental disorder (Coryell et al. 1993; Judd et al. 2000; Wells et al. 1989). Recently, a large multiwave psychiatric epidemiologic survey in 4,796 Dutch adults from the general population who completed three measurement waves in a period of 3 years found evidence of trait and state effects as well, but not scar effects. Major depression episodes had temporary (*state*) but not enduring (*scar*) effects on self-reported role functioning (Ormel et al. 2004). According to the authors, the findings are best explained by synchrony of change between depression and role functioning, superimposed on trait vulnerability that expresses itself in, among others, premorbid role dysfunction. The scarring reported in previous studies may well reflect trait vulnerability and residual symptom effects. Nonetheless, the issue of residual disability remains controversial.

18.4.4. Public Health and the Organization of Health Care

Although understanding of the causal relationships between mental disorder and disability is far from perfect, there is now substantial evidence that effective treatment of mental disorder reduces social role disability, at least for depression. The public health challenge is now to organize health care systems so that they are capable of delivering effective treatment to all persons with depressive illness in the population that need treatment. Effective treatments are not sufficient; we also need effective health care systems capable of disseminating those treatments on a population basis (Wagner, Austin, & VonKorff 1996). Beyond that, there remains an urgent need for greater understanding of the mechanisms and effective management of disability due to mental disorders than currently exists.

18.5. CONCLUSIONS

Four key findings emerged from the aforementioned analyses. First, respondents generally attributed more disability to their mental than physical disorders. Second, the higher disability of the mental than physical disorders held as strongly in developing as in developed countries. Third, the higher aggregate disability of mental than physical disorder was much more pronounced for disability in social and personal relationships than in productive (work and housework) roles. Fourth, the proportion of cases in treatment at the time of interview was much lower for mental than physical disorders in developed countries and even more so in developing countries both in the total sample and when we focused exclusively on cases rated severely disabling.

Given this greater disability of mental than physical disorders, it is disturbing to find that only a minority of even severe cases of mental disorder receive treatment and that treatment was substantially more common among comparably severe physical disorders. In combination with the burden of disability that mental disorders produce, the low treatment rates call for more attention to mental disorders.

ACKNOWLEDGMENT

Some material in this chapter appeared in Ormel et al. (2008). This material is reprinted with the permission of the *British Journal of Psychiatry*.

REFERENCES

American Psychiatric Association. (1994). *Diagnostic and Statistical Manual of Mental Disorders (DSM-IV)*, 4th ed. Washington, DC: American Psychiatric Association.

Andrews, G., Henderson, S., & Hall, W. (2001). Prevalence, comorbidity, disability and service utilisation. Overview of the Australian National Mental Health Survey. *British Journal of Psychiatry*, **178**, 145–53.

Aneshensel, C. S., Frerichs, R. R., & Huba, G. J. (1984). Depression and physical illness: A multiwave, nonrecursive causal model. *Journal of Health and Social Behavior*, **25**, 350–71.

Baker, M., Stabile, M., & Deri, C. (2001). What do self-reported, objective, measures of health measure? *Journal of Human Resources*, **39**, 1067–193.

Barsky, A. J., Goodson, J. D., Lane, R. S., & Cleary, P. D. (1988). The amplification of somatic symptoms. *Psychosomatic Medicine*, **50**, 510–19.

Bergmann, M. M., Byers, T., Freedman, D. S., & Mokdad, A. (1998). Validity of self-reported diagnoses leading to hospitalization: A comparison of self-reports with hospital records in a prospective study of American adults. *American Journal of Epidemiology*, **147**, 969–77.

Bertani, A., Perna, G., Migliarese, G., Di Pasquale, D., Cucchi, M., Caldirola, D., & Bellodi, L. (2004). Comparison of the treatment with paroxetine and reboxetine in panic disorder: A randomized, single-blind study. *Pharmacopsychiatry*, **37**, 206–10.

Berto, P., D'Ilario, D., Ruffo, P., Di Virgilio, R., & Rizzo, F. (2000). Depression: Cost-of-illness studies in the international literature: A review. *Journal of Mental Health Policy and Economics*, **3**, 3–10.

Bijl, R. V., & Ravelli, A. (2000). Current and residual functional disability associated with psychopathology: Findings from the Netherlands Mental Health Survey and Incidence Study (NEMESIS). *Psychological Medicine*, **30**, 657–68.

Buist-Bouwman, M. A., de Graaf, R., Vollebergh, W. A., & Ormel, J. (2005). Comorbidity of physical and mental disorders and the effect on workloss days. *Acta Psychiatrica Scandinavica*, **111**, 436–43.

Centers for Disease Control and Prevention. (2004). *Health*. United States: Center for Disease Control.

Connor, K. M., & Davidson, J. R. (2001). SPRINT: A brief global assessment of post-traumatic stress disorder. *International Clinical Psychopharmacology*, **16**, 279–84.

Coryell, W., Scheftner, W., Keller, M., Endicott, J., Maser, J., & Klerman, G. L. (1993). The enduring psychosocial consequences of mania and depression. *American Journal of Psychiatry*, **150**, 720–7.

Coulehan, J. L., Schulberg, H. C., Block, M. R., Madonia, M. J., & Rodriguez, E. (1997). Treating depressed primary care patients improves their physical, mental, and social functioning. *Archives of Internal Medicine*, **157**, 1113–20.

Davidson, J., Yaryura-Tobias, J., DuPont, R., Stallings, L., Barbato L. M., Van Der Hoop, R. G., & Li, D. (2004). Fluvoxamine-controlled release formulation for the treatment of generalized social anxiety disorder. *Journal of Clinical Psychopharmacology*, **24**, 118–25.

Druss, B. G., Rosenheck, R. A., & Sledge, W. H. (2000). Health and disability costs of depressive illness in a major U.S. corporation. *American Journal of Psychiatry*, **157**, 1274–8.

Goetzel, R. Z., Hawkins, K., Ozminkowski, R. J., & Wang, S. (2003). The health and productivity cost burden of the "top 10" physical and mental health conditions affecting six large U.S. employers in 1999. *Journal of Occupational and Environmental Medicine*, **45**, 5–14.

Hambrick, J. P., Turk, C. L., Heimberg, R. G., Schneier, F. R., & Liebowitz, M. R. (2004).

Psychometric properties of disability measures among patients with social anxiety disorder. *Journal of Anxiety Disorders*, 18, 825–39.

Haro, J. M., Arbabzadeh-Bouchez, S., Brugha, T. S., de Girolamo, G., Guyer, M. E., Jin, R., Lepine, J. P., Mazzi, F., Reneses, B., Vilagut, G., Sampson, N. A., & Kessler, R. C. (2006). Concordance of the Composite International Diagnostic Interview Version 3.0 (CIDI 3.0) with standardized clinical assessments in the WHO World Mental Health Surveys. *International Journal of Methods in Psychiatric Research*, 15, 167–80.

Hays, R. D., Wells, K. B., Sherbourne, C. D., Rogers, W., & Spritzer, K. (1995). Functioning and well-being outcomes of patients with depression compared with chronic general medical illnesses. *Archives of General Psychiatry*, 52, 11–19.

Hudson, J. I., Perahia, D. G., Gilaberte, I., Wang, F., Watkin, J. G., & Detke, M. J. (2007). Duloxetine in the treatment of major depressive disorder: An open-label study. *BMC Psychiatry*, 7, 43.

Hyman, S., Chisholm, D., Kessler, R. C., Patel, V., & Whiteford, H. (2006). Mental disorders. In *Disease Control Priorities in Developing Countries*, ed. D. T. Jamison, J. G. Breman, A. R. Measham, G. Alleyne, M. Claeson, D. B. Evans, P. Jha, A. Mills, & P. Musgrove, pp. 605–625. New York: Oxford University Press.

International Diabetes Federation. (2005). *2005 Diabetes Atlas*, 3rd ed. Brussels: International Diabetes Federation.

Judd, L. L., Akiskal, H. S., Zeller, P. J., Paulus, M., Leon, A. C., Maser, J. D., Endicott, J., Coryell, W., Kunovac, J. L., Mueller, T. I., Rice, J. P., & Keller, M. B. (2000). Psychosocial disability during the long-term course of unipolar major depressive disorder. *Archives of General Psychiatry*, 57, 375–80.

Katschnig, H., Freeman, H., & Sartorius, N. (1997). *Quality of Life in Mental Disorders*. Chichester, England: John Wiley and Sons.

Katzelnick, D. J., Simon, G. E., & Pearson, S. D. (2000). Randomized trial of a depression management program in high utilizers of medical care. *Archives of Family Medicine*, 9, 345–51.

Kessler, R. C., Bergland, P., Chiu, W. T., Demler, O., Heeringa, S., Hiripi, E., Jin, R., Pennell, B.-E., Walters, E. E., Zaslavsky, A., & Zheng, H. (2004). The US National Comorbidity Survey Replication (NCS-R): Design and field procedures. *International Journal of Methods in Psychiatric Research*, 13, 69–92.

Kessler, R. C., Chiu, W. T., Demler, O., Merikangas, K. R., & Walters, E. E. (2005). Prevalence, severity, and comorbidity of 12-month DSM-IV disorders in the National Comorbidity Survey Replication. *Archives of General Psychiatry*, 62, 617–27.

Kessler, R. C., & Frank, R. G. (1997). The impact of psychiatric disorders on work loss days. *Psychological Medicine*, 27, 861–73.

Kessler, R. C., Ormel, J., Demler, O., & Stang, P. E. (2003). Comorbid mental disorders account for the role impairment of commonly occurring chronic physical disorders: Results from the National Comorbidity Survey. *Journal of Occupational and Environmental Medicine*, 45, 1257–66.

Kessler, R. C., & Ustun, T. B. (2004). The World Mental Health (WMH) survey initiative version of the World Health Organization (WHO) Composite International Diagnostic Interview (CIDI). *International Journal of Methods in Psychiatric Research*, 13, 93–121.

King, H., & Rewers, M. (1993). Global estimates for prevalence of diabetes mellitus and impaired glucose tolerance in adults. WHO Ad Hoc Diabetes Reporting Group. *Diabetes Care*, 16, 157–77.

Kish, L., & Frankel, M. R. (1974). Inferences from complex samples. *Journal of the Royal Statistical Society*, 36, 1–37.

Knight, M., Stewart-Brown, S., & Fletcher, L. (2001). Estimating health needs: The impact of a checklist of conditions and quality of life measurement on health information derived from community surveys. *Journal of Public Health Medicine*, 23, 179–86.

Kriegsman, D. M., Penninx, B. W., van Eijk, J. T., Boeke, A. J., & Deeg, D. J. (1996). Self-reports and general practitioner information on the presence of chronic diseases in community dwelling elderly. A study on the accuracy of patients' self-reports and on determinants of inaccuracy. *Journal of Clinical Epidemiology*, 49, 1407–17.

Leon, A. C., Olfson, M., Portera, L., Farber, L., & Sheehan, D. V. (1997). Assessing psychiatric impairment in primary care with the Sheehan Disability Scale. *International Journal of Psychiatry in Medicine*, 27, 93–105.

Maetzel, A., & Li, L. (2002). The economic burden of low back pain: A review of studies published between 1996 and 2001. *Best Practice and Research Clinical Rheumatology*, 16, 23–30.

Manuel, D. G., Schultz, S. E., & Kopec, J. A. (2002). Measuring the health burden of chronic disease and injury using health adjusted life expectancy and the Health Utilities Index. *Journal of Epidemiology and Community Health*, **56**, 843–50.

Merikangas, K. R., Ames, M., Cui, L., Stang, P. E., Ustun, T. B., Von Korff, M., & Kessler, R. C. (2007). The impact of comorbidity of mental and physical conditions on role disability in the US adult household population. *Archives of General Psychiatry*, **64**, 1180–8.

Mintz, J., Mintz, L. I., Arruda, M. J., & Hwang, S. S. (1992). Treatments of depression and the functional capacity to work. *Archives of General Psychiatry*, **49**, 761–8.

Moussavi, S., Chatterji, S., Verdes, E., Tandon, A., Patel, V., & Ustun, B. (2007). Depression, chronic diseases, and decrements in health: Results from the World Health Surveys. *Lancet*, **370**, 851–8.

Murray, C. J. L., & Lopez, A. D. (1996). *The Global Burden of Disease: A Comprehensive Assessment of Mortality and Disability from Diseases, Injuries and Risk Factors in 1990 and Projected to 2020*. Cambridge, MA: Harvard University Press.

Mynors-Wallis, L., Gath, D. H., Lloyd-Thomas, A. R., & Tomlinson, D. (1995). Randomised controlled trial comparing problem solving treatment with amitriptyline and placebo for major depression in primary care. *British Medical Journal*, **310**, 441–5.

Nathan, P. E., & Gorman, J. M. (1998). *A Guide to Treatment That Works*. Oxford: Oxford University Press.

National Center for Health Statistics. (1994). Evaluation of National Health Interview Survey diagnostic reporting. *Vital Health Statistics 2*, **120**, 1–116.

Ormel, J., Kempen, G. I., Deeg, D. J., Brilman, E. I., van Sonderen, E., & Relyveld, J. (1998). Functioning, well-being, and health perception in late middle-aged and older people: Comparing the effects of depressive symptoms and chronic medical conditions. *Journal of the American Geriatrics Society*, **46**, 39–48.

Ormel, J., Oldehinkel, A. J., Nolen, W. A., & Vollebergh, W. (2004). Psychosocial disability before, during, and after a major depressive episode: A 3-wave population-based study of state, scar, and trait effects. *Archives of General Psychiatry*, **61**, 387–92.

Ormel, J., Petukhova, M., Chatterji, S., Aguilar-Gaxiola, S., Alonso, J., Angermeyer, M. C., Bromet, E. J., Burger, H., Demyttenaere, K., de Girolamo, G., Haro, J. M., Hwang, I., Karam, E., Kawakami, N., Lépine, J. P., Medina-Mora, M. E., Posada-Villa, J., Sampson, N., Scott, K., Üstün, T. B., Von Korff, M., Williams, D. R., Zhang, M., & Kessler, R. C. (2008). Disability and treatment of specific mental disorders across the world. *The British Journal of Psychiatry*, **192**, 368–75.

Ormel, J., Rijsdijk, F. V., Sullivan, M., van Sonderen, E., & Kempen, G. I. (2002). Temporal and reciprocal relationship between IADL/ADL disability and depressive symptoms in late life. *Journal of Gerontology*, **57B**, 338–47.

Ormel, J., VonKorff, M., Ustun, T. B., Pini, S., Korten, A., & Oldehinkel, T. (1994). Common mental disorders and disability across cultures. Results from the WHO Collaborative Study on Psychological Problems in General Health Care. *The Journal of the American Medical Association*, **272**, 1741–8.

Ormel, J., Von Korff, M., Van Den Brink, W., Katon, W., Brilman, E., & Oldehinkel, T. (1993). Depression, anxiety, and social disability show synchrony of change in primary care patients. *American Journal of Public Health*, **83**, 385–90.

Pallanti, S., Bernardi, S., & Quercioli, L. (2006). The Shorter PROMIS Questionnaire and the Internet Addiction Scale in the assessment of multiple addictions in a high-school population: Prevalence and related disability. *CNS Spectrum*, **11**, 966–74.

Pisani, P., Bray, F., & Parkin, D. M. (2002). Estimates of the world-wide prevalence of cancer for 25 sites in the adult population. *International Journal of Cancer*, **97**, 72–81.

Reed, S. D., Lee, T. A., & McCrory, D. C. (2004). The economic burden of allergic rhinitis: A critical evaluation of the literature. *Pharmacoeconomics*, **22**, 345–61.

Reijneveld, S. A., & Stronks, K. (2001). The validity of self-reported use of health care across socioeconomic strata: A comparison of survey and registration data. *International Journal of Epidemiology*, **30**, 1407–14.

Roglic, G., Unwin, N., Bennett, P. H., Mathers, C., Tuomilehto, J., Nag, S., Connolly, V., & King, H. (2005). The burden of mortality attributable to diabetes: Realistic estimates for the year 2000. *Diabetes Care*, **28**, 2130–5.

Schoenborn, C. A., Adams, P. F., & Schiller, J. S. (2003). Summary health statistics for the U.S. population: National Health Interview Survey, 2000. *Vital Health Statistics*, **10**, 1–83.

Spitzer, R. L., Kroenke, K., Linzer, M., Hahn, S. R., Williams, J. B., deGruy, F. V., III, Brody, D., & Davies, M. (1995). Health-related quality of life in primary care patients with mental disorders. Results from the PRIME-MD 1000 Study. *The Journal of the American Medical Association*, 274, 1511–17.

Sprangers, M. A., de Regt, E. B., Andries, F., van Agt, H. M., Bijl, R. V., de Boer, J. B., Foets, M., Hoeymans, N., Jacobs, A. E., Kempen, G. I., Miedema, H. S., Tijhuis, M. A., & deHaes H. C. (2000). Which chronic conditions are associated with better or poorer quality of life? *Journal of Clinical Epidemiology*, 53, 895–907.

Thompson, C., Kinmonth, A. L., Stevens, L., Peveler, R. C., Stevens, A., Ostler, K. J., Pickering, R. M., Baker, N. G., Henson, A., Preece, J., Cooper, D., & Campbell, M. J. (2000). Effects of a clinical-practice guideline and practice-based education on detection and outcome of depression in primary care: Hampshire Depression Project randomised controlled trial. *Lancet*, 355, 185–91.

Tiemens, B. G., Ormel, J., Jenner, J. A., Van Der Meer, K., Van Os, T. W., Van Den Brink, R. H., Smit, A., & Van DenBrink, W. (1999). Training primary-care physicians to recognize, diagnose and manage depression: Does it improve patient outcomes? *Psychological Medicine*, 29, 833–45.

Tylee, A., Gastpar, M., Lepine, J. P., & Mendlewicz, J. (1999). DEPRES II: A patient survey of the symptoms, disability and current management of depression in the community. *International Clinical Psychopharmacology*, 3, 139–51.

Ustun, T. B., & Sartorius, N. (1995). *Mental Illness in General Health Care: An International Study.* New York: John Wiley and Sons.

Verbrugge, L. M., & Patrick, D. L. (1995). Seven chronic conditions: Their impact on US adults' activity levels and use of medical services. *American Journal of Public Health*, 85, 173–82.

Von Korff, M., Ormel, J., Katon, W., & Lin, E. H. B. (1992). Disability and depression in medical patients: A longitudinal analysis. *Archives of General Psychiatry*, 49, 91–100.

Wagner, E. H., Austin, B. T., & VonKorff, M. (1996). Organizing care for patients with chronic illness. *The Milbank Quarterly*, 74, 511–44.

Wang, P. S., Beck, A., Berglund, P., Leutzinger, J. A., Pronk, N., Richling, D., Schenk, T. W., Simon, G., Stang, P., Ustun. T. B., & Kessler, R. C. (2003) Chronic medical conditions and work performance in the health and work performance questionnaire calibration surveys. *Journal of Occupational and Environmental Medicine*, 45, 1303–11.

Ware, J. E., Jr., Brook, R. H., Rogers, W. H., Keeler, E. B., Davies, A. R., Sherbourne, C. D., Goldberg, G. A., Camp, P., & Newhouse, J. P. (1986). Comparison of health outcomes at a health maintenance organisation with those of fee-for-service care. *Lancet*, 1, 1017–22.

Wells, K. B., & Sherbourne, C. D. (1999). Functioning and utility for current health of patients with depression or chronic medical conditions in managed, primary care practices. *Archives of General Psychiatry*, 56, 897–904.

Wells, K. B., Stewart, A., Hays, R. D., Burnham, A., Rogers, W., Daniels, M., Berry, S., Greenfield, S., & Ware, J. (1989). The functioning and well-being of depressed patients. *The Journal of the American Medical Association*, 262, 914–19.

Wiersma, D., DeJong, A., & Ormel, J. (1988). The Groningen Social Disabilities Schedule: Development, relationship with I.C.I.D.H., and psychometric properties. *International Journal of Rehabilitation Research*, 11, 213–24.

World Bank. (2003). *World Development Indicators 2003.* Washington, DC: The World Bank.

World Health Organization. (1980). *International Classification of Impairments, Disabilities and Handicaps.* Geneva, Switzerland: World Health Organization.

World Health Organization. (2001). *International Classification of Functioning, Disability and Health: ICF.* Geneva: World Health Organization.

19 The Joint Association of Mental and Physical Conditions with Disability

KATE M. SCOTT

19.1. INTRODUCTION

We now know that disability is a common consequence of both physical and mental disorders. Those studies that have assessed the relative level of disability associated with physical and mental conditions have found mental disorders to be at least as disabling as common chronic physical conditions (Armenian et al. 1998; Hays et al. 1995; Ormel et al. 1998; Wells et al. 1989b). But we also know that mental and physical disorders co-occur at greater than chance levels (Buist-Bouwman et al. 2005a; Dew 1998; Scott et al. 2007; Wells, Golding, & Burnam 1989a), and this raises an important question: What is the nature of the joint impact of mental and physical conditions on disability? Is it the case that the disability associated with each condition adds together so that an individual with mental–physical comorbidity is doubly disabled relative to an individual with just one condition? Or, does the overlap in some symptoms between mental and physical conditions mean that their combination does not have an additive effect on disability? A third possibility, and the most concerning from a clinical point of view, is that the presence of one condition (say, mental disorder) exacerbates the effect of the other (the physical condition) on disability. In this third scenario, the joint effect of mental–physical comorbidity on disability would be greater than the sum of the individual effects.

Analytically, these different possibilities are expressed in terms of the distinction between "additive" and "interactive" models of comorbidity (Schettini & Frank 2004). An additive model of mental–physical comorbidity would suggest that mental and physical conditions have independent effects on functioning which add together when they occur jointly, so the combined effect is approximately equal to the sum of the parts. An interactional model suggests that comorbidity is associated with significantly greater (or lesser) levels of dysfunction than predicted by a simple sum of the disabling effects of the individual disorders.

Some studies have researched the joint effects of mental and physical disorder on disability and found them to be greater than the effects of either condition alone, but have not investigated whether the nature of the joint effect is additive or interactive (Druss et al. 2000; Sareen et al. 2006). Of the research that has distinguished between additive and interactive models, some has concluded that mental and physical conditions have mostly additive effects on disability (Buist-Bouwman et al. 2005b; Ormel et al. 1998; Stein et al. 2006; Wells et al. 1989a). But other research has found interactive (synergistic) effects of mental and physical conditions (Kessler et al. 2001, 2003; Egede 2004; Schmitz et al. 2007). Adding to the variability in results, a recent study by Merikangas et al. (2007) observed a number of significant interactions between mental and physical conditions in predicting days out of role that were nearly all negative.

There is a statistical issue that may be part of the explanation for the divergent findings from prior research. Researchers in this area typically use either linear regression or logistic regression modeling to analyze their data. Linear regression models the influence of multiple variables on an additive scale, and interaction effects are therefore assessed in terms of whether the combined effect of variables is significantly greater or lesser than the added individual effects. Logistic regression by contrast uses a multiplicative scale, so interaction effects are modeled in terms of whether the combined effect of variables is significantly greater or lesser than the multiplied individual effects. The underlying model of how mental and physical disorders might combine is considered to be additive (Ahlbom & Alfredsson 2005), and the interaction of mental and physical disorders should therefore be assessed as a departure from additivity, not multiplicativity (Ahlbom & Alfredsson 2005; Andersson et al. 2005). The use of logistic regression is more likely to result in no interactions or negative interactions relative to using linear regression, unless the logistic regression analyses are modified to assess interaction on an additive scale (Ahlbom & Alfredsson 2005; Andersson et al. 2005; Schmitz et al. 2007). In this study on the World Mental Health (WMH) Surveys, we used such a modified logistic regression approach.

Four groups were compared in terms of their association with disability: those with mental disorder in the absence of a given physical disorder; those with physical disorder in the absence of mental disorder; those with both; and those with neither. Six common physical conditions were investigated: arthritis, heart disease, respiratory disease, chronic back or neck pain, chronic headache, and diabetes. The mental disorders investigated included those in the depressive–anxiety spectrum. The objective was to ascertain whether the joint effect of mental and physical conditions on the probability of severe disability was greater than, lesser than, or approximately equal to the sum of the individual effects.

19.2. APPROACH

19.2.1. Mental Disorder Status

This study includes 12-month anxiety disorders (generalized anxiety disorder, panic disorder and/or agoraphobia, posttraumatic stress disorder, and social phobia) and depressive disorders (dysthymia and major depressive disorder). Anxiety and depressive disorders were aggregated into a single category on the basis of prior findings from the WMH Surveys that anxiety disorders and depressive disorders have equal and independent relationships with a wide range of chronic physical conditions (Scott et al. 2007).

19.2.2. Disability

Disability was assessed with the WMH Survey version of the World Health Organization Disability Assessment Schedule (WHODAS-II), referred to here as the WMH WHODAS. This instrument assesses disability in several domains: role impairment, mobility, self-care, social functioning, and cognitive functioning, and was administered as a generic section to all participants in the part 2 subsample, asking about disability in the past 30 days attributable to health – emotional or mental health – problems. More detail on the WMH WHODAS is provided elsewhere (Scott et al. 2006; Von Korff et al. 2008). In addition to domain scores, a global score can be calculated as an aggregation of domain scores; the global score is used in this chapter. Higher scores (on a 0–100 scale) indicate greater disability. Due to the pronounced skew in the

WHODAS distribution, it was dichotomized for the current analyses, defined as a score on or above the 90th percentile of the WMH WHODAS distribution in each country (i.e., capturing the most disabled 10% of the population). This was done in order to ensure that the presence of disability in this chapter would indicate those with more clinically relevant impairment.

19.2.3. Analysis Methods

The prevalence of a WMH WHODAS score on or above the 90th percentile was calculated for those with a given physical condition (in the absence of mental disorder), for those with mental disorder (in the absence of the physical condition), for those with both mental disorder and the physical condition, and for those with neither, on a country-by-country basis. These prevalence estimates do not control for age and sex differences across the disorder groups. The country-specific results for two of the physical conditions (back or neck pain and heart disease) are shown here, which are indicative of the results for all the physical conditions.

Analyses assessing the interaction of mental disorder and a given physical condition were carried out on the pooled data set (i.e., all countries combined). For the (additive) interaction tests, the two risk factors (mental disorder and a physical condition) were coded into three dummy variables (Andersson et al. 2005): (1) those with mental disorder in the absence of the physical condition (MD); (2) those with a given physical condition in the absence of mental disorder (PC); (3) those with both mental disorder and the physical condition (MD + PC). The group with neither mental disorder nor the physical condition was the common reference category. These dummy variables were entered simultaneously into logistic regression models on the pooled WMH data set, predicting a WMH WHODAS score on or above the 90th percentile, controlling for age, sex, and education (with the exception that France did not collect information on education). A separate model was run for each of the six physical conditions. We assessed whether odds of disability for MD + PC were significantly greater than, lesser than, or equal to the sum of the separate odds for MD and PC. The results from these analyses are expressed as a "synergy index" (SI), adopting the following formula: $SI = [OR_{MD+PC} - 1]/[(OR_{MD} - 1) + (OR_{PC} - 1)]$. If there is no additive interaction, $SI = 1$, and a value greater than 1 indicates a positive synergistic effect (Andersson et al. 2005).

19.3. FINDINGS

19.3.1. Disability Prevalence – Country-Specific Results

Results for two conditions (back or neck pain and heart disease) are shown in Figures 19.1 and 19.2. Two features stand out from the figures. First, generally speaking, those without either the physical or the mental condition were least likely to be represented among the most disabled 10%, while those with both mental disorder and back or neck pain were most likely to be among the most disabled. These results were not adjusted for age and sex, and given that mental disorders decrease with age and physical conditions increase with age, this means that the distinction between the four groups in terms of their disability status is not as clear-cut as it would be with age adjustment.

The second characteristic feature of these figures is that there is a good deal of variability across countries. Although there are likely to be some substantive reasons for this, it is also partly a function of the fact that some of the surveys had quite low prevalence of mental disorders, and so smaller numbers still in the group with both physical and mental

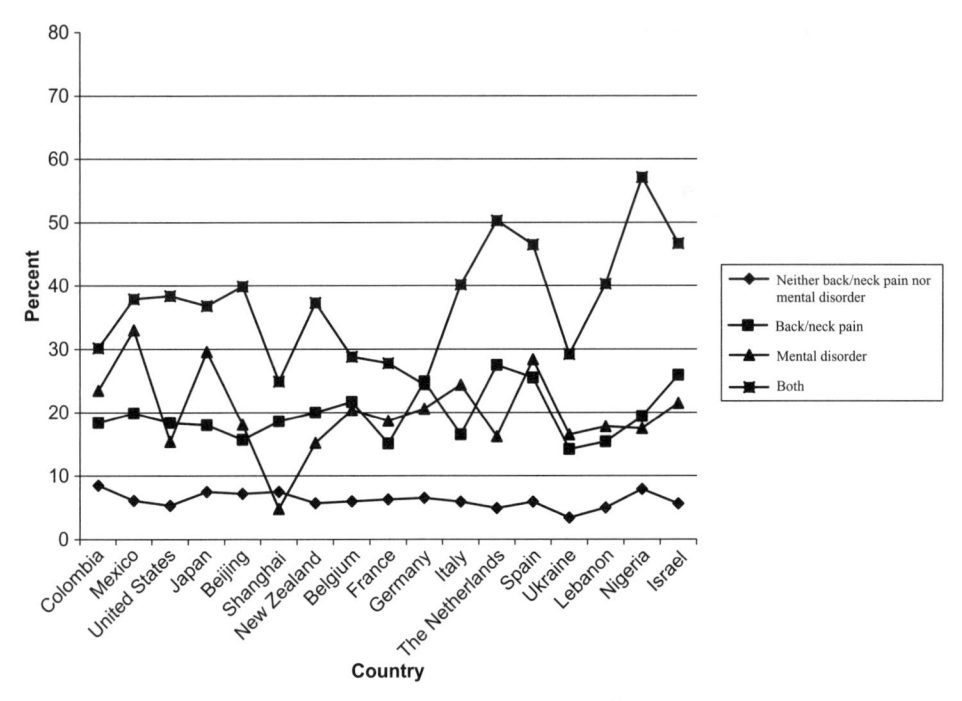

The Joint Association of Mental and Physical Conditions with Disability 233

Figure 19.1. Percent in top 10% of WMH WHODAS distribution with mental disorder, chronic back or neck pain, both, or neither.

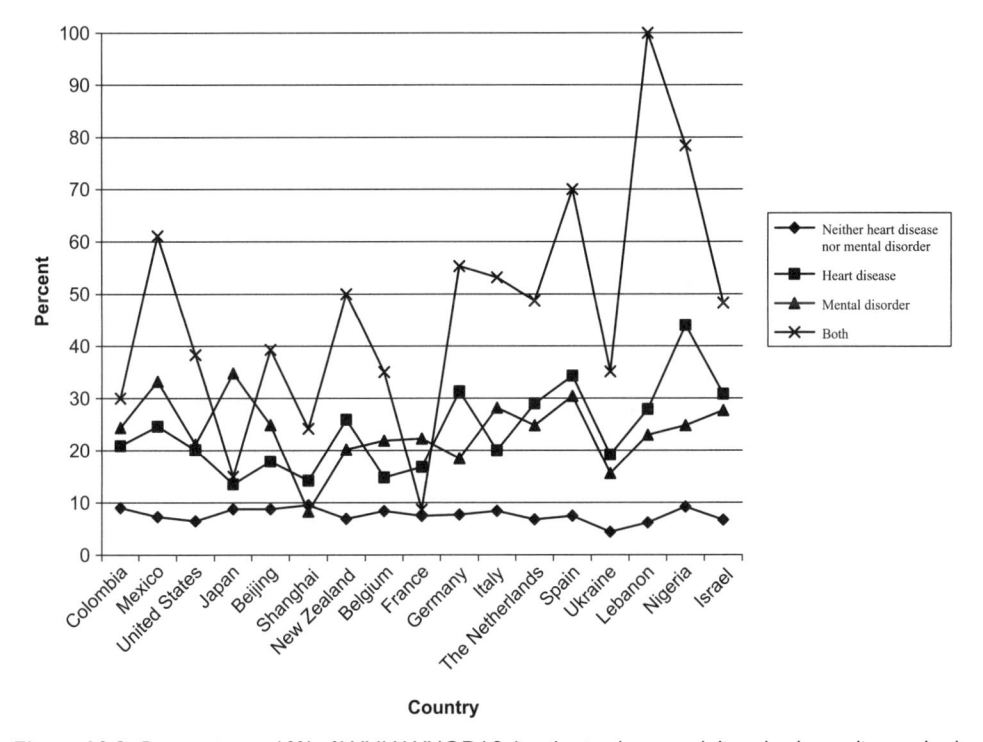

Figure 19.2. Percent in top 10% of WMH WHODAS distribution by mental disorder, heart disease, both, or neither.

Table 19.1. Odds of WMH WHODAS disability score on or above 90th percentile, pooled data (n = 42,697)

Physical condition	OR (95% CI)			
	Physical condition (PC)[a]	Mental disorder (MD)[b]	Mental disorder + physical condition (MD + PC)	Synergy index (SI)[c]
Diabetes	1.8 (1.5, 2.1)*	3.8 (3.5, 4.2)*	8.8 (6.9, 11.1)*	2.2 (1.6, 2.9)*
Respiratory disease	2.0 (1.7, 2.3)*	3.9 (3.6, 4.3)*	6.1 (5.0, 7.4)*	1.3 (1.0, 1.7)*
Headache	2.4 (2.1, 2.7)*	3.8 (3.5, 4.2)*	6.6 (5.8, 7.6)*	1.3 (1.1, 1.6)*
Heart disease	2.7 (2.3, 3.2)*	4.0 (3.7, 4.3)*	6.9 (5.7, 8.4)*	1.2 (1.0, 1.6)
Arthritis	2.5 (2.2, 2.8)*	4.0 (3.5, 4.4)*	8.1 (7.0, 9.3)*	1.6 (1.3, 1.9)*
Back or neck pain	3.4 (3.0, 3.8)*	4.0 (3.6, 4.5)*	9.2 (8.1, 10.4)*	1.5 (1.3, 1.8)*

[a] The specified physical condition in the absence of mental disorder.
[b] Mental disorder: either a 12-month depressive or 12-month anxiety disorder, or both, in the absence of the specified physical condition.
[c] SI = [OR_{MD+PC} − 1]/[(OR_{MD} − 1) + (OR_{PC} − 1)]. If there is no additive interaction, SI = 1, and a value greater than 1 indicates a positive synergistic effect.
* $p < .05$.

conditions, leading to potentially unstable estimates. For this reason the estimates based on the pooled data set are likely to be the more reliable.

19.3.2. Pooled Estimates

The odds of severe disability in the three groups (MD, PC, and MD + PC), plus the synergy index, are given in Table 19.1 for all six physical conditions. There are several results of note here. If one compares across the first two columns of data it is apparent that the odds of severe disability were generally greater for mental disorder (in the absence of a given physical condition) than they were for the physical condition (in the absence of mental disorder). Second, the third column of data shows that the odds of disability were always greater for those with both mental disorder and the physical condition, relative to either condition alone. The third and most important result is that for all conditions except heart disease there was a significant synergy index; that is, the odds of severe disability were significantly greater than the sum of the odds for the single conditions (the equivalent to a positive interaction on an additive scale). For heart disease, the synergy index was lower than that for the other conditions, but there was a trend toward synergy in the effect of mental disorder and heart disease on disability. This suggests that in the presence of mental disorder, the effect of a given physical condition on disability is increased relative to the effect the physical condition has when occurring alone (or vice versa).

19.4. DISCUSSION

So, what is the nature of the joint impact of mental and physical conditions on disability? Greater than additive, it would appear. Three key findings emerged: First, those with mental disorders were more likely to be severely disabled than those with the six physical conditions investigated here. Second, those with comorbid mental and physical conditions were more likely to be severely disabled than those with either condition alone. Third, mental–physical comorbidity exerted synergistic effects, with the odds of severe disability among those with both mental disorder and a physical condition (with the exception of heart disease) being significantly greater than the sum of the odds of the single conditions.

The finding of a synergistic effect of mental–physical comorbidity is consistent with earlier research that also found positive interactions (Kessler et al. 2001, 2003; Egede 2004; Schmitz et al. 2007), though, as noted earlier, at least as many studies have found only additive effects. There are many methodological differences across studies that may account for the fact that some studies found evidence of synergy and others found only additive effects, but one such methodological feature noted earlier is that studies using logistic regression, when this is adapted to assess interactions additively (e.g., Egede 2004; Schmitz et al. 2007; and the current study), are more likely to observe synergistic effects than when interactions are tested using multiplicative models (e.g., Stein et al. 2006).

What is unique about the current study is that this is the first to sample from both developing and developed countries and to use a measure of severe disability rather than any disability days (which can be influenced by brief inconsequential illness). Other important methodological features of this study are that it included the full adult age range and used diagnoses of depression and anxiety disorders based on the full Composite International Diagnostic Interview (CIDI), rather than a short form or a scale measure of depression symptoms. It is interesting that the degree of synergistic effect we observed was generally lower than that found by Schmitz et al. (2007), the study probably most comparable to what we have done here; this may be explained in part by some of the methodological features just mentioned.

The important question then is as follows: how might mental and physical conditions combine together in a synergistic fashion – how could the presence of one amplify the disability impact of the other? In fact, there are a number of candidate mechanisms, including biological, behavioral, and psychological factors. There may be an underlying shared pathophysiology, such as that associated with the functioning of the autonomic nervous system (through the sympathetic–adrenal–medullary (SAM) system) and the neuroendocrine system (through the hypothalamic–pituitary–adrenocortical (HPA) axis). Disturbances in both these systems have been associated with depression and anxiety disorders (Goodyer 2007; Heim & Nemeroff 1999; McEwen 2003) and with a range of physical disorders mediated by metabolic, cardiovascular, and immune systems (Chrousos & Kino 2007; Cohen, Janicki-Deverts, & Miller 2007; McEwen 1998). The cumulative effect of physiological dysregulation across multiple systems associated with stress has been proposed as a form of "allostatic load" on the body and brain (McEwen 1998). Interestingly in the context of the current results, a study by Karlamanagla et al. (2002) found that a summary measure of allostatic load predicted functional decline over and above individual physiological markers, lifestyle and demographic variables, and baseline levels of functioning. Allostatic load may therefore be one mechanism through which the combined effect of different morbidities on functioning may be greater than the sum of the individual effects.

Beyond direct biological mechanisms, it is also clear that the presence of a disorder such as depression can exacerbate the effect of a chronic physical condition on disability through the effect depression has on reducing treatment adherence and engaging in poorer health behaviors (such as smoking and sedentary behavior) (Cohen & Rodriguez 1995; Evans et al. 2005). Depression co-occurring with chronic pain is also known to affect the perception and appraisal of pain and the ability to cope with it (Campbell, Clauw, & Keefe 2003; Van Puymbroeck, Zautra, & Harakas 2007). It is also possible that the presence of a chronic physical condition may amplify the disabling effect of a mental disorder, for example, in increasing the sense of hopelessness and helplessness that are among the incapacitating features of depression.

It has been observed that the relationship between mental and physical disorders is frequently bidirectional (Cohen & Rodriguez 1995; Dew 1998; Kiecolt-Glaser et al. 2002) and it may be that bidirectionality itself contributes to the synergistic effect of these conditions on disability. Depression, for example, may facilitate the development of diabetes through the metabolic effects of HPA axis hyperactivity, but then the resulting disability and lifestyle changes required by the advent of diabetes can maintain or exacerbate the depression. Hence, a self-perpetuating feedback loop between mental and physical disorders can develop; their comorbidity then operates to increase the morbidity of each disorder, and so too the associated disability.

Clearly then, this is an issue with clinical ramifications. Schettini and Frank (2004) take the view that if two conditions have additive effects on disability, this may indicate that both need to be targeted for treatment in order to reduce their joint disability burden, and if two conditions have synergistic effects, novel treatments need to be designed and targeted to particular comorbidities. At the very least, these and other similar results present a strong case for the need to treat both conditions. This may seem obvious, but in fact it is not the position always adopted by clinicians when confronted with mental–physical comorbidity. For example, some physicians in medical settings take the view that mental disorder is an understandable consequence of physical disease that does not require a specific treatment focus (Evans et al. 2005). Similarly, some mental health clinicians consider that "living with a mental illness is generally such a struggle that physical health is of lesser importance" (Hyland et al. 2003). The current research suggests that such attitudes may unhelpfully prolong the disability the individual experiences.

These findings need to be interpreted within the context of some limitations specific to this study. First, the cross-sectional nature of the surveys means that it cannot be assumed that the disability measured here is a consequence of either the mental or physical conditions reported. Second, the analyses of each physical condition did not control for comorbidity with other physical conditions. Additionally, mental disorders not included in the depression–anxiety spectrum were not controlled for in the analyses. This may mean that the distinctions between the groups are less clear-cut than their labeling implies, but it is unlikely to have affected the pattern of results. Lastly, the cutpoint for defining disability (above the 90th percentile of the WMH WHODAS for each country) may not mean the same thing in different countries. The proportion of each country with any disability on the WMH WHODAS showed considerable cross-national variation (data not shown), so it is possible that the nature of the disability experienced by the 10% most disabled in a given population would also vary. Nonetheless, the general patterning of results (those with both conditions more likely to be severely disabled relative to either condition alone) was observed across the majority of countries.

In conclusion, the WMH Surveys found that the joint effect of mental and physical conditions on the probability of severe disability was synergistic, such that the combined effect of mental and physical conditions was significantly greater than the summed effects of the individual conditions. There are a number of possible biological, behavioral, and psychological mechanisms that may contribute to this effect. Treating clinicians need to rise to the challenge of according both mental and physical conditions equal priority, especially when they co-occur in the same individual, in order to adequately manage the resulting disability.

ACKNOWLEDGMENT

Some material in this chapter appeared in Scott et al. (2009). This material is reprinted with the permission of *Psychological Medicine*.

REFERENCES

Ahlbom, A., & Alfredsson, L. (2005). Interaction: A word with two meanings creates confusion. *European Journal of Epidemiology*, 20, 563–4.

Andersson, T., Alfredsson, L., Kallberg, H., Zdravkovic, S., & Ahlbom, A. (2005). Calculating measures of biological interaction. *European Journal of Epidemiology*, 20, 575–9.

Armenian, H. K., Pratt, L. A., Gallo, J., & Eaton, W. W. (1998). Psychopathology as a predictor of disability: A population-based follow-up study in Baltimore, Maryland. *American Journal of Epidemiology*, 148, 269–75.

Buist-Bouwman, M. A., de Graaf, R., Vollebergh, W. A., Alonso, J., Bruffaerts, R., & Ormel, J. (2005a). Functional disability of mental disorders and comparison with physical disorders: A study among the general population of six European countries. *Acta Psychiatrica Scandinavica*, 113, 492–500.

Buist-Bouwman, M. A., de Graaf, R., Vollebergh, W. A. M., & Ormel, J. (2005b). Comorbidity of physical and mental disorders and the effect on work-loss days. *Acta Psychiatrica Scandinavica*, 111, 436–43.

Campbell, L. C., Clauw, D. J., & Keefe, F. J. (2003). Persistent pain and depression: A biopsychosocial perspective. *Biological Psychiatry*, 54, 399–409.

Chrousos, G. P., & Kino, T. (2007). Glucocorticoid action networks and complex psychiatric and/or somatic disorders. *Stress*, 10, 213–19.

Cohen, S., Janicki-Deverts, D., & Miller, G. E. (2007). Psychological stress and disease. *Journal of the American Medical Association*, 298, 1685–7.

Cohen, S., & Rodriguez, M. S. (1995). Pathways linking affective disturbances and physical disorders. *Health Psychology*, 14, 374–80.

Dew, M. A. (1998). Psychiatric disorder in the context of physical illness. In *Adversity, Stress and Psychopathology*, ed. B. P. Dohrenwend, pp. 177–218. New York: Oxford University Press.

Druss, B. G., Marcus, S. C., Rosenheck, R. A., Olfson, M., Tanielian, M. A., & Pincus, H. A. (2000). Understanding disability in mental and general medical conditions. *American Journal of Psychiatry*, 157, 1485–91.

Egede, L. E. (2004). Diabetes, major depression, and functional disability among US adults. *Diabetes Care*, 27, 421–8.

Evans, D. L., Charney, D. S., Lewis, L., Golden, J. M., Ranga Rama Krishnan, K., Nemeroff, C. B., Bremner, J. D., Carney, R. M., Coyne, J. C., Delong, M. R., Frasure-Smith, N., Glassman, A. H., Gold, P. W., Grant, I., Gwyther, L., Ironson, G., Johnson, R. L., Kanner, A. M., Katon, W. J., Kaufmann, P. G., Keefe, F. J., Ketter, T., Laughren, T. P., Leserman, J., Lyketsos, C. G., McDonald, W. M., McEwan, B. S., Miller, A. H., Musselman, D., O'Connor, C., Petitto, J. M., Pollock, B. G., Robinson, R. G., Roose, S. P., Rowland, J., Sheline, Y., Sheps, D. S., Simon, G., Spiegel, D., Stunkard, A., Sunderland, T., Tibbits, P., & Valvo, W. J. (2005). Mood disorders in the medically ill: Scientific review and recommendations. *Biological Psychiatry*, 58, 175–89.

Goodyer, I. M. (2007). The hypothalamic-pituitary-adrenal axis: Cortisol, DHEA and mental and behavioral function. In *Depression and Physical Illness*, ed. A. Steptoe, pp. 280–98. London: Cambridge University Press.

Hays, R. D., Wells, K. B., Sherbourne, C. D., Rogers, W., & Spritzer, K. (1995). Functioning and well-being outcomes of patients with depression compared with chronic general medical illnesses. *Archives of General Psychiatry*, 52, 11–19.

Heim, C., & Nemeroff, C. B. (1999). The impact of early adverse experiences on brain systems involved in the pathophysiology of anxiety and affective disorders. *Biological Psychiatry*, 46, 1509–22.

Hyland, B., Judd, F., Davidson, S., Jolley, D., & Hocking, B. (2003). Case managers' attitudes to the physical health of their patients. *Australian and New Zealand Journal of Psychiatry*, 37, 710–14.

Karlamangla, A. S., Singer, B. H., McEwen, B. S., Rowe, J. W., & Seeman, T. E. (2002). Allostatic load as a predictor of functional decline: MacArthur studies of successful aging. *Journal of Clinical Epidemiology*, 55, 696–710.

Kessler, R. C., Greenberg, P. E., Mickelson, K. D., Meneades, L. M., and Wang, P. S. (2001). The effects of chronic medical conditions on work loss and work cutback. *Journal of Occupational and Environmental Medicine*, **43** (3), 218–25.

Kessler, R. C., Ormel, J., Demler, O., & Stang, P. E. (2003). Comorbid mental disorders account for the role impairment of commonly occurring chronic physical disorders: Results from the National Comorbidity Survey. *Journal of Occupational and Environmental Medicine*, **45**, 1257–66.

Kiecolt-Glaser, J. K., McGuire, L., Robles, T. F., & Glaser, R. (2002). Emotions, morbidity, and mortality: New perspectives from psychoneuroimmunology. *Annual Review of Psychology*, **53**, 83–107.

McEwen, B. S. (1998). Protective and damaging effects of stress mediators. *New England Journal of Medicine*, **338**, 171–9.

McEwen, B. S. (2003). Mood disorders and allostatic load. *Biological Psychiatry*, **54**, 200–7.

Merikangas, K. R., Ames, M., Cui, L., Stang, P. D., Ustun, B., Von Korff, M., & Kessler, R. (2007). The impact of comorbidity of mental and physical conditions on role disability in the US adult household population. *Archives of General Psychiatry*, **64**, 1180–8.

Ormel, J., Kempen, G. I. J. M., Deeg, D. J. H., Brilman, E. I., Sonderen, E., & Relyveld, J. (1998). Functioning, well being, and health perception in late middle-aged and older people: Comparing the effects of depressive symptoms and chronic medical conditions. *American Geriatrics Society*, **46**, 39–48.

Sareen, J., Jacobi, F., Cox, B. J., Belik, S.-L., Clara, I., & Stein, M. B. (2006). Disability and poor quality of life associated with comorbid anxiety disorders and physical conditions. *Archives of Internal Medicine*, **166**, 2109–16.

Schettini Evans, A., & Frank, S. J. (2004). Adolescent depression and externalizing problems: Testing two models of comorbidity in an inpatient sample. *Adolescence*, **39**, 1–18.

Schmitz, N., Wang, J., Malla, A., & Lesage, A. (2007). Joint effect of depression on chronic conditions on disability: Results from a population-based study. *Psychosomatic Medicine*, **69**, 10.

Scott, K., McGee, M., Wells, J., & Oakley Browne, M. (2006). Disability in Te Rau Hinengaro: The New Zealand Mental Health Survey (NZMHS). *Australian and New Zealand Journal of Psychiatry*, **40**, 889–95.

Scott, K. M., Bruffaerts, R., Tsang, A., Ormel, J., Alonso, J., Angermeyer, M. C., Benjet, C., Bromet, E., de Girolamo, G., de Graaf, R., Gasquet, I., Gureye, O., Haro, J. M., He, Y., Kessler, R. C., Levinson, D., Mneimneh, Z. N., Oakley Browne, M. A., Posada-Villa, J., Stein, D. J., Takeshima, T., & Von Korff, M. (2007). Depression-anxiety relationships with chronic physical conditions: Results from the World Mental Health surveys. *Journal of Affective Disorders*, **103**, 113–20.

Scott, K. M., Von Korff, M., Alonso, J., Angermeyer, M. C., Bromet, E., Fayyad, J., de Girolamo, G., Demyttenaere, K., Gasquet, I., Gureje, O., Haro, J. M., He, Y., Kessler, R. C., Levinson, D., Medina Mora, M. E., Oakley Browne, M., Ormel, J., Posada-Villa, J., Watanabe, M., & Williams, D. (2009). Mental–physical co-morbidity and its relationship with disability: Results from the World Mental Health Surveys. *Psychological Medicine*, **39**, 33–43.

Stein, M. B., Cox, B. J., Afifi, T. O., Belik, S.-L., & Sareen, J. (2006). Does co-morbid depressive illness magnify the impact of chronic physical illness: A population-based perspective. *Psychological Medicine*, **36**, 587–96.

Van Puymbroeck, C. M., Zautra, A. J., & Harakas, P. P. (2007). Chronic pain and depression: Twin burdens of adaptation. In *Depression and Physical Illness*, ed. A. Steptoe, pp. 145–64. London: Cambridge University Press.

Von Korff, M., Crane, P. K., Alonso, J., Vilagut, G., Angermeyer, M. C., Bruffaerts, R., de Girolamo, G., Gureje, O., de Graaf, R., Huang, Y., Iwata, N., Karam, E. G., Kovess, V., Lara, C., Levinson, D., Posada-Villa, J., Scott, K. M., & Ormel, J. (2008). Modified WHODAS-II provides valid measure of global disability but filter items increased skewness. *Journal of Clinical Epidemiology*, **61**, 1132–43.

Wells, K. B., Golding, J. M., & Burnam, M. A. (1989a). Affective, substance use, and anxiety disorders in persons with arthritis, diabetes, heart disease, high blood pressure, or chronic lung conditions. *General Hospital Psychiatry*, **11**, 320–7.

Wells, K. B., Stewart, A., Hays, R. D., Burnam, M. A., Rogers, W., Daniels, M., Berry, S., Greenfield, S., & Ware, J. (1989b). The functioning and well-being of depressed patients. *The Journal of the American Medical Association*, **262**, 914–19.

20 Disability in "Pure" versus "Comorbid" Mental and Physical Conditions

PAUL K. CRANE

20.1. INTRODUCTION

Chronic conditions are associated with disability – this is not a surprise. Nor is it a surprise that individuals with any particular chronic condition often have more than one chronic condition; comorbidity may be the rule rather than the exception for many chronic conditions. Few studies have investigated whether disability associated with chronic conditions may be attributable to the chronic condition itself or to concurrent comorbid conditions. Similarly, the role of economic development in disability related to chronic conditions has rarely been evaluated.

These questions were addressed with data from the World Mental Health (WMH) Survey Initiative. Five prototypic chronic conditions were compared, representing one mental, two pain, and two physical conditions: depression/anxiety, back/neck pain, head pain, diabetes, and heart disease. Survey respondents who endorsed any of these conditions were classified into the "comorbid condition" category if they had any of a large number of comorbid conditions. If respondents did not endorse any of the comorbid conditions, they were classified into the "pure condition" category. Then the proportions of individuals with "pure" versus "comorbid" conditions were compared who endorsed any disability as measured by the World Health Organization's Disability Assessment Schedule – II (WHODAS-II) as modified for use in the World Mental Health Surveys (WMH WHODAS); the proportion of individuals who endorsed difficulties in four specific WMH WHODAS domains: social functioning, communication, movement, and self-care; and the mean number of reported disability days. Disability days represent a composite summary of the number of days out of the last 30 for which the respondent was completely disabled plus fractions of days for which the respondent was partially disabled.

20.2. APPROACH

20.2.1. Disability Measures

The WMH WHODAS assessed five domains of functioning: understanding and communicating, self-care, getting around, getting along with others, and life activities. In the first four domains, there was a filter question, a series of specific items with severity ratings, and a question about days in the last month that these kinds of interference occurred. The fifth domain, life activities, consisted of a series of questions about activity limitation days in the prior month.

20.2.2. Scoring the WMH WHODAS

The WHO has not yet adopted a standardized approach to scoring the WHODAS-II, although it is generally scored on a 0–100 scale, with higher scores indicating greater disability. A score of 100 indicates the maximum possible score, and intermediate scores indicate the percent of the maximum possible score. For the understanding and communicating, getting around, self-care, and getting along with others domains, the WMH WHO-DAS was scored by estimating (on a 0–100 scale) the percent of the maximum possible score that was observed for the sum of the severity items and the percent of the maximum number of days of activity limitation in the prior month. These two scores were multiplied and then divided by 100 so that the resulting score ranged from 0 to 100, where 100 would signify the maximum possible disability. The proportion of participants were determined in each group with nonzero scores in each of these domains. For the life activities domain, a weighted sum of activity limitation days in the prior month was estimated. The following terms were added together: (1) the number of days totally unable to carry out normal activities in the prior month; (2) one-half the number of days of reduced activities; (3) one-half the number of days of reduced quality or care in work activities; and (4) one-quarter the number of days requiring extreme effort to perform at one's usual level. If this sum exceeded 30, it was recoded to equal 30 so that the sum had a range from zero to 30.

20.2.3. Chronic Condition Assessment

The WMH version of the CIDI was used to determine 12-month and lifetime prevalence of various mental disorders. Self-reported items assessed the 12-month prevalence of chronic pain conditions and the lifetime presence of chronic physical diseases. More detailed information on the methods used to determine the presence of physical conditions is provided in Chapter 4.

20.2.4. Prototypic Chronic Conditions Definitions

We defined depression/anxiety as 12-month prevalence of depression, dysthymia, generalized anxiety disorder, social phobia, panic, agoraphobia without panic, and/or posttraumatic stress disorder. We defined back/neck and head pain as 12-month prevalence of these conditions. Diabetes and heart disease were defined as lifetime prevalence of these disorders under the assumption that they were also present in the prior 12 months.

20.2.5. "Pure" versus "Comorbid" Chronic Conditions Definitions

Comorbid chronic conditions included any of the five prototypic chronic conditions plus cancer, asthma, other lung disorders, epilepsy, stroke, HIV, and ulcers. Participants who reported only one of these prototypic conditions and none of the other chronic physical diseases listed above were classified as having a "pure" chronic condition. Participants with any prototypic condition who had either another prototypic condition or any of the other chronic physical conditions listed previously were classified as having a "comorbid" chronic condition.

20.2.6. Data Analysis

Unweighted counts of numbers of participants with pure and comorbid prototypic conditions were added across developing and developed countries. Proportions of participants in each of these groups with nonzero scores for overall disability and for each disability domain were determined. Mean disability days, as defined earlier, were also determined across each of these groups.

20.3. FINDINGS

Numbers of participants with pure and comorbid conditions, along with demographic characteristics, are provided in Table 20.1. Comorbid prototypic conditions were much more prevalent than pure prototypic conditions in both developing and developed countries, ranging from two out of three cases of depression/anxiety to four out of five or more cases of heart disease. The proportion of participants with "pure" headache who were female was similar to the proportion of participants with comorbid headache. For the other conditions, the proportion of participants with comorbid conditions who were female was greater than the proportion of participants with "pure" conditions in both developed and developing countries. Not surprisingly, participants with pure conditions tended to be younger than participants with comorbid conditions. Comparing each of the prototypic conditions, there were not marked differences in the percent of participants who had educational attainment exceeding the median level for their country in developing countries, while in developed countries persons with comorbid conditions were somewhat less likely to have educational attainment above their country's median level.

Proportions of participants with pure conditions from developed and developing countries who had difficulties in each disability domain are shown in Figure 20.1. Overall proportions of participants who had difficulties in each disability domain were lower in developing countries than in developed countries across all prototypic conditions. Difficulties with self-care were uncommon across all prototypic conditions. For depression, higher proportions of participants had difficulties in communication than difficulties in social role functioning or movement. A similar pattern was seen for head pain. For back pain, diabetes, and heart disease, higher proportions of participants indicated problems with movement than with the other domains.

Proportions of participants with comorbid conditions from developing countries who had difficulties in each disability domain are shown in Figure 20.2. As was observed among persons with pure conditions, the overall proportions of participants with comorbid conditions who had difficulties in each disability domain were lower in developing countries than in developed countries across all prototypic conditions. Patterns across disability domains were similar to those seen in developed countries. Comparing Figures 20.1 and 20.2, much higher proportions of participants with comorbid conditions had difficulties in each domain relative to those with pure conditions.

Figure 20.3 compares the proportion of participants with pure versus comorbid conditions from developed and developing countries that reported disability in any of the five domains (i.e., with any global disability). The presence of any global disability was higher among persons from developed countries than developing countries for both those with pure and those with comorbid conditions. As might be expected, persons with comorbid conditions were much more likely to have any global disability than persons with pure conditions.

The mean number of disability days among participants with pure and comorbid conditions from developed and developing countries are shown in Figure 20.4. The same pattern was observed. Across all conditions the proportion with any disability and the number of disability days were higher in the developed than the developing world. Consistent with the results for WHODAS domains, the proportion with any disability and the mean number of disability days was higher for those

Table 20.1. Descriptive characteristics by developing versus developed world and by pure versus comorbid diseases

Chronic disorder	"Pure" n (%)	"Comorbid" n (%)	Total	Female "Pure" (%)	Female "Comorbid" (%)	Age >40 "Pure" (%)	Age >40 "Comorbid" (%)	Educ. "Pure" (%)	Educ. "Comorbid" (%)
				Developing world					
Depression/anxiety	517 (31)	1,166 (69)	1,683	54	72	34	54	47	45
Back pain	616 (23)	2,013 (77)	2,629	49	66	50	67	54	49
Head pain	414 (20)	1,640 (80)	2,054	72	73	30	61	41	46
Diabetes	122 (30)	285 (70)	407	50	62	74	80	49	52
Heart disease	157 (15)	907 (85)	1,064	44	68	69	82*	52	55
				Developed world					
Depression/anxiety	1,769 (33)	3,651 (67)	5,420	61	66	36	57	45	42
Back pain	1,229 (20)	4,789 (80)	6,018	46	60	60	73	52	45
Head pain	842 (21)	3,162 (79)	4,004	72	71	36	58	48	41
Diabetes	404 (23)	1,368 (77)	1,772	47	53	88	91	54	43
Heart disease	422 (20)	1,692 (80)	2,114	34	48	90	95	56	44

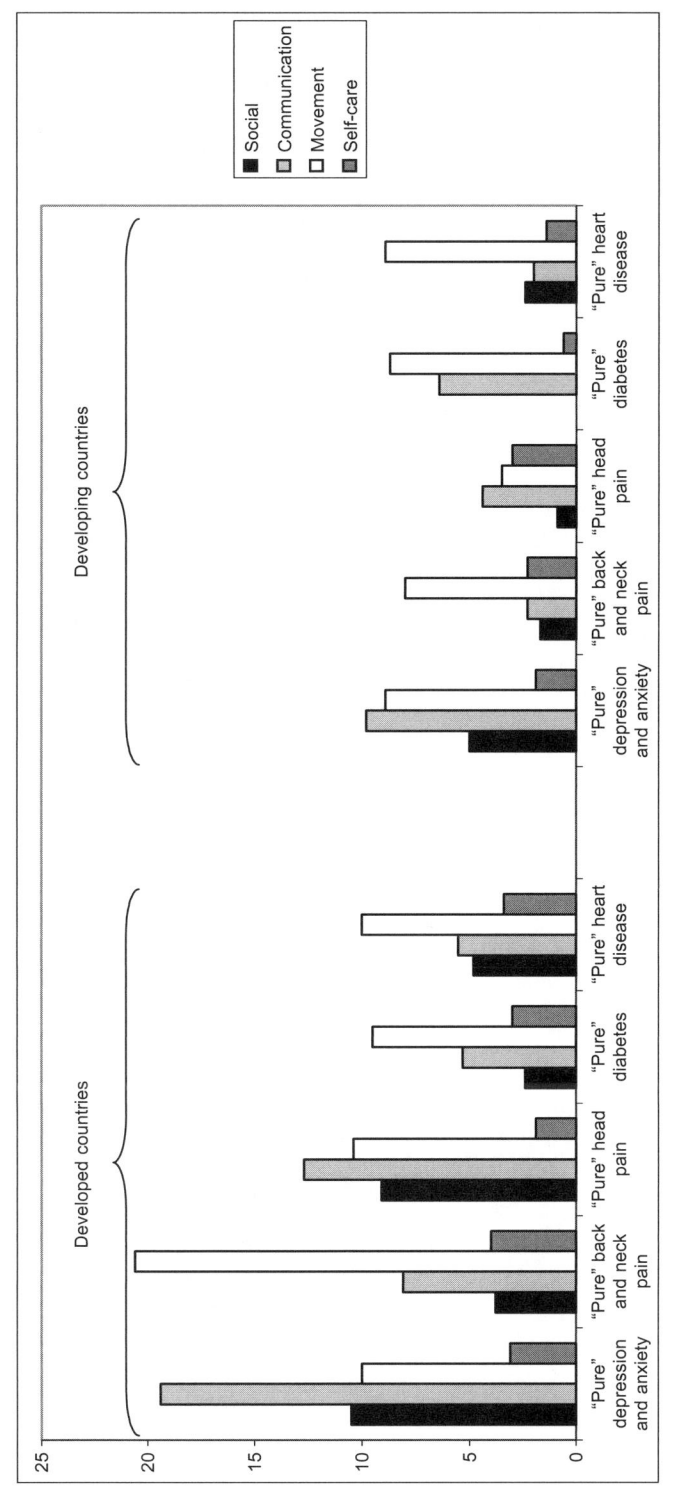

Figure 20.1. Proportion of participants with "pure" chronic disorders who endorsed disability in four WHODAS domains in developed and developing countries.

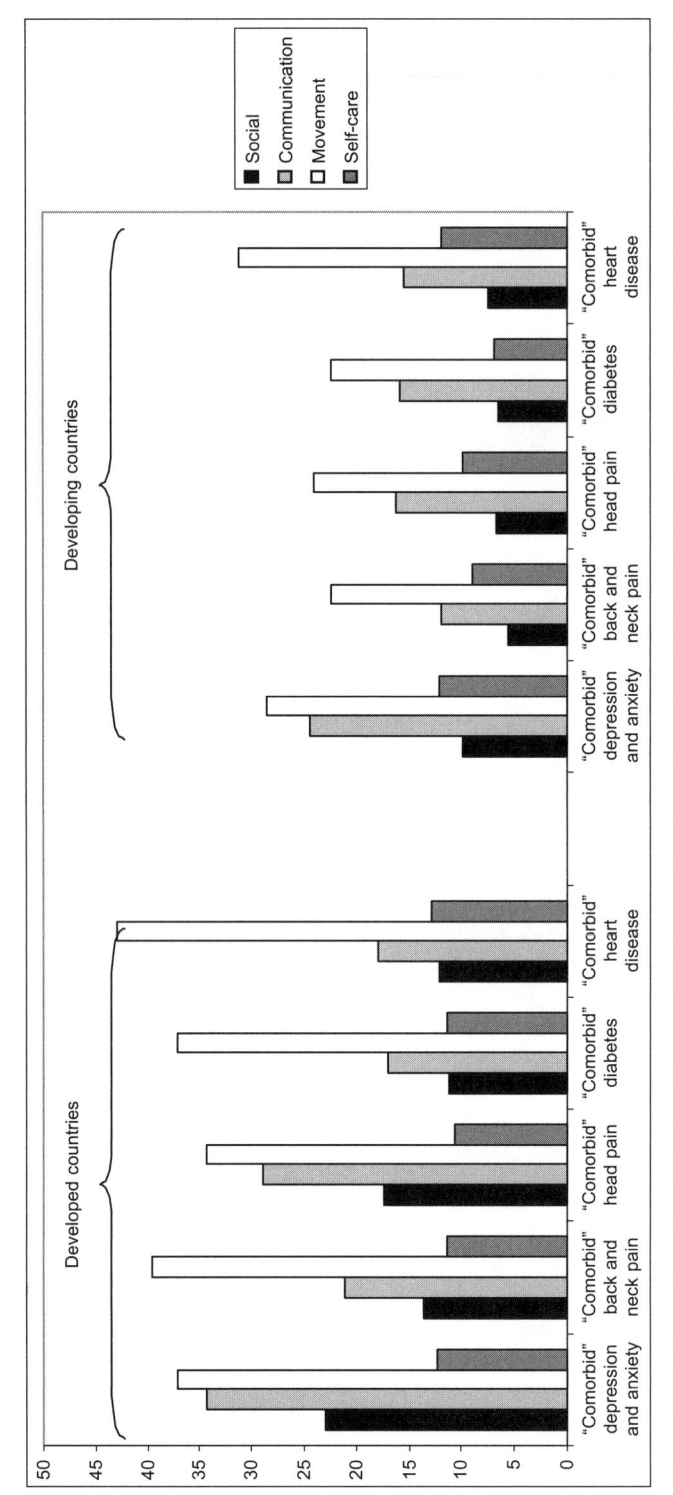

Figure 20.2. Proportion of participants with comorbid chronic disorders who endorsed disability in four WHODAS domains in developed and developing countries.

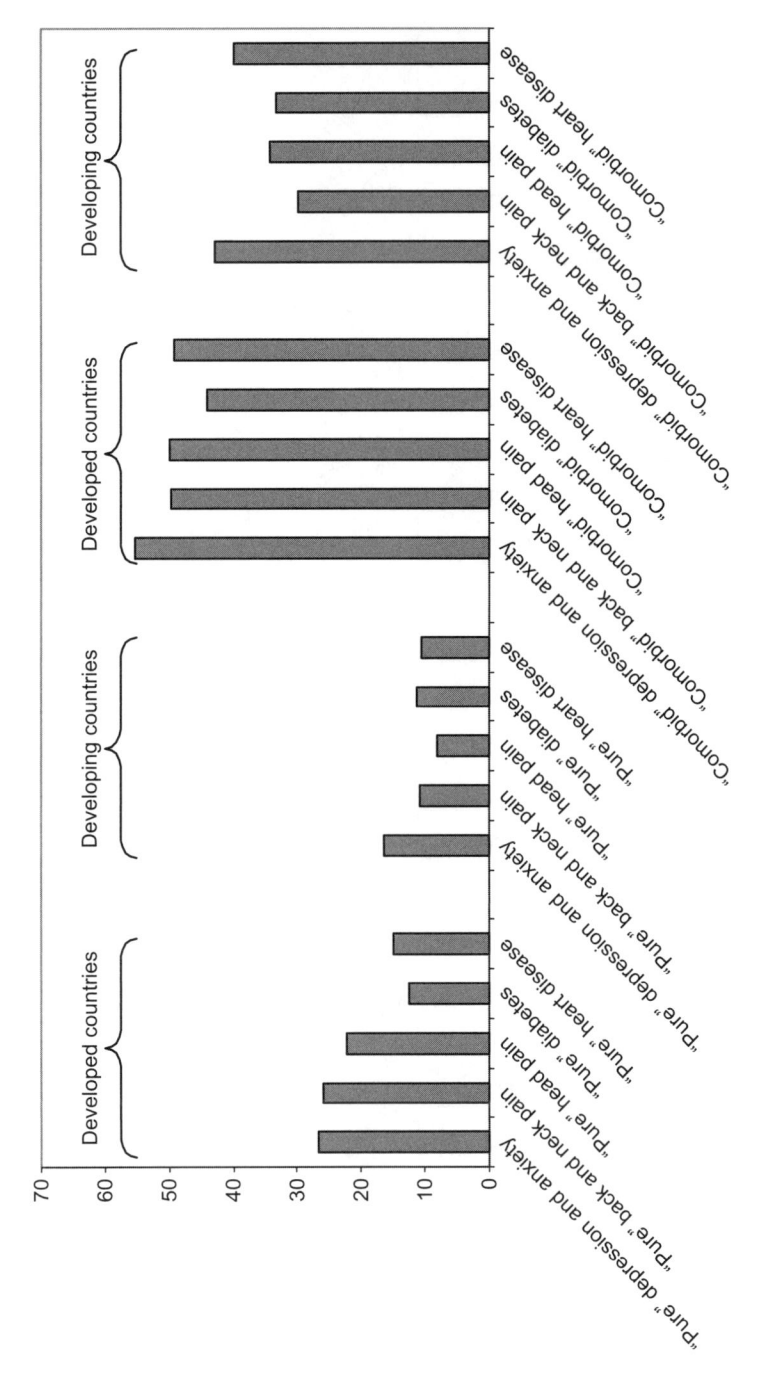

Figure 20.3. Proportion of participants with any global disability as measured by the WHODAS, stratified by "pure" versus "comorbid" condition and developed versus developing countries.

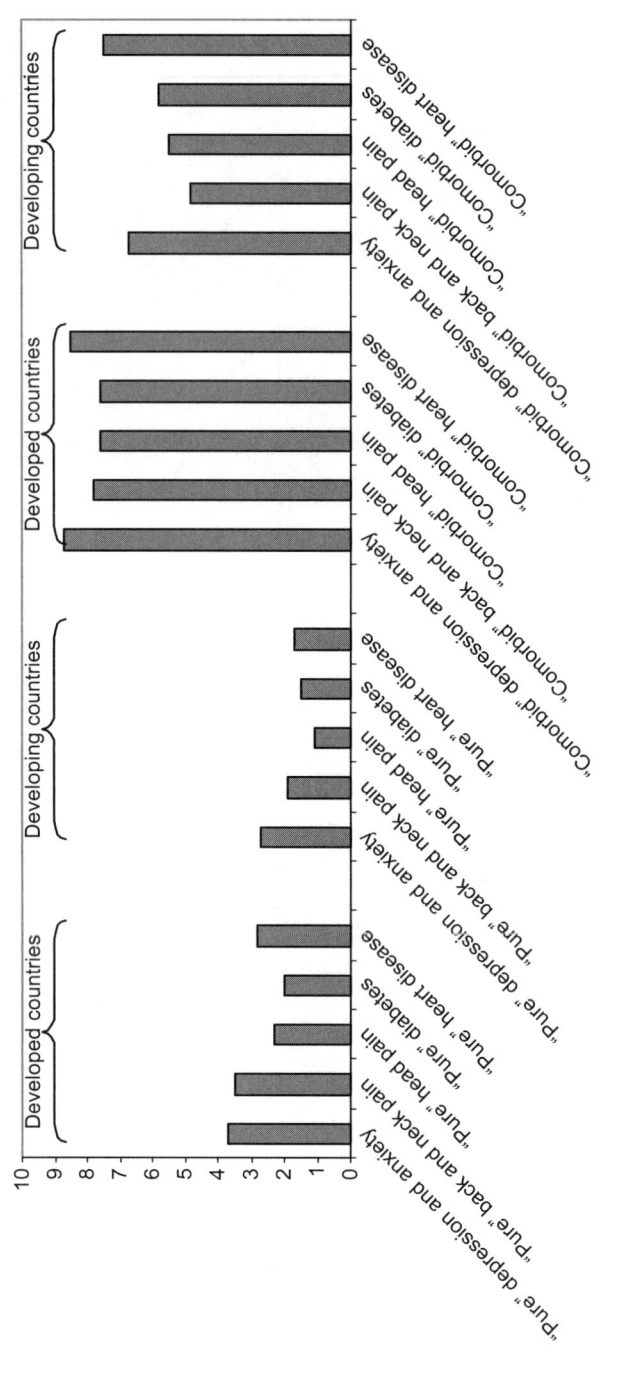

Figure 20.4. Mean number of disability days for participants, stratified by "pure" versus "comorbid" condition and developed versus developing countries.

with comorbid prototypic conditions than those with pure prototypic conditions.

20.4. DISCUSSION

For each of the five prototypic chronic conditions examined, "pure" conditions were much less prevalent than were comorbid conditions. This makes attribution of disability (or other factors) to the specific prototypic condition difficult in small samples that may have few individuals with "pure" conditions. For the five conditions considered here, in representative cross-sectional samples, two out of three to more than four out of five individuals with each condition had at least one other comorbid chronic condition. These findings are consistent with a study that found that individuals with disabilities typically had comorbid conditions (Kinne, Patrick, & Doyle 2004). The WMH Survey Initiative has very large samples, facilitating analyses that may not be possible in smaller studies.

Across all prototypic conditions, the proportion of individuals endorsing each WHODAS subdomain was markedly higher among those with comorbid than those with "pure" conditions. Likewise, higher proportions of respondents endorsed global disability, and average disability days were higher for those with comorbid conditions compared to those with "pure" conditions. This finding is not surprising, but serves to validate the belief that for each of these prototypic chronic conditions, having one or more comorbid conditions is associated with additional disability. Similar findings for headache were found in a study using WMH Survey data based on the U.S. sample (Saunders et al. 2008), as well as another analysis of WMH Survey data finding that depression's largest impacts on overall health occurred when depression was comorbid with other conditions (Moussavi et al. 2007). Data from the pain literature suggest that comorbid conditions lead to greater endorsement of pain and higher physical impact from pain (Leong et al. 2007). The present investigation builds on those by confirming their findings across developed and developing samples, and across five prototypic psychiatric, pain, and physical conditions.

Across all prototypic conditions, the proportion of individuals endorsing each WHODAS subdomain was higher in developed than in developing countries. Similarly, higher proportions of respondents with these conditions endorsed global disability, and average disability days were higher for respondents in developed than in developing countries. There are at least two potential explanations for these findings. One potential explanation is that the meaning of these disabilities differs with country development status – that is, for a given level of actual disability, someone in the developed world would be more likely to endorse some level of disability than someone in the developing world. This concept is referred to as differential item functioning (DIF) (Camilli & Shepard 1994; Holland & Wainer 1993). A second potential explanation is that for a given severity of a chronic condition, there are aspects to life in the developed world that are more difficult than they would be in the developing world. A third possible factor is that persons with chronic conditions from developed countries tended to be somewhat older than persons with chronic conditions from developing countries. Additional investigations as to the sources of these differences would be of great importance. Developing countries may be able to avoid the disability associated with chronic conditions in the developed world, while developed countries may have opportunities to reduce disability associated with chronic conditions.

Individuals with chronic conditions were especially likely to endorse problems with mobility. There were two notable exceptions: participants with "pure" depression/anxiety and with "pure" headache were more likely to endorse problems with communication than with mobility. In contrast, participants with comorbid depression/anxiety or headache endorsed mobility problems more commonly than they endorsed communication problems. This finding may be due to conditions comorbid with depression/anxiety or head pain, producing problems with mobility rather than depression/anxiety or headache themselves, though this cross-sectional study cannot be conclusive on that point. For the other prototypic chronic conditions evaluated here, the relative importance of the different disability domains was similar for those with "pure" as for those with comorbid conditions, except that proportions of participants endorsing each WHODAS domain were much higher among those with comorbid than those with "pure" conditions.

In summary, we were able to differentiate between individuals with "pure" and those with comorbid chronic conditions using data from a large international study. Pure disorders were much less common than comorbid disorders in both developed and developing countries. Proportions of individuals with "pure" conditions who endorsed each WHODAS domain were lower than proportions of individuals with comorbid conditions. Across conditions, whether "pure" or comorbid, proportions endorsing nonzero levels of each disability domain were higher in developed than in developing countries. Mobility was the most commonly endorsed disability domain across conditions, with the notable exceptions of "pure" depression/anxiety and headache. These findings emphasize the importance of comorbid conditions on disability associated with each condition and suggest interesting further lines of analysis to determine why chronic conditions appear more disabling in the developed than in the developing world.

REFERENCES

Camilli, G., & Shepard, L. A., eds. (1994). *Methods for Identifying Biased Test Items. Measurement Methods for the Social Sciences.* Thousand Oaks, CA: Sage Publications.

Holland, P. W., & Wainer, H., eds. (1993). *Differential Item Functioning.* Hillsdale, NJ: Erlbaum.

Kinne, S., Patrick, D. L., & Doyle, D. L. (2004). Prevalence of secondary conditions among people with disabilities. *American Journal of Public Health,* **94**, 443–5.

Leong, I. Y., Farrell, M. J., Helme, R. D., & Gibson, S. J. (2007). The relationship between medical comorbidity and self-rated pain, mood disturbance, and function in older people with chronic pain. *Journals of Gerontology. Series A, Biological Sciences and Medical Sciences,* **62**, 550–5.

Moussavi, S., Chatterji, S., Verdes, E., Tandon, A., Patel, V., & Ustun, B. (2007). Depression, chronic diseases, and decrements in health: Results from the World Health Surveys. *Lancet,* **370**, 851–8.

Saunders, K., Merikangas, K., Low, N. C., Von Korff, M., & Kessler, R. C. (2008). Impact of comorbidity on headache-related disability. *Neurology,* **70**, 538–47.

21 Labor Force Participation, Unemployment, and Mental–Physical Comorbidity

MICHAEL R. VON KORFF

21.1. INTRODUCTION

High labor force participation and low unemployment among working-age adults are needed to support the societal needs of young, elderly, and disabled citizens for education, health care, long-term care, and income maintenance services. Sustaining employment is also critical to the health and well-being of individuals and their families. Beyond the economic consequences for families of loss of income and work-related benefits, health-related effects of unemployment include increased mortality, physical and psychological health problems, and greater use of health care services (Jin, Shah, & Svoboda 1995; Mathers & Schofield 1998; Morris & Cook 1991).

As the national populations in most countries age, and the prevalence of chronic physical diseases and comorbid mental disorders increases, the challenges of maximizing labor force participation and minimizing unemployment among working-age adults grow. Chronic physical disease and psychological illness are associated with increased unemployment, disability claims, and absence from work (De Buck et al. 2006; Goetzel et al. 2003; Lerner et al. 2004; Lotter et al. 2006; Rytsala et al. 2007; Wedegartner et al. 2007). Chronic physical conditions and psychological illness are also associated with reduced performance at work (Adler et al. 2006; Dewa & Lin 2000; Kessler et al. 2006; Lim, Sanderson, & Andrews 2000; Sanderson et al. 2007; Smit et al. 2006; Wang et al. 2004; Wang, Simon, & Kessler 2004). Randomized controlled trials have found that effective treatment of psychological disorders can reduce work loss and, possibly, improve work performance (Rollman et al. 2006; Rost, Smith, & Dickinson 2004; Wang et al. 2007; Wells et al. 2000). However, there is almost no information on the implications of chronic physical conditions and psychological disorders for unemployment in developing countries.

Even though the co-occurrence of mental disorders and chronic physical conditions is common among working-age adults, the implications of mental–physical comorbidity for labor force participation and unemployment have not been extensively studied. Available evidence suggests that psychological illness is strongly associated with unemployment among persons with comorbid chronic physical disease. For example, Von Korff et al. (2005) found that among persons with diabetes, depression was a stronger predictor of unemployment and work disability than were clinical measures of diabetes severity and diabetes complications. There are no population-based studies assessing the independent and joint effects of chronic physical illnesses and psychological disorders on labor force participation and unemployment in either developed or developing countries. Income maintenance programs, work demands, and the cultural context of work differ between developed and developing countries. For that reason, it is of considerable interest to understand whether mental–physical comorbidity shows differences in its association with labor force participation and unemployment between developed and developing countries.

In this chapter, population-based rates of labor force participation and unemployment are compared for persons with both a chronic physical illness and a depressive/anxiety disorder, for persons with either a chronic physical illness or a depressive/anxiety disorder (but not both), and for persons with neither. Using data from the World Mental Health (WMH) Surveys Initiative, these analyses provide the first population-based comparison of labor force participation and unemployment rates by health status comparing populations from developed and developing countries.

21.2. APPROACH

In each of the surveys of the WMH Survey Initiative, participants were asked about their current employment situation. Labor force participation and unemployment were analyzed among persons between 18 and 59 years of age (inclusive). Older persons and students were excluded. Participants were classified as employed if they said their current occupational status was employed, self-employed, laid-off, maternity leave, or illness/sick leave. Participants were classified as unemployed if they said their current occupational status was looking for work, unemployed, disabled, or other. Homemakers and retired persons were not counted as being either employed or unemployed. The labor force participation rate was defined as the number of persons who were employed divided by the number of persons who were employed, unemployed, retired, or homemakers. The unemployment rate was defined as the number of persons unemployed divided by the number of persons who were either employed or unemployed (as defined previously).

Labor force participation rates and unemployment rates are reported for each participating survey, for developed and developing countries separately, and for all countries combined. The association of mental–physical comorbidity with labor force participation and unemployment was assessed using logistic regression after adjusting for age, sex, education (above or below the median for each country), and country. Chronic physical illness was considered present among persons reporting any of the following chronic physical conditions: heart disease, diabetes, asthma, chronic obstructive pulmonary disease, tuberculosis, cancer, ulcers, epilepsy, HIV/AIDS, arthritis, back pain, headache, or other chronic pain. Psychological illness was considered present among persons meeting *Diagnostic and Statistical Manual of Mental Disorders, Fourth Edition* (DSM-IV) diagnostic criteria for major depression, dysthymia, generalized anxiety disorder, panic disorder, agoraphobia, posttraumatic stress disorder, or social phobia. For chronic pain and the psychological disorders, the conditions were reported present in the prior year.

Logistic regression models were used to compare risks (as measured by odds ratios) of not being a labor force participant (excluding students from the analysis) and risks of being unemployed among persons who were labor force participants by physical and mental disorder status. Each survey participant was classified as having neither a physical nor a psychological disorder, a physical disorder only, or a psychological disorder only, or as having both physical and psychological disorder. The odds ratios were adjusted for age, sex, relative educational level (above or below the country median), and country. Since a question about educational attainment was not included in the French survey, persons from France were not included in these analyses.

Table 21.1. Percent of population in labor force (employed, laid-off, on sick leave, or on maternity leave) among persons aged 18–59 years (excluding students)

Country	Labor force participation N	Percent
Nigeria	1,568	83.3
Shanghai	560	79.4
Beijing	712	75.6
Ukraine	1,076	74.4
Mexico	2,079	64.1
Lebanon	775	60.3
Colombia	2,134	59.5
South Africa	3,895	37.2
All developing	*12,799*	*59.5*
New Zealand	5,646	84.9
The Netherlands	833	84.5
France	1,087	84.1
Japan	563	83.7
United States	4,574	81.4
Belgium	770	81.4
Germany	943	78.3
Israel	3,631	74.5
Italy	1,301	72.8
Spain	1,346	70.7
All developed	*20,694*	*79.9*
All countries	*33,493*	*72.0*

21.3. FINDINGS

Among both developed and developing countries, there was notable variation in labor force participation rates (Table 21.1). Among the developed countries, 83% of working-age adults in New Zealand were labor force participants, compared to 70% in Spain. Labor force participation exceeded 80% in Nigeria, compared to 37% in South Africa. The labor force participation rate in developing countries averaged 59.5%, compared to a mean of 79.9% in developed countries. However, South Africa had a markedly lower labor force participation rate than the other developing countries participating in the WMH Surveys. The median labor force participation rate was 81.4% in developed countries versus 69.3% in developing countries, reflecting a general trend toward lower labor force participation rates in developing than developed countries.

While the overall rate of unemployment was twice as high in the developing countries (22.8%) than in the developed countries (11.2%), the unemployment rate in South Africa was considerably higher than the unemployment rates in the other developing countries (Table 21.2). The difference in median unemployment rates between developed and developing countries was modest. Among the developing countries, the median unemployment rate was 13.5%, while among the developed countries it was only slightly lower (12.0%).

In both developed and developing countries, labor force participation rates were lower

Table 21.2. Percent of labor force participants who are unemployed among persons aged 18–59 years (excluding students)

Country	Unemployed N	Percent
Mexico	1,273	7.1
Shanghai	488	11.6
Lebanon	477	12.0
Ukraine	905	13.5
Nigeria	1,522	13.6
Beijing	601	14.3
Colombia	1,513	17.8
South Africa	2,657	47.9
All developing	*9,436*	*22.8*
New Zealand	4,812	5.3
Japan	493	5.9
The Netherlands	740	7.4
France	1,001	9.7
Italy	1,059	12.0
Belgium	695	12.1
Spain	1,059	12.2
United States	4,227	12.5
Germany	835	13.2
Israel	3,373	18.6
All developed	*18,294*	*11.2*
All countries	*27,730*	*15.3*

Table 21.3. Labor force participation rate and unemployment rate by mental–physical comorbidity status for developed and developing countries

	Neither	Physical only	Mental only	Both
Labor force participation rate (%)				
Developed	83.0	78.7	77.2	68.8
Developing	63.6	56.4	51.4	44.8
All	75.0	70.2	69.7	61.7
Unemployment rate (%)				
Developed	8.7	11.7	14.8	22.1
Developing	21.1	23.9	30.8	32.7
Both	13.4	15.9	18.8	24.6

and unemployment rates were higher among persons with chronic physical conditions and psychological disorders (Table 21.3). In general, labor force participation rates were considerably lower, and unemployment rates higher, among persons with both mental and physical disorders, compared to persons with physical morbidity only or with psychological morbidity only. In developing countries, the unemployment rate among persons with mental–physical comorbidity was only slightly higher than the unemployment rate among persons with noncomorbid psychological illness. In contrast, unemployment rates among persons with a mental disorder, with and without a comorbid physical disorder, were considerably higher than those among persons with chronic physical disease only.

Gender-specific labor force participation and unemployment rates by mental–physical comorbidity status are given in Table 21.4

Table 21.4. Labor force participation rate and unemployment rate and mental–physical comorbidity status for developed and developing countries by gender

	Neither	Physical only	Mental only	Both
		Males		
Labor force participation rate (%)				
Developed	90.7	87.5	87.0	73.3
Developing	74.5	69.5	60.3	58.7
Both	83.9	81.2	78.6	69.7
Unemployment rate (%)				
Developed	7.8	10.4	12.3	23.7
Developing	24.0	27.6	37.9	36.9
Both	14.6	16.3	20.2	26.8
		Females		
Labor force participation rate (%)				
Developed	74.2	70.9	70.7	66.3
Developing	50.6	47.4	44.0	39.7
Both	64.6	61.1	63.5	57.7
Unemployment rate (%)				
Developed	9.8	13.1	16.8	21.1
Developing	15.4	19.9	20.7	30.1
Both	11.7	15.4	17.6	23.3

Table 21.5. Odds ratios for not being in the labor force and for unemployment (excluding students) by mental–physical comorbidity for developed and developing countries, controlling for age, sex, education, and country (France excluded)

	Neither	Physical only	Mental only	Both	p-value
Not in labor force					
Developed	1.0	1.2 (1.1, 1.4)	1.4 (1.2, 1,7)	2.1 (1.8, 2.3)	$p < .0001$
Developing	1.0	1.0 (0.9, 1.2)	1.2 (0.9, 1.6)	1.2 (0.9, 1.4)	$p = .39$
Unemployment					
Developed	1.0	1.5 (1.3, 1.7)	1.9 (1.5, 2.4)	3.3 (2.8, 3.8)	$p < .0001$
Developing	1.0	1.1 (0.9, 1.2)	1.3 (1.0, 1.8)	1.4 (1.1, 1.9)	$p = .02$

for developed and developing countries. The sex-specific trends in labor force participation and unemployment rates by mental–physical comorbidity status were generally similar among males and females. However, among females in developing countries, labor force participation rates did not differ appreciably among persons with physical versus psychological disorders.

Multivariate analyses adjusting for age, sex, education, and country showed that relative to persons with neither mental nor physical morbidity, the odds ratios of not being in the labor force were doubled among persons with mental–physical comorbidity residing in developed countries (Table 21.5). There was a smaller increase in risk of not being in the labor force among persons with physical morbidity only and with mental morbidity only in developed countries. In contrast, differences in risk of not being in the labor force did not differ significantly by mental–physical comorbidity status in developing countries. The difference in risk of unemployment by mental–physical comorbidity status was smaller in developing than in developed countries. Persons with both mental and physical morbidity had more than a three fold excess in risk of unemployment in developed countries, compared to a 1.4-fold increase in developing countries (Table 21.5).

21.4. DISCUSSION

In the countries included in the WMH Survey Initiative, comorbidity of mental disorders and chronic physical conditions was associated with increased risk of unemployment in both developed and developing countries. This risk differential was greater in developed countries than in developing countries. Mental–physical comorbidity was also associated with reduced labor force participation in developed countries, but not in developing countries (albeit the trend was in the same direction). In developed countries, the presence of psychological disorder in the absence of a physical disorder was associated with increased risk of not being in the labor force and of unemployment among labor force participants. This was also true for chronic physical conditions in the absence of comorbid psychological disorder, but the risk differentials were smaller. These results point to the importance of the co-occurrence of mental and physical disorders as possible determinants of employment status in both developed and developing countries. The apparently weaker association of mental–physical comorbidity in developing countries is an intriguing observation that merits further research.

The implications of mental–physical comorbidity for work productivity are potentially large. In developed countries among persons with neither physical nor psychological illness, 77% of working-age adults were currently employed (i.e., 83.0% labor force participation rate × 92.3% current employment rate). In contrast, among working-age adults with both physical and psychological illness in developed countries, only 54% were currently employed (68.8% × 77.9%). The corresponding figures for developing countries were 50% for persons without physical or mental disorder compared to 30% for persons with both mental and physical disorders. These rates highlight the potential importance for national economic well-being of understanding how to maximize the work abilities of persons with comorbid mental and physical disorders.

In a cross-sectional survey, it is not possible to determine whether differences in psychological status are a cause or a consequence of unemployment. While there is substantial evidence from other research supporting the deleterious effects of depressive and anxiety disorders on work disability, the results reported here are consistent with psychological illness causing or resulting from reduced labor force participation and increased unemployment. However, in either case, the increased prevalence of psychological disorder and comorbid physical illness among unemployed persons is likely to be an important consideration in designing programs to return people to work.

In conclusion, reduced labor force participation and increased unemployment was most strongly associated with comorbid psychological and physical disorders. The strength of this association was stronger in developed than in developing countries. However, in both developed and developing countries, among working-age adults, the percent of the population that is currently working is substantially lower among persons with comorbid mental and physical disorders.

REFERENCES

Adler, D. A., McLaughlin, T. J., Rogers, W. H., Chang, H., Lapitsky, L., & Lerner, D. (2006). Job performance deficits due to depression. *American Journal of Psychiatry*, **163**, 1569–76.

De Buck, P. D., de Bock, G. H., van Dijk, F., van den Hout, W. B., Vandenbroucke, J. P., & Vliet Vlieland, T. P. (2006). Sick leave as a predictor of job loss in patients with chronic arthritis. *International Archives of Occupational and Environmental Health*, **80**, 160–70.

Dewa, C. S., & Lin, E. (2000). Chronic physical illness, psychiatric disorder and disability in the workplace. *Social Science and Medicine*, **51**, 41–50.

Goetzel, R. Z., Hawkins, K., Ozminkowski, R. J., & Wang, S. (2003). The health and productivity cost burden of the "top 10" physical and mental health conditions affecting six large U.S. employers in 1998. *Journal of Occupational and Environmental Medicine*, **45**, 5–14.

Jin, R. L., Shah, C. P., & Svoboda, T. J. (1995). The impact of unemployment on health: A review of the evidence. *Canadian Medical Association Journal*, **153**, 529–40.

Kessler, R. C., Akiskal, H. S., Ames, M., Birnbaum, H., Greenberg, P., Hirschfeld, R. M., Jin, R., Merikangas, K. R., Simon, G. E., & Wang, P. S. (2006). Prevalence and effects of mood disorders on work performance in a nationally representative sample of U.S. workers. *American Journal of Psychiatry*, **163**, 1561–8.

Lerner, D., Adler, D. A., Chang, H., Lapitsky, L., Hood, M. Y., Perissinotto, C., Reed, J., McLaughlin, T. J., Berndt, E. R., & Rogers, W. H. (2004). Unemployment, job retention, and productivity loss among employees with depression. *Psychiatric Services*, **55**, 1371–8.

Lim, D., Sanderson, K., & Andrews, G. (2000). Lost productivity among full-time workers with mental disorders. *Journal of Mental Health Policy and Economics*, **3**, 139–46.

Lotter, F., Franche, R. L., Hogg-Johnson, S., Burdorf, A., & Pole, J. D. (2006). The prognostic value of depressive symptoms, fear-avoidance, and self-efficacy for duration of lost-time benefits in workers with musculoskeletal disorders. *Journal of Occupational and Environmental Medicine*, **63**, 794–801.

Mathers, C. D., & Schofield, D. J. (1998). The health consequences of unemployment: The evidence. *Medical Journal of Australia*, **168**, 178–82.

Morris, J. K., & Cook, D. G. (1991). A critical review of the effect of factory closures on health. *British Journal of Industrial Medicine*, **48**, 1–8.

Rollman, B. L., Belnap, B. H., Mazumdar, S., Houck, P. R., Zhu, F., Gardner, W., Reynolds, C. F., III, Schulberg, H. C., & Shear, M. K. (2006). A randomized trial to improve the quality of treatment for panic and generalized anxiety disorders in primary care. *Archives of General Psychiatry*, **62**, 1332–41.

Rost, K., Smith, J. L., & Dickinson, M. (2004). The effect of improving primary care depression management on employee absenteeism and productivity: A randomized trial. *Medical Care*, **42**, 1202–10.

Rytsala, H. J., Melartin, T. K., Leskela, U. S., Sokero, T. P., Lestela-Mielonen, P. S., & Isometsa, E. T. (2007). Predictors of long-term work disability in major depressive disorder: A prospective study. *Acta Psychiatrica Scandinavica*, **115**, 206–13.

Sanderson, K., Tilse, E., Nicholson, J., Oldenburg, B., & Graves, N. (2007). Which presenteeism measures are more sensitive to depression and anxiety? *Journal of Affective Disorders*, **101**, 65–74.

Smit, F., Cuijpers, P., Oostenbrink, J., Batelaan, N., de Graaf, R., & Beekman, A. (2006). Costs of nine common mental disorders: Implications for curative and preventive psychiatry. *Journal of Mental Health Policy and Economics*, **9**, 193–200.

Von Korff, M., Katon, W., Lin, E. H., Simon, G., Ciechanowshi, P., Ludman, E., Oliver, M., Rutter, C., & Young, B. (2005). Work disability among individuals diabetes. *Diabetes Care*, **28**, 1326–32.

Wang, P. S., Beck, A., Berglund, P., Leutzinger, J. A., Pronk, N., Richling, D., Schenk, T. W., Simon, G., Stang, P., Ustun, T. B., & Kessler, R. C. (2003). Chronic medical conditions and work performance in the health and work performance questionnaire calibration surveys. *Journal of Occupational and Environmental Medicine*, **45**, 1303–11.

Wang, P. S., Beck, A. L., Berglund, P., McKenas, D. K., Pronk, N. P., Simon, G. E., & Kessler, R. C. (2004). Effects of major depression on moment-in-time work performance. *American Journal of Psychiatry*, **161**, 1885–91.

Wang, P. S., Simon, G., & Kessler, R. C. (2003). The economic burden of depression and the cost-effectiveness of treatment. *International Journal of Methods for Psychiatric Research*, **12**, 22–33.

Wang, P. S., Simon, G. E., Avorn, J., Azocar, F., Ludman, E. J., McCulloch, J., Petukhova, M. Z., & Kessler, R. C. (2007). Telephone screening, outreach, and care management for depressed workers and impact on clinical and work productivity outcomes: A randomized controlled trial. *The Journal of the American Medical Association*, **298**, 1401–11.

Wedegartner, F., Sittaro, N. A., Emrich, H. M., & Dietrich, D. E. (2007). Disability caused by affective disorders – What do the Federal German Health report data teach us? *Psychiatrische Praxis*, **34**, S252–5.

Wells, K. B., Sherbourne, C., Schoenbaum, M., Duan, N., Meredith, L., Unutzer, J., Miranda, J., Carney, M. F., & Rubenstein, L. V. (2000). Impact of disseminating quality improvement programs for depression in managed primary care: A randomized controlled trial. *The Journal of the American Medical Association*, **12**, 212–20.

22 Perceived Stigma and Mental–Physical Comorbidity

JORDI ALONSO, ANDREA BURON, AND GEMMA VILAGUT

22.1. INTRODUCTION

"Stigma" is a social construction that defines individuals in terms of a distinguishing characteristic or mark and devalues them as a consequence (Dinos et al. 2004). The presence of stigmatizing attitudes and discriminating behaviors has been applied to many health circumstances, from urinary incontinence to leprosy, cancer, or AIDS. The general public, however, seems to disapprove of persons with mental illness more than of persons with physical disabilities (Corrigan et al. 2000, 2003; Hinshaw & Cicchetti 2000; Rusch, Angermeyer, & Corrigan 2005; Socall & Holtgraves 1992).

Research on health-related stigmatization can be traced back to the mid-twentieth century. Goffman (1963) defined stigma as "an attribute that is deeply discrediting" that reduces the bearer "from a whole and usual person to a tainted, discounted one," and also as the relationship between "an attribute and a stereotype," permeating social interactions and motivating the stigmatized individual to hide the mark. Other similar definitions have been proposed more recently, such as "a characteristic of a person that is contrary to a norm of a social unit" (Link & Pehlan 2001; Stafford & Scott 1986); "stigmatized people possess some attribute that convey a social identity that is devalued in a particular social context" (Crocker, Major, & Steele 1998; Link & Pehlan 2001); and a "relationship between an attribute and a stereotype to produce a definition of stigma as a mark that links a person with undesirable characteristics" (Jones et al. 1984; Link & Pehlan 2001). In light of these varying definitions, the conceptualization of stigma is not viewed as definite (Link & Phelan 2001).

All definitions proposed have three things in common: namely, that stigma is a mark or label; it arises from society and individuals' interactions (the "stigmatizers" and the "stigmatized"); and it has negative consequences for the bearer of the stigma. Several authors have classified stigma into "public stigma" and "self-stigma." *Public stigma* comprises reactions of the general public toward a group based on stigma about that group, whereas *self-stigma* refers to the reactions of individuals who belong to a stigmatized group and turn the stigmatizing attitudes against themselves (Rusch et al. 2005).

In his review about the measurement of stigma, Link et al. (2004) find a wide range of approaches, from surveys to qualitative studies. Most of the research involved nonexperimental surveys with vignettes, in which standardized questions about a picture depicting someone with mental illness were asked to respondents. Experimental studies with vignettes, in which the investigator randomly assigned the manipulated variable to study groups, as well as qualitative studies, have been less often employed to study stigma. According to Link et al. (2004), the varying definitions of stigma, as well as the differences in research methods employed, have resulted in considerable variability in findings. Stereotyping and the expectations of status loss and discrimination have been the most frequently studied dimensions of stigma. Behaviors indicative of the presence of mental illness as a stimulus and the presence of emotional reactions were also quite often assessed. Other components of stigma that have been studied include labeling and behavioral responses to stigma. The majority of studies have focused on the general population, assessing the opinions of, for example, the general adult population or college students about their feelings and experiences with mentally ill people in their community.

The other group that has been quite widely studied is professionals in general and psychiatrists in particular. This research has explored the professionals themselves, as well as their opinions of self-perceived stigma and its impact on the mentally ill (Angermeyer 2003). Patients' families and caregivers have also been studied in depth to assess the burden experienced, including stigma, and their psychological well-being. Quite surprisingly, people with mental disorders have not been studied directly very often. When they have, the research has most often focused on a specific type of disorder such as schizophrenia or depression or a selected psychiatric institution (Angermeyer 2003).

The World Mental Health (WMH) Survey Initiative assessed both mental disorders and chronic physical conditions. Among persons with significant activity limitations due to psychological and/or physical illness, the WMH Surveys also asked several questions about health-related stigma. Thus, the WMH Surveys provide a unique opportunity to assess health-related stigma in developed and developing countries worldwide. In this chapter we assess the prevalence of stigma among individuals with moderate-to-high disability and its association with chronic physical conditions and mental disorders in the 17 countries participating in the WMH Surveys. In addition, we assessed the impact of health-related stigma among individuals with mental disorders in a subset of six European countries participating in the ESEMeD (European Study of the Epidemiology of Mental Disorders) surveys (Alonso et al. 2007).

22.2. APPROACH

22.2.1. Measurement of Stigma in the WMH

Perceived health-related stigma was assessed with two items from the World Health Organization Disability Assessment Schedule – II (WHODAS-II) (Epping-Jordan & Ustun 2000): "How much *embarrassment* did you experience because of your health problems during the past 30 days?" and "How much *discrimination* or *unfair treatment* did you experience because of your heath problems during the past 30 days?" For both questions, response options included the following: "None, a little, some, a lot, or extreme." Individuals endorsing at least "a little" embarrassment and at least "a little" discrimination were considered to have health-related stigma. Because stigma related to health problems is most relevant to persons with significant health problems, the stigma questions were only administered to individuals who reported significant (i.e., reporting at least "moderate") activity limitation due to health problems in the month prior to the interview (in one or more of these functions: cognition, mobility, self-care, and social).

We recognize that the measure of stigma in the WMH Surveys was incomplete in at least two ways: First, perceived stigma was assessed only with two items instead of more complex measures used in studies focused largely on perceived stigma. Given the scope of the WMH Surveys, the number of questions that could be devoted to assessing stigma was necessarily limited, which can have implications for measurement error in assessment of perceived stigma. Second, stigma questions were administered only to those individuals who reported significant health-related activity limitation in the month before the interview. The underlying assumption was that questions about perceived stigma are not particularly salient to individuals who do not experience activity limitations. Recognizing these limitations, this study is the first cross-national study to collect information among individuals in the general population with and without chronic physical conditions and mental disorders.

22.2.2. Mental Disorders and Chronic Conditions in WMH Surveys

Disorders considered in the analyses reported here include anxiety disorders (generalized anxiety disorder, panic disorder and/or agoraphobia, posttraumatic stress disorder, and social phobia) and mood disorders (dysthymia and major depressive disorder). The analyses in this chapter concern persons with (1) an anxiety disorder in the absence of comorbid mood disorder, (2) a mood disorder in the absence of comorbid anxiety disorder, or (3) comorbid mood and anxiety disorder. All disorders considered referred to the 12 months prior to the interview.

22.2.3. Chronic Physical Conditions

The physical conditions in the analyses reported here include stroke, heart attack or heart disease, asthma or chronic obstructive pulmonary disease (COPD), diabetes, ulcer, HIV/AIDS, epilepsy, tuberculosis, and cancer. The numbers of chronic physical disorders were grouped as 0, 1, and >2. (Heart attack and heart disease were counted as one condition, as were asthma and COPD.)

22.2.4. Impact of Stigma

For some countries, quality-of-life data were collected, permitting analyses of the association of stigma and health status. Quality of life was measured through the 12-item short-form (SF-12) health survey, which refers to the previous 4 weeks and has two component summary scores: the physical component score (PCS) and the mental component score (MCS). The PCS and MCS scales were scored using norm-based methods with the item weights from the general U.S. population and a linear t-score transformation with a mean of 50 and a standard deviation of 10. Scores greater than 50 are better and those lesser than 50 are worse than the U.S. population mean. This information was collected in the six ESEMeD countries: Belgium, France, Germany, Italy, the Netherlands, and Spain (Alonso et al. 2009).

Other variables used to evaluate the impact of health-related stigma included work and role limitation in the month prior to the interview were assessed by the WHODAS-II. A work lost days (WLD) index was obtained as the weighted sum of (1) the number of days totally unable to work or carry out normal activities in the prior month; (2) one-half the number of days of reduced work and activities; (3) one-half the number of days of reduced quality or care in work activities; and (4) one-quarter the number of days requiring extreme effort to perform at one's usual level. If this sum exceeded 30, it was recoded to equal 30 so that the sum had a range from 0 to 30. The scores were linearly transformed to a 0–100 range.

Based on another question of the WHODAS-II about days with social difficulties in the previous 30 days, a social limitation index was computed dividing the number of days with difficulties by 30 and multiplied by 100. People who did not report any difficulties were computed as 0 days. The range of the index was 0–100; the higher the number the more the social limitation.

Finally, interference with help-seeking behavior was also assessed. Respondents were asked whether they had delayed help-seeking for their mental health, had not sought professional help, or had quit treatment because they were concerned either *about what people would think* or that *people could found out that they were in treatment* for their mental health.

22.2.5. Analyses

Odds ratios for the association of chronic physical conditions and mental disorders with stigma were estimated via logistic regression, with the presence of perceived stigma as the dependent variable. Predictors included age (four levels), gender, education level (completed secondary education or not), number of chronic physical conditions (0, 1, and >2), and number and type of mental disorders (none, only mood, only anxiety, and comorbid mood and anxiety). Information on education was not available for France. We did not perform logistic regression analyses for countries if fewer than 20 people reported stigma.

Data are presented for each survey and for all countries combined, for surveys in developing countries with a World Development Index <0.90 (i.e., Beijing, Colombia, Lebanon, Mexico, Nigeria, Ukraine, and Shanghai), and for developed countries.

To estimate the independent association of perceived stigma with quality of life, work and role limitation, and social limitation, a series of least-square multivariate linear regression models were developed with data from the six European (ESEMeD) countries: Belgium, France, Germany, Italy, the Netherlands, and Spain. Sociodemographic and other variables were included as the independent variables. Dependent variables were, respectively, the SF-12 Physical and Mental Component Scores, the WLD index, and the social difficulties index. Nonstandardized regression coefficients indicate the adjusted difference in mean outcome scores between the categories while controlling for all other variables.

22.3. FINDINGS

22.3.1 Prevalence of Perceived Stigma

Table 22.1 shows the weighted proportion of the adult population with significant activity limitations. It is among these individuals that the questions about stigma were asked. Table 22.1 also shows the proportions reporting health-related embarrassment, health-related discrimination, and perceived stigma defined by the presence of both embarrassment and discrimination. The prevalence of significant activity limitation ranged from 4.6 to 24.1%. Among those with significant activity limitations, embarrassment (range 15.2–87.4%) was more common than was perceived discrimination (range 6.2–37.7%). Among persons with significant activity limitations, perceived stigma was relatively common: 13.5% in the overall sample (22.1% in developing and 11.7% in developed countries).

Mean age was similar among those with and without perceived stigma. Male gender and lower education levels tended to be more common among persons reporting perceived stigma than among those not reporting it. The prevalence of perceived stigma among persons with and without chronic physical disease and among persons with and without a mental disorder is provided in Table 22.2. Except in three countries with small numbers of respondents with significant activity limitations (Beijing, Shanghai, and Lebanon), the prevalence of health-related stigma was greater among persons with a mental disorder (prevalence for all countries: 21.9%) than

Table 22.1. Sample characteristics and population estimates of the prevalence of perceived stigma, chronic physical condition, and mental disorder by country

Country	Sample size (N)	Response rate (%)	Activity limitation (N%)		Embarrassment (%)	Discrimination (%)	Perceived stigma[a] (%)	Chronic physical condition (%)	Mental disorder (%)
The Americas									
Colombia	4,426	87.7	173	5.0	33.6	23.8	17.8	37.8	29.8
Mexico	5,782	76.6	185	4.6	45.1	25.6	21.0	27.3	32.2
United States	9,282	70.9	1,154	16.2	31.1	13.8	8.5	53.2	36.5
Asia									
Japan	2,436	56.4	97	7.5	48.4	9.9	8.7	39.7	11.2
Beijing	2,633	74.8	69	5.0	36.2	20.2	12.4	39.4	17.7
Shanghai	2,568	74.6	41	6.5	44.3	37.7	22.4	49.6	5.2
Lebanon	2,857	70.0	198	13.5	25.3	14.8	9.2	28.3	20.4
Israel	4,859	79.3	1,089	22.6	53.8	24.6	20.2	49.4	20.4
Oceania									
New Zealand	12,992	73.3	1,393	14.5	31.9	14.6	8.7	46.9	28.2
Europe									
Belgium	2,419	50.6	205	13.7	37.7	14.8	12.5	38.2	22.1
France	2,894	45.9	244	13.1	76.7	13.0	12.8	31.8	25.9
Germany	3,555	57.8	219	13.5	19.6	6.2	3.2	49.3	13.6
Italy	4,712	71.3	215	10.0	37.8	13.5	13.1	35.3	18.9
The Netherlands	2,372	56.4	291	20.3	20.7	15.3	6.7	45.7	20.2
Spain	5,473	78.6	376	10.3	15.2	11.7	8.2	41.4	20.5
Ukraine	4,725	78.3	506	24.1	87.4	32.4	32.1	59.2	28.6
Africa									
Nigeria	6,752	79.3	1,089	22.6	23.4	17.5	9.7	25.3	7.8
All countries			6,574	13.5	41.0	18.0	13.5	46.6	25.5
Developing countries			1,291	8.6	56.0	26.2	22.1	44.4	24.7
Developed countries			5,283	15.5	37.8	16.3	11.7	47.1	25.6

Note: Data taken from *The World Mental Health Surveys.*
[a] Stigma was considered present when both embarrassment and discrimination were reported.

Table 22.2. Percent prevalence (and 95% confidence intervals) of perceived stigma according to chronic physical condition and mental disorder status among persons with significant activity limitation

	% (95% CI)			
	Chronic physical condition		**Mental disorder**	
Country	**Absent**	**Present**	**Absent**	**Present**
The Americas				
Colombia	12.5 (7.8, 19.6)	26.6 (17.1, 38.8)	12.1 (6.2, 22.3)	31.4 (18.9, 47.3)
Mexico	20.4 (12.6, 31.2)	22.6 (14.7, 33.2)	12.3 (6.6, 21.7)	39.2 (27.8, 52.0)
United States	6.8 (4.9, 9.4)	10.0 (7.2, 13.8)	3.7 (2.2, 6.2)	16.9 (12.9, 21.9)
Asia				
Japan	9.1 (4.3, 18.5)	8.0 (2.3, 24.6)	6.3 (3.3, 11.7)	27.8 (11.2, 54.0)
Beijing	11.5 (4.8, 25.1)	13.8 (5.3, 31.8)	12.6 (6.2, 23.9)	11.5 (3.4, 32.8)
Shanghai	2.9 (0.4, 17.0)	42.2 (10.1, 82.6)	22.5 (6.9, 53.1)	21.9 (2.4, 75.8)
Lebanon	9.4 (3.3, 24.0)	5.7 (1.8, 16.9)	10.8 (6.0, 18.7)	2.9 (1.0, 8.1)
Israel	17.1 (14.0, 20.7)	23.4 (19.8, 27.3)	17.4 (14.9, 20.3)	30.9 (24.7, 7.8)
Oceania				
New Zealand	9.1 (6.6, 12.6)	8.1 (5.8, 11.3)	5.8 (3.9, 8.6)	16.0 (12.2, 20.5)
Europe				
Belgium	12.7 (6.9, 22.2)	12.1 (5.3, 25.4)	10.2 (5.1, 19.4)	20.6 (10.2, 37.1)
France	7.6 (3.4, 16.4)	24.0 (10.0, 47.4)	9.2 (3.0, 25.1)	23.2 (11.9, 40.3)
Germany	3.6 (1.8, 7.3)	2.9 (1.1, 7.6)	0.7 (0.4, 1.5)	19.3 (9.9, 34.4)
Italy	12.0 (6.7, 20.5)	15.0 (8.0, 26.3)	10.3 (5.6, 18.3)	24.9 (15.4, 37.6)
The Netherlands	7.7 (3.3, 16.9)	5.5 (2.6, 11.3)	6.0 (2.6, 13.2)	9.3 (4.4, 18.7)
Spain	8.5 (4.6, 15.2)	7.7 (3.4, 16.4)	5.5 (2.5, 11.4)	18.7 (12.5, 26.9)
Ukraine	30.3 (21.1, 41.3)	33.4 (26.4, 41.3)	30.0 (22.1, 39.3)	37.5 (31.1, 44.4)
Africa				
Nigeria	9.9 (5.7, 16.5)	9.2 (2.7, 26.8)	7.6 (4.2, 13.4)	35.2 (13.8, 64.7)
All countries	11.8 (10.6, 13.3)	15.5 (13.8, 17.3)	10.6 (9.4, 12.0)	21.9 (19.8, 24.1)
Developing countries	18.3 (14.6, 22.7)	28.2 (22.9, 34.2)	19.2 (15.4, 23.6)	31.2 (26.8, 36.0)
Developed countries	10.5 (9.2, 12.0)	13.0 (11.5, 14.8)	8.8 (7.7, 10.1)	20.0 (17.7, 22.5)

Note: Data taken from *The World Mental Health Surveys.*

among persons without a mental disorder (10.6%). In contrast, the prevalence of perceived stigma among persons with a chronic physical condition (15.5%) relative to those without (11.8%) was smaller. Of course, comparison of prevalence rates of perceived stigma among persons with and without chronic physical disease and persons with and without a mental disorder is not meaningful without controlling for differences in age, sex, educational attainment, and comorbidity.

The association of chronic physical disease and mental disorder status with perceived stigma, controlling for age, sex, education, and comorbidity, is presented in Table 22.3. Compared to those without a chronic physical condition, perceived stigma was somewhat more likely to be reported by those with two or more chronic physical conditions (pooled odds ratios of 1.3 for a single chronic condition and 1.4 for multiple chronic conditions).

In contrast, perceived stigma was much more likely to occur among individuals with mental disorders in comparison to those without mental disorders. As shown in Table 22.3 and Figure 22.1, there was an increased

Table 22.3. Odds ratios (and confidence intervals) for perceived stigma according to the number of chronic physical conditions and mental disorder status, controlling for age, sex, and education, among people with significant activity limitation

	Chronic physical condition		Mental disorder		
			\(Reference = None\)		
Country	One	Two or more	Anxiety only	Mood only	Comorbid mood and anxiety
All countries	1.3 (1.0, 1.6)*	1.4 (1.1, 1.8)*	1.8 (1.3, 2.4)*	2.3 (1.8, 3.0)*	3.4 (2.7, 4.2)*[a]
Developing countries	1.7 (1.0, 2.8)*	1.3 (0.8, 2.1)	2.0 (1.1, 3.5)*	1.8 (1.2, 2.7)*	3.3 (2.1, 5.2)*
Developed countries	1.1 (0.9, 1.5)	1.6 (1.2, 2.1)*	1.9 (1.4, 2.6)*	2.5 (1.8, 3.3)*	3.6 (2.7, 4.6)*

Note: Data taken from *The World Mental Health Surveys*. Country not included if fewer than 20 people have stigma.
[a] Pooled odds ratios (ORs) for comorbid mood and anxiety disorders are significantly greater than the pooled OR for noncomorbid mood and noncomorbid anxiety.
* $p < .05$.

occurrence of stigma for persons with an anxiety disorder in the absence of a mood disorder (OR = 1.8; Figure 22.1) and for persons with a mood disorder in the absence of an anxiety disorder (OR = 2.3; Figure 22.2). Among persons with comorbid mood and anxiety mental disorders, the increased risk of stigma was greater still (OR = 3.4; Figure 22.3). The pattern of association of perceived stigma with anxiety and depressive disorders was similar in both developed and developing countries.

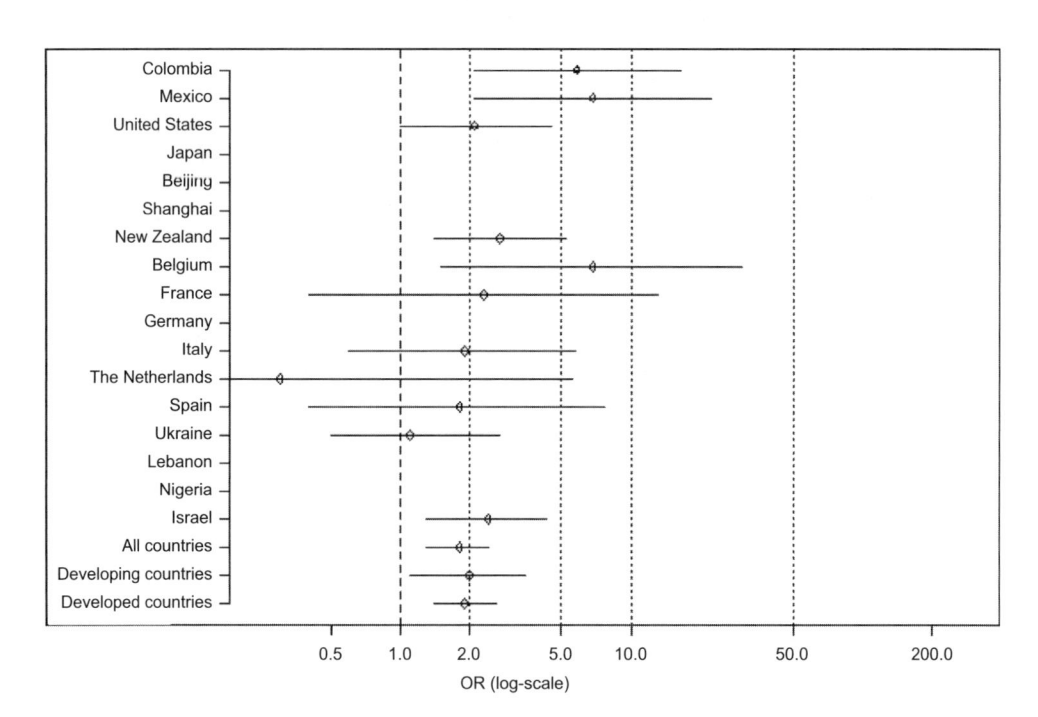

Figure 22.1. Anxiety disorders, but not mood disorders.

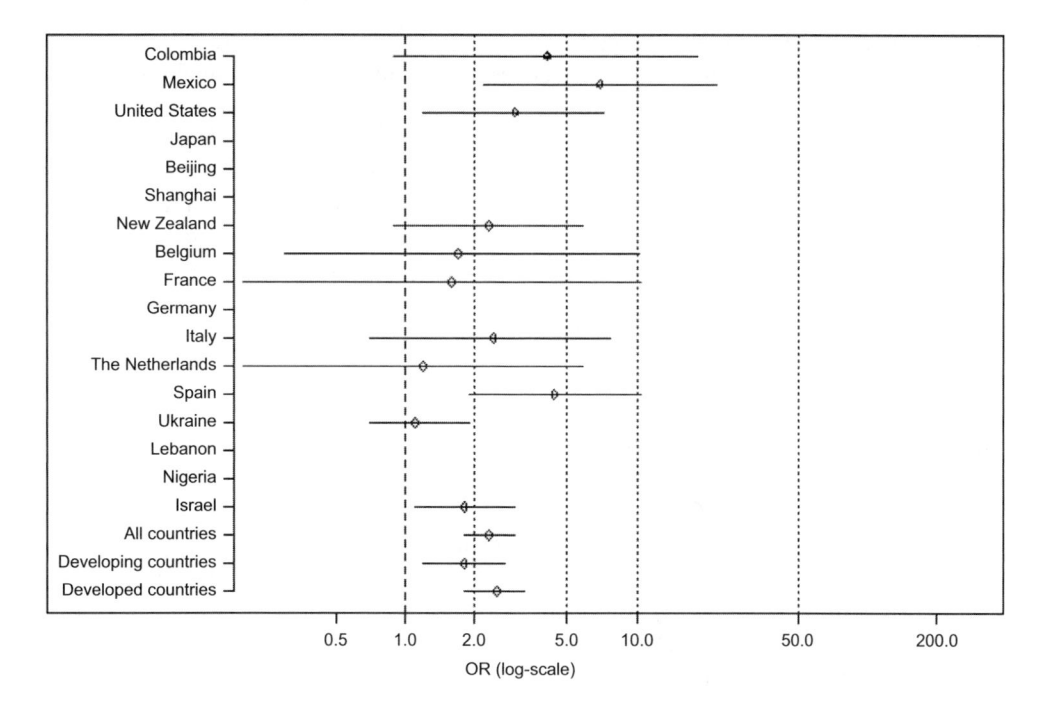

Perceived Stigma and Mental–Physical Comorbidity

Figure 22.2. Mood disorders, but not anxiety disorders.

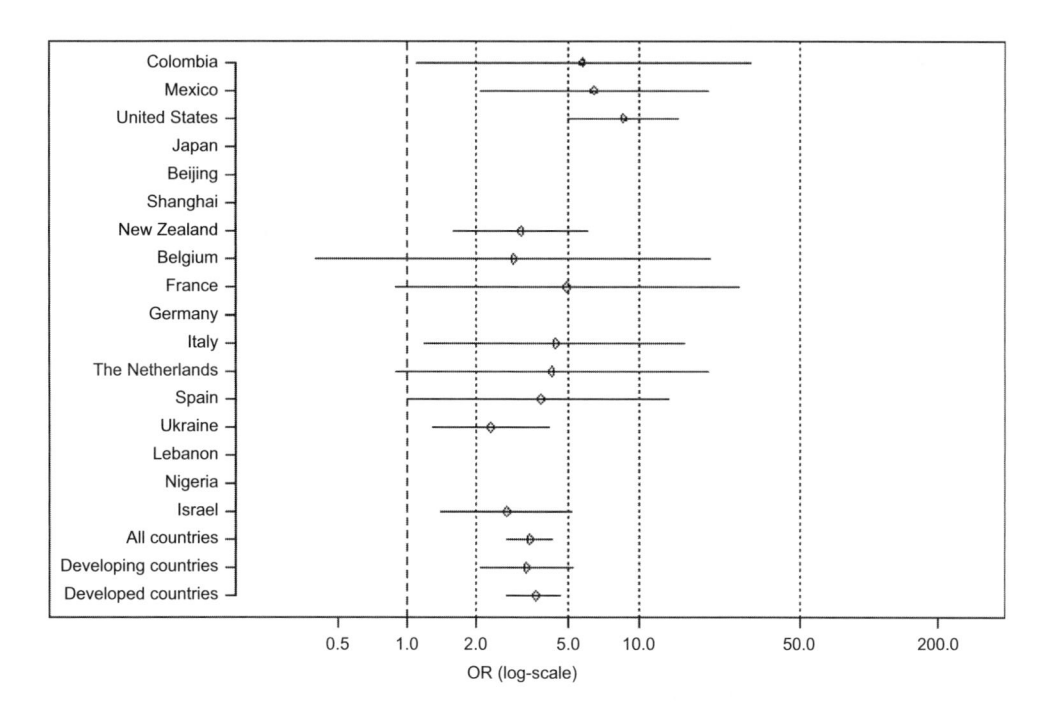

Figure 22.3. Comorbid anxiety and mood disorders.

We assessed whether the presence of comorbid mood and anxiety disorder was more strongly associated with perceived stigma than that of noncomorbid mood and noncomorbid anxiety disorder (country-specific estimates not shown). In the pooled analysis, the risk of perceived stigma was significantly lower (OR = 0.7, 95% CI = 0.5–0.9) for persons with mood disorder only and for persons with anxiety disorder only (OR = 0.5, 95% CI = 0.4–0.7) relative to persons with comorbid mood and anxiety disorder. Thus, the presence of comorbid mood and anxiety disorder was associated with significantly greater likelihood of perceived stigma than among persons with noncomorbid mood or anxiety disorders. We also assessed whether persons with a mental disorder without a comorbid physical disorder were more likely to report perceived stigma than persons with a physical disorder without a mental disorder. In a pooled analysis, persons with a mood or an anxiety disorder that was not comorbid with a physical disorder were more likely to report stigma (OR = 1.9, 95% CI = 1.2–2.4) relative to persons with a chronic physical disorder that was not comorbid with a mental disorder.

22.3.2. Impact of Perceived Stigma among Individuals with Mental Disorders

In a subgroup of the study sample (respondents from the six European countries of the ESEMeD project), information on the quality of life, work and role limitations, social difficulties, and interference with help-seeking behavior were also analyzed. In the bivariate analysis, all individuals with mental disorders showed lower quality of life, as indicated by the SF-12 PCS and MCS scores, 10 or more points below the general population mean. Moreover, individuals with perceived stigma scored, on average, about 6 additional points lower on the PCS and almost 5 points lower on the MCS than those without stigma. Similarly, the WLD index was almost 20 points higher among those with stigma, though this difference was not significant. The mean social limitation index for those with perceived stigma was 40.4, significantly higher than those without stigma (10.2). No significant differences among those with and those without perceived stigma were found for interference with seeking services.

Results of the multivariate analyses are summarized in Figure 22.4. These analyses indicate that stigma was significantly associated with lower (less favorable) SF-12 PCS scores (-4.65; $p < .05$), while the decrement in MCS (-3.70) was nonsignificant. Perceived stigma was also associated with a significantly higher proportion of WLD index (14.62; $p < .05$) and of social limitation (28.09; $p < .001$).

22.4. DISCUSSION

Our results show that among persons with significant activity limitations, perceived stigma is commonly reported, where stigma is defined by the presence of both embarrassment and perceived discrimination. Despite between-country variation in the prevalence of perceived stigma, mental disorders – particularly comorbid depression and anxiety – showed a robust association with stigma, while chronic physical disorders showed a relatively weak association. Thus, mental disorders appear to be a more important correlate of perceived stigma than do chronic physical conditions among persons in the general population with significant activity limitations in both developed and developing countries.

Our results also show that perceived stigma is relatively common among individuals with mental disorders and significant disability. Among these individuals, perceived stigma is more frequent among those with less education, those married, and those unemployed.

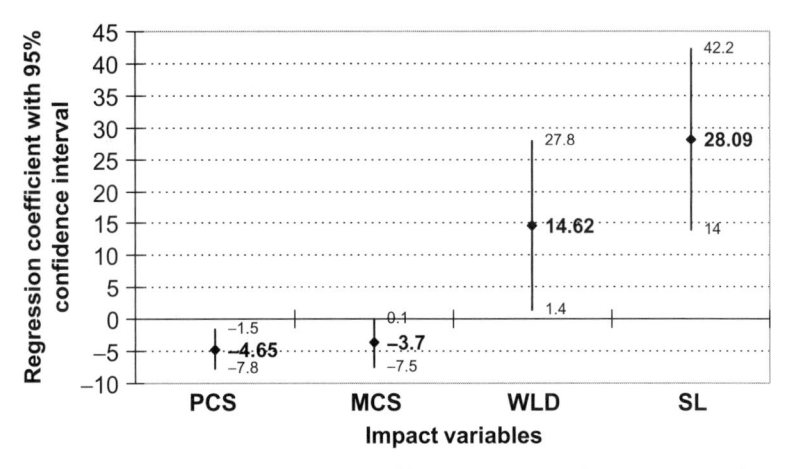

Figure 22.4. Impact of stigma over the physical (PCS) and mental (MCS) components of quality of life, work lost days (WLD) index, and social limitation (SL) index among individuals with mental disorders and significant disability in the six ESEMeD countries (including Belgium, France, Germany, Italy, the Netherlands, and Spain) ($N = 815$). Values are regression coefficients and the interval are 95% confidence intervals.

And it is associated with significantly worse physical quality of life, more work and role limitation, and more social limitation than the other individuals with mental disorders (but no perceived stigma).

To our knowledge, the data collected in the WMH Surveys Initiative allowed us to obtain the first international population-based results to assess the differential prevalence of stigma among individuals with mental disorders or physical conditions. And the WMH Surveys also allowed us to be able to assess the impact of perceived stigma among people with mental disorders. The frequency and impact of perceived stigma suggest that it might be necessary to systematically address it when evaluating individuals with common mental disorders.

Some implications follow from the findings summarized here. There is need that health care providers and other stakeholders be aware of the negative consequences of stigma. It is necessary to increase the society's awareness of this reality and decreasing prejudices in the areas of employment and education. On the other hand, more research is needed in assessing the associations described in this chapter. There is need for longitudinal studies with focus on the evolution of stigma and health and social outcomes. And it would be important to apply qualitative approaches to examine these relationships.

ACKNOWLEDGMENT

Some material in this chapter appeared in Alonso et al. (2008) and (2009). This material is reprinted with the permission of *Acta Psychiatrica Scandinavica* and *Journal of Affective Disorders*.

REFERENCES

Alonso, J., Buron, A., Rojas-Farreras, S., de Graaf, R., Haro, J. M., de Girolamo, G., Bruffaerts, R., Kovess, V., Matschinger, H., & Vilagut, G. (In press). Perceived stigma among individuals with common mental disorders. Journal of Affective Disorders.

Alonso, J., Buron, A., Bruffaerts, R., He, Y., Posada-Villa, J., Lepine, J. P., Angermeyer, M. C., Levinson, D., de Girolamo, G., Tachimori, H., Mneimneh, Z. N., Medina-Mora, M. E., Ormel, J., Scott, K. M., Gureje, O., Haro, J. M., Gluzman, S., Lee, S., Vilagut, G., Kessler, R. C., Von Korff, M., & World Mental Health Consortium. (2008).

Association of perceived stigma and mood and anxiety disorders: Results from the World Mental Health Surveys. *Acta Psychiatrica Scandinavica*, **118**, 305–14.

Alonso, J., Codony, M., Kovess-Masfety, V., Angermeyer, M. C., Katz, S. J., Haro, J. M., De Girolamo, G., De Graaf, R., Demyttenaere, K., Vilagut, G., Almansa, J., Lépine, J. P., & Brugha, T. S. (2007). Population level of unmet need for mental health care in Europe. Results from the European Study of Epidemiology of Mental Disorders (ESEMeD) Project. *British Journal of Psychiatry*, **190**, 299–306.

American Psychiatric Association. (1994). *Diagnostic and Statistical Manual of Mental Disorders, Fourth Edition (DSM-IV)*. Washington, DC: American Psychiatric Association.

Angermeyer, M. C. (2003). [The stigma of mental illness from the patient's view – An overview]. [Article in German]. *Psyciatrische Praxis*, **30**, 358–66.

Bowling, A. (2005). Just one question: If one question works, why ask several? *Journal of Epidemiology and Community Health*, **59**, 342–5.

Corrigan, P., Thompson, V., Lambert, D., Sangster, Y., Noel, J. G., & Campbell, J. (2003). Perceptions of discrimination among persons with serious mental illness. *Psychiatric Services*, **54**, 1105–10.

Corrigan, P. W. (2004). Target-specific stigma change: A strategy for impacting mental illness stigma. *Psychiatric Rehabilitation Journal*, **28**, 113–21.

Corrigan, P. W., River, L. P., Lundin, R. K., Wasowki, K. U., Campion, J., Mathisen, J., Goldstein, H., Bergman, M., Gagnon, C., & Kubiak, M. A. (2000). Stigmatizing attributions about mental illness. *Journal of Community Psychology*, **28**, 91–102.

Corrigan, P. W., & Watson, A. C. (2002). Understanding the impact of stigma on people with mental illness. *World Psychiatry*, **1**, 16–20.

Crocker, J., Major, B., & Steele, C. (1998). Social stigma. In *The Handbook of Social Psychology*, 4th ed., vol. **2**, ed. D. Gilbert, S. T. Fiske, & G. Linzdey, p. 505. New York: McGraw-Hill.

Dietrich, S., Beck, M., Bujantugs, B., Kenzine, D., Matschinger, H., & Angermeyer, M. C. (2004). The relationship between public causal beliefs and social distance toward mentally ill people. *Australian and New Zealand Journal of Psychiatry*, **38**, 348–54.

Dinos, S., Stevens, S., Serfaty, M., Weich, S., & King, M. (2004). Stigma: The feelings and experiences of 46 people with mental illness. *British Journal of Psychiatry*, **184**, 176–81.

Epping-Jordan, J., & Ustun, T. (2000). The WHO-DAS II: Levelling the playing field for all disorders. In *WHO Mental Health Bulletin*. Geneva: World Health Organization.

Goffman, E. (1963). *Stigma. Notes on the Management of Spoiled Identity*. New Jersey: Prentice Hall.

Haro, J. M., Arbabzadeh-Bouchez, S., Brugha, T. S., de Girolamo, G., Guyer, M. E., Jin, R., Lepine, J. P., Mazzi, F., Reneses, B., Vilagut, G., Sampson, N. A., & Kessler, R. C. (2006). Concordance of the Composite International Diagnostic Interview Version 3.0 (CIDI 3.0) with standardized clinical assessments in the WHO World Mental Health Surveys. *International Journal of Methods in Psychiatric Research*, **15**, 167–80.

Hinshaw, S. P., & Cicchetti, D. (2000). Stigma and mental disorder: Conceptions of illness, public attitudes, personal disclosure, and social policy. *Development and Psychopathology*, **12**, 555–98.

Jones, E., Farina, A., Hastorf, A., Markus, H., Miller, D. T., & Scott, R. (1984). *Social Stigma: The Psychology of Marked Relationships*. New York: Freeman.

Kessler, R. C., & Ustun, T. B. (2004). The World Mental Health (WMH) Survey Initiative Version of the World Health Organization (WHO) Composite International Diagnostic Interview (CIDI). *International Journal of Methods in Psychiatric Research*, **13**, 93–121.

Link, B. G., Cullen, F. T., Struening, E., Shrout, P. E., & Dohrenwend, B. P. (1989). A modified labelling theory approach to mental disorders: An empirical assessment. *American Sociological Review*, **54**, 400–23.

Link, B. G., & Phelan, J. C. (2001). Conceptualizing stigma. *Annual Review of Sociology*, **27**, 363–85.

Link, B. G., Struening, E. L., Rahav, M., Phelan, J. C., & Nuttbrock, L. (1997). On stigma and its consequences: Evidence from a longitudinal study of men with dual diagnoses of mental illness and substance abuse. *Journal of Health and Social Behavior*, **38**, 177–90.

Link, B. G., Yang, L. H., Phelan, J. C., & Collins, P. Y. (2004). Measuring mental illness stigma. *Schizophrenia Bulletin*, **30**, 511–41.

National Center for Health Studies. (1994). Evaluation of National Health Interview Survey diagnostic reporting. *Vital Health Statistics 2*, **120**, 1–116.

Perry, B. L., Pescosolido, B. A., Martin, J. K., McLeod, J. D., & Jensen, P. S. (2007). Comparison of public attributions, attitudes, and stigma in regard to depression among children and adults. *Psychiatric Services*, **58**, 632–5.

Pescosolido, B. A., Monahan, J., Link, B. G., Stueve, A., & Kikuzawa, S. (1999). The public's view of the competence, dangerousness, and need for legal coercion of persons with mental health problems. *American Journal of Public Health*, **89**, 1339–45.

Research Triangle Institute. (2004). *SUDAAN Language Manual, Release 9.0*. Research Triangle Park, NC: Research Triangle Institute.

Rusch, N., Angermeyer, M. C., & Corrigan, P. W. (2005). Mental illness stigma: Concepts, consequences, and initiatives to reduce stigma. *European Psychiatry*, **20**, 529–39.

Sartorius, N. (2006). Lessons from a 10-year global programme against stigma and discrimination because of an illness. *Psychology, Health and Medicine*, **11**, 383–8.

Sartorius, N., & Schultze, H. (2005). *Reducing the Stigma of Mental Illness: A Report from a Global Association*. Cambridge: Cambridge University Press.

Sirey, J. A., Bruce, M. L., Alexopoulos, G. S., Perlick, D. A., Friedman, S. J., & Meyers, B. S. (2001). Stigma as a barrier to recovery: Perceived stigma and patient-rated severity of illness as predictors of antidepressant drug adherence. *Psychiatric Services*, **52**, 1615–20.

Socall, D. W., & Holtgraves, T. (1992). Attitudes toward the mentally ill: The effects of label and beliefs. *The Sociological Quarterly*, **33**, 435–45.

Stafford, M. C., & Scott, R. R. (1986). Stigma deviance and social control: Some conceptual issues. In *The Dilemma of Difference*, ed. S. C. Ainlay, G. Becker, & L. M. Coleman, pp. 77–91. New York: Plenum.

Thornicroft, G., Rose, D., Kassam, A., & Sartorius, N. (2007). Stigma: Ignorance, prejudice or discrimination? *British Journal of Psychiatry*, **190**, 192–3.

Van Brakel, W. H. (2006). Measuring health-related stigma – A literature review. *Psychology, Health and Medicine*, **11**, 307–34.

Wahl, O. F. (1999). Mental health consumers' experience of stigma. *Schizophrenia Bulletin*, **25**, 467–78.

Wait, S., & Harding, E. (2006). *Moving to Social Integration of People with Severe Mental Illness: From Policy to Practice*. United Kingdom: International Longevity Centre.

Wittchen, H. U., & Jacobi, F. (2005). Size and burden of mental disorders in Europe – A critical review and appraisal of 27 studies. *European Neuropsychopharmacology*, **15**, 357–76.

Wolter, K. M. (1985). *Introduction to Variance Estimation*. New York: Springer-Verlag.

World Health Organization. (2001). *The World Health Report 2001 Mental Health: New Understanding, New Hope*. Geneva: WHO Library Cataloguing.

23 How Physical Comorbidity Affects Treatment of Major Depression in Developing and Developed Countries

OYE GUREJE

23.1. INTRODUCTION

Depression is often comorbid with physical disorders. Several studies suggest that persons with depression have elevated risk of co-occurring chronic pain and a range of chronic medical conditions such as metabolic, respiratory, and cardiovascular disorders (Brown, Khan, & Mahadi 2000; Eaton 2002; Gureje 2007; Rudish & Nemeroff 2003). Earlier reports have been strengthened by the findings of the World Mental Health (WMH) Surveys, which have shown that the comorbidity of depression and physical conditions is not limited to one type of chronic pain or physical disease and that such comorbidity cuts across countries at different developmental stages (Demyttenaere et al. 2007; Gureje et al. 2008; Ormel et al. 2007). The co-occurrence of depression with a physical disorder is commonly associated with a greater burden of disability than the presence of depression or physical disorder alone. For example, concurrent pain and depression have a much greater impact than either disorder alone on functional status (Bair et al. 2003).

A significant proportion of persons with depression fail to receive any treatment for their condition. This unmet need for care exists everywhere in the world but is particularly large in developing countries (Wang et al. 2007a). Paradoxically, even though the co-occurrence of depression with physical disorder often increases health care utilization, comorbidity is associated with a lower likelihood of treatment for depression. Several studies have found that the presence of a physical condition distracts physicians from the recognition and treatment of comorbid depression (Jones & Doebbeling 2007; Kessler et al. 1999; Tylee 2006). Previous studies examining the effect of comorbid physical disorders on the recognition and treatment of depression have been conducted in clinical settings. These cross-sectional studies have taken a "snapshot" of the likelihood that a patient's particular consultation would lead to the recognition of his or her depression. In effect, we know about the outcome of only one interaction between the clinician and the patient with comorbid conditions, not what happens with multiple consultations. Since persons with chronic physical conditions seek health care more often, it is plausible that the likelihood of comorbid depression being detected would be greater across multiple consultations, even if depression was less likely to be recognized and treated at any single consultation.

Previous studies about the effect of physical comorbidity on recognition and treatment of depression have been conducted in developed countries of Western Europe and North America. It is unclear whether comorbid physical conditions have the same effect on recognition in developing countries where the pattern of doctor–patient interaction may be different and where the organization of the health care service is certainly different. For example, there is evidence that the extent to which patients with depression will present to clinicians with physical problems may vary considerably between clinics based on whether patients receive more or less personalized care (Simon et al. 1999). This evidence also suggests that such styles of care provision differ broadly between clinics in developed and developing countries, with the former more likely to provide personalized care and the latter less likely to do so (Gureje 2004).

In this chapter, data from the WMH Surveys are used to address the question of whether, among respondents in the community, the co-occurrence of physical disorders and depression reduces or increases the likelihood of the depression receiving treatment in the prior year.

23.2. APPROACH

The analyses reported in this chapter include only persons meeting criteria for major depression in the prior 12 months. A full account of the methods used to assess major depression is provided in Chapter 4. Among persons meeting criteria for major depression in the past year, the following questions were used to determine whether they had received treatment for depression in the prior 12 months:

- Did you ever in your life talk to a medical doctor or other professional about your sadness/discouragement/lack of interest? (By "professional" we mean psychologists, counselors, spiritual advisors, herbalists, acupuncturists, and other healing professionals.)
- Did you receive treatment for your sadness/discouragement/lack of interest at any time in the past 12 months?

Persons who give affirmative responses to both these questions, and who met diagnostic criteria for major depression, were counted as cases of major depression that were treated in the prior year. The analytic objective was to assess whether the presence of chronic physical disease and/or chronic pain influenced the likelihood of major depression being treated in the prior year.

The association of chronic physical disease and chronic pain with the likelihood of major depression being treated was assessed for the following chronic diseases and chronic pain conditions:

- *Chronic physical diseases:* Asthma or chronic obstructive pulmonary disease, heart disease (including myocardial infarction), diabetes, ulcers, tuberculosis, epilepsy, cancer, and HIV/AIDS
- *Chronic pain conditions:* Back/neck pain, headache, arthritis/rheumatism, and other chronic pain conditions

For both chronic physical disease and chronic pain conditions, the number of conditions present was counted and classified as none, one, or two or more.

The analyses reported here use data from developing countries (Colombia, Mexico, China (Beijing and Shanghai), Lebanon, and Nigeria) and from developed countries (New Zealand, Japan, Israel, and the United States). Countries that did not ask questions needed to determine whether depression was treated in the prior 12 months were not included in these analyses. Since the number of cases of major depression available for analysis was limited within individual surveys, the analyses reported here focus on the percent of major depression cases treated in developed and developing countries.

For developing and developed countries, the percent of major depression cases treated and the standard error of the estimates are reported overall by the numbers of chronic physical diseases and chronic pain conditions present. In order to assess whether

Table 23.1. Number of cases of major depression (unweighted) and the percent of major depression cases treated (weighted estimate) by survey

Survey	Number of cases of major depression	Percent of major depression cases treated
Developing countries		
Colombia	276	13.7
Mexico	259	11.9
Beijing	59	0.0
Shanghai	30	0.0
Lebanon	40	5.7
Nigeria	73	9.5
Developed countries		
United States	793	39.1
Japan	53	21.3
New Zealand	890	49.2
Israel	290	27.3

the presence of chronic physical disease and/or chronic pain was associated with either increased or reduced likelihood of treatment of major depression, logistic regression analyses were carried out. In these analyses, persons with major depression were classified as treated or not. The association of number of chronic physical diseases (none, one, or two or more) and number of chronic pain conditions (none, one, or two or more) with major depression treatment status was evaluated controlling for age, gender, and educational attainment. Educational attainment was classified as either above or below the median education level within each country. Odds ratios are reported based on these analyses in which the reference groups are persons with no chronic physical disease and persons with no chronic pain condition.

23.3. FINDINGS

Table 23.1 shows the weighted estimates or the proportion of treated cases for each of the surveys. A striking observation is the large difference between developed and developing countries. The treated cases in the four developed countries constituted between 21.3 and 49.2% of all cases, while in developing countries the range was from 0.0 to 13.7%. Tables 23.2 and 23.3 show the proportions of respondents with treated depression relative to the presence of comorbid chronic physical conditions and chronic pain in developing and developed countries. While the presence of comorbid chronic disease or chronic pain seems to increase the likelihood of depression being treated in developed countries, the reverse seems to be the case in developing countries.

Tables 23.4 and 23.5 present the results of multivariate analyses testing whether the probability of treatment of depression differs significantly when depression is comorbid with physical conditions. These analyses control for age, sex, and high versus low education. Table 23.4 shows that in developed countries, persons whose depression was comorbid with two or more chronic physical diseases were more likely to receive mental health treatment compared to those with noncomorbid depression. No such relationship was observed in developing countries. On the other hand, Table 23.5 shows that in developing countries, persons whose depression was comorbid with one chronic pain condition were significantly less likely than those with noncomorbid depression to receive mental health treatment, while there was a trend in the same direction among persons with two or more pain conditions. In a further exploration of this latter finding, the analysis was conducted separately for males and females. In the sex-specific analyses, it was found that this significant association was observed only among females, not in males. The odds ratio for treatment among females with comorbid depression was

How Physical Comorbidity Affects Treatment of Major Depression

Table 23.2. Percent (and standard error) of adults with major depression in the prior 12 months who have received treatment for depression in the prior 12 months (developed and developing countries)

	No chronic disease	One chronic disease	Two or more chronic diseases	All persons	Number with major depression
Developing countries	12.1% (2.0)	7.7% (2.1)	10.7% (5.4)	11.0% (1.6)	737
Developed countries	37.6% (1.6)	42.9% (2.5)	44.7% (3.7)	39.9% (1.3)	2,026

Chronic physical diseases include asthma or chronic obstructive pulmonary disease, heart disease (including myocardial infarction), diabetes, ulcers, tuberculosis, epilepsy, cancer, and HIV/AIDS.

Table 23.3. Percent (and standard error) of adults with major depression in the prior 12 months who have received treatment for depression in the prior 12 months by number of chronic pain conditions (developed and developing countries)

	No chronic pain	One chronic pain	Two or more chronic pains	All persons	Number with major depression
Developing countries	14.1% (2.5)	7.2% (2.0)	9.8% (2.7)	11.0% (1.6)	737
Developed countries	38.7% (2.1)	38.5% (2.4)	43.2% (2.4)	39.9% (1.3)	2,026

Chronic pain conditions include back/neck pain, headache, arthritis/rheumatism, and other chronic pain.

Table 23.4. Odds ratio (and 95% confidence interval) for the association of number of chronic physical diseases with treatment of depression in the prior 12 months among adults with major depression in the prior 12 months (developed and developing countries)

	No chronic disease	One chronic disease	Two or more chronic diseases
Developing countries	1.0	0.6 (0.3, 1.2)	0.9 (0.2, 3.4)
Developed countries	1.0	1.2 (1.0, 1.6)	1.4* (1.0, 2.0)

Odds ratios estimated by logistic regression adjusted for age, gender, number of pain conditions, and high versus low education relative to country-specific median level of education.

Chronic physical diseases include asthma or chronic obstructive pulmonary disease, heart disease (including myocardial infarction), diabetes, ulcers, tuberculosis, epilepsy, cancer, and HIV/AIDS.

* $p < .05$.

Table 23.5. Odds ratio (and 95% confidence interval) for the association of number of chronic pain conditions with treatment of depression in the prior 12 months among adults with major depression in the prior 12 months (developed and developing countries)

	No chronic pain	One chronic pain	Two or more chronic pains
Developing countries	1.0	0.5* (0.3, 1.0)	0.7 (0.3, 1.4)
Developed countries	1.0	1.0 (0.7, 1.5)	1.1 (0.8, 1.4)

Odds ratios estimated by logistic regression adjusted for age, gender, number of pain conditions, and high versus low education relative to country-specific median level of education.

Chronic pain conditions include back/neck pain, headache, arthritis/rheumatism, and other chronic pain.

* $p < .05$.

0.3 (95% CI = 0.1–0.6), while for males it was 1.2 (95% CI = 0.4–3.6). No relationship between presence of comorbid chronic pain and treatment of depression was found in developed countries.

23.4. DISCUSSION

There were several important results of the analyses reported in this chapter. Depression was less likely to be treated in developing countries, but physical comorbidity status influenced likelihood of mental health treatment. The presence of multiple chronic physical conditions increased the likelihood of receiving treatment for depression among persons living in developed countries. In developing countries, on the other hand, the presence of chronic pain condition reduced the likelihood of treatment of depression – an observation that held only among females.

The finding that persons with depression were less likely to receive treatment in developing compared to developed countries is in accord with previous findings. As noted in a previous report from the WMH Surveys, even though a gap exists between need and service for mental health conditions in most countries, developed and developing, the latter show a more striking level of unmet need across most mental disorders (Wang et al. 2007a, 2007b). A recent publication has reviewed the major barriers to mental health service delivery in low- and middle-income countries (Saraceno et al. 2007).

The observation that persons with chronic physical diseases are more likely to receive treatment for a co-occurring depression than persons with no physical conditions in developed countries is, on initial consideration, contrary to previous reports. Prior literature has found that the recognition and treatment of depression is less likely among persons with physical complaints and conditions.

For example, when patients with depression present with multiple physical complaints or provide nonpsychological attributions for their symptoms, their depression is much less likely to be recognized by clinicians (De Wester 1996; Kessler et al. 1999; Kirmayer et al. 1993). Similar observations have been made in regard to chronic medical diseases. There is evidence, for example, that even though depression is twice as likely to occur among patients with diabetes compared to the general population, depression is recognized among only about 25% of the former compared to about 50% of the latter (Goldman, Nielsen, & Champion 1999; Rubin et al. 2004). Studies conducted in primary care settings in which a cross-sectional assessment of the likelihood of depression recognition is studied may capture the outcome of one consultation. It is possible, however, that the likelihood of recognition of depression increases with multiple consultations. Patients with chronic physical diseases in the community are more likely to make multiple consultations over a 1-year time span. Our observation that the presence of chronic physical disease increased the likelihood of treatment of co-occurring depression in developed countries may therefore reflect the effect of such multiple consultations in the community. This observation was made in developed countries, but not in developing countries. It should be noted that this observation for developed countries does not imply that the increased treatment rates for depression are commensurate with the increased number of health care visits. We do not know how many such visits were made before co-occurring depression was detected and treated. The fact that persons with chronic pain, who may also tend to have increased numbers of health care visits, were not more likely to receive treatment for comorbid depression suggests that the increased treatment of depression among persons with chronic disease may not have been due to increased numbers of visits alone.

On the other hand, we found that the presence of chronic pain was associated with reduced likelihood of treatment for comorbid depression in developing countries, but not in developing countries. This observation accords with previous findings that physical conditions may detract clinicians from the presence of a co-occurring depression, thus leading to lack of recognition and failure to treat. The pattern of health care delivery in developing countries leads to an overall poorer recognition and treatment of depression. When it is comorbid with physical complaints, it is possible that physical comorbidity distracts clinicians, resulting in even lower rates of detection and treatment of depression. Previous studies have indicated that the organization of services in general health care settings in developing countries, where most people with depression receive care (Wang et al. 2007a, 2007b), is impersonal, with less likelihood of treatment continuity and record-keeping (Gureje 2004; Simon et al. 1999). In such settings, it is unlikely that repeated or multiple visits would ameliorate the problem of poor recognition and treatment of depression.

In conclusion, this report shows that persons with depression comorbid with chronic diseases in developed countries are more likely to receive treatment for depression, possibly as a result of multiple consultations. The low level of treatment for depression in developing countries seemed to be made worse by the presence of chronic pain conditions, a finding that was observed only among females. Further research is needed to understand how comorbid physical conditions influence recognition and treatment of mental disorders in developed and developing countries, at the time of a particular encounter and over more extended periods of time.

REFERENCES

Bair, M. J., Robinson, R. L., Katon, W., & Kroenke, K. (2003). Depression and pain comorbidity: A literature review. *Archives of Internal Medicine*, **163**, 2433–45.

Brown, E., Khan, D. A., & Mahadi, S. (2000). Psychiatric hospital in inner city outpatients with moderate or severe asthma. *International Journal of Psychiatry in Medicine*, **30**, 295–7.

De Wester, J. N. (1996). Recognizing and treating the patient with somatic manifestations of depression. *Journal of Family Practice*, **43**, S3–15.

Demyttenaere, K., Bruffaerts, R., Lee, S., Posada-Villa, J., Kovess, V., Angermeyer, M. C., Levinson, D., de Girolamo, G., Nakane, H., Mneimneh, Z., Lara, C., de Graaf, R., Scott, K. M., Gureje, O., Stein, D. J., Haro, J. M., Bromet, E. J., Kessler, R. C., Alonso, J., & Von Korff, M. (2007). Mental disorders among persons with chronic back or neck pain: Results from the World Mental Health Surveys. *Pain*, **129**, 332–42.

Eaton, W. W. (2002). Epidemiologic evidence on the comorbidity of depression and diabetes. *Journal of Psychosomatic Research*, **53**, 903–6.

Goldman, L. S., Nielsen, N. H., & Champion, H. C. (1999). Awareness, diagnosis, and treatment of depression. *Journal of General Internal Medicine*, **14**, 569–80.

Gureje, O. (2004). What can we learn from a cross-national study of somatic distress? *Journal of Psychosomatic Research*, **56**, 409–12.

Gureje, O. (2007). Psychiatric aspects of pain. *Current Opinion in Psychiatry*, **20**, 42–6.

Gureje, O., Von Korff, M., Kola, L., Demyttenaere, K., He, Y., Posada-Villa, J., Lepine, J. P., Angermeyer, M. C., Levinson, D., de Girolamo, G., Iwata, N., Karam, A., Guimaraes Borges, G. L., de Graaf, R., Browne, M. O., Stein, D. J., Haro, J. M., Bromet, E. J., Kessler, R. C., & Alonso, J. (2008). The relation between multiple pains and mental disorders: Results from the World Mental Health Surveys. *Pain*, **135**, 82–91.

Jones, L. E., & Doebbeling, C. C. (2007). Depression screening disparities among veterans with diabetes compared with the general veteran population. *Diabetes Care*, **30**, 2216–21.

Kessler, D., Lloyd, K., Lewis, G., & Gray, D. P. (1999). Cross sectional study of symptom attribution and recognition of depression and anxiety in primary care. *British Medical Journal*, **318**, 436–9.

Kirmayer, L. J., Robbins, J. M., Dworkind, M., & Yaffe, M. J. (1993). Somatization and the recognition of depression and anxiety in primary care. *American Journal of Psychiatry*, **150**, 734–41.

Ormel, J., Von Korff, M., Burger, H., Scott, K. M., Demyttenaere, K., Huang, Y. Q., Posada-Villa, J., Pierre Lepine, J., Angermeyer, M. C., Levinson, D., de Girolamo, G., Kawakami, N., Karam, E., Medina-Mora, M. E., Gureje, O., Williams, D., Haro, J. M., Bromet, E. J., Alonso, J., & Kessler, R. C. (2007). Mental disorders among persons with heart disease – Results from World Mental Health surveys. *General Hospital Psychiatry*, **29**, 325–34.

Rubin, R. R., Ciechanowski, P., Egede, L. E., Lin, E. H., & Lustman, P. J. (2004). Recognizing and treating depression in patients with diabetes. *Current Diabetes Reports*, **4**, 119–25.

Rudish, B., & Nemeroff, C. B. (2003). Epidemiology of comorbid coronary artery disease and depression. *Biological Psychiatry*, **54**, 227–40.

Saraceno, B., van Ommeren, M., Batniji, R., Cohen, A., Gureje, O., Mahoney, J., Sridhar, D., & Underhill, C. (2007). Barriers to improving mental health services in low and middle income countries. *Lancet*, **370**, 1164–74.

Simon, G. E., Von Korff, M., Piccinelli, M., Fullerton, C., & Ormel, J. (1999). An international study of the relation between somatic symptoms and depression. *New England Journal of Medicine*, **341**, 1329–35.

Tylee, A. (2006). Identifying and managing depression in primary care in the United Kingdom. *The Journal of Clinical Psychiatry*, **67**, 41–5.

Wang, P. S., Aguilar-Gaxiola, S., Alonso, J., Angermeyer, M. C., Borges, G., Bromet, E. J., Bruffaerts, R., de Girolamo, G., de Graaf, R., Gureje, O., Haro, J. M., Karam, E. G., Kessler, R. C., Kovess, V., Lane, M. C., Lee, S., Levinson, D., Ono, Y., Petukhova, M., Posada-Villa, J., Seedat, S., & Wells, J. E. (2007a). Worldwide use of mental health services for anxiety, mood and substance disorders: Results from 17 countries in the WHO World Mental Health (WMH) Surveys. *Lancet*, **370**, 841–50.

Wang, P. S., Angermeyer, M., Borges, G., Bruffaerts, R., Tat Chiu, W., Girolamo, G., Fayyad, J., Gureje, O., Haro, J. M., Huang, Y., Kessler, R. C., Kovess, V., Levinson, D., Nakane, Y., Oakley Brown, M. A., Ormel, J. H., Posada-Villa, J., Aguilar-Gaxiola, S., Alonso, J., Lee, S., Heeringa, S., Pennell, B. E., Chatterji, S., & Üstün, T. B. (2007b). Delay and failure in treatment seeking after first onset of mental disorders in the WHO World Mental Health (WMH) Survey Initiative. *World Psychiatry*, **6**, 177–85.

24 Mental–Physical Comorbidity and Predicted Mortality

HUIBERT BURGER

24.1. INTRODUCTION

The increased mortality risk associated with mental disease is well established (Bruce et al. 1994). In particular, depression has shown to be a risk factor for cardiovascular mortality, but also for mortality from other causes (Mykletun et al. 2007; Penninx et al. 1999; Schulz, Drayer, & Rollman 2002). Although the pathways from depression to premature death have not been fully elucidated, it is presently acknowledged that a substantial amount of excess mortality results from the association of depression with cardiovascular disease (Thomas, Kalaria, & O'Brien 2004), or its risk factors including diabetes (Knol et al. 2007) and hypertension (Meyer et al. 2004). This is because cardiovascular diseases and diabetes are still important causes of premature death; in fact, they are among the top 10 leading causes of death (Mathers & Loncar 2006). In addition, and not entirely independently from cardiovascular disease, a considerable part of the extra morbidity and mortality in depression may be due to behavioral risk factors. Notably, smoking, which has prevalence as high as 50% among individuals with depression, compared to less than 25% in the general population (Kalman, Morissette, & George 2005), and has well-established detrimental health effects (Peto et al. 1992). Therefore, smoking behavior may be responsible for a substantial portion of the excess cardiovascular mortality and all-cause mortality in depression but perhaps also in anxiety disorders.

Although there is growing evidence that depression is an independent risk factor for mortality, it is not known to what extent this excess mortality can be explained by the association of depression with chronic cardiovascular conditions and smoking. Recent research has shown that the association of chronic physical conditions is stronger for comorbid anxiety and depression than for one of these mental disorders alone (Scott et al. 2007; Stordal et al. 2003), so the association of anxiety disorders with excess mortality due to comorbid chronic disease is also of interest. Research evidence regarding the pathways from psychological illness to excess mortality is scarce (Mykletun et al. 2007).

The aim of the analyses presented here is to estimate the impact of the association of major depression and anxiety disorders with smoking, diabetes mellitus, a history of myocardial infarction, and hypertension on the risk of mortality in persons older than 50 years. This was done using data from the World Mental Health (WMH) Surveys carried out in 17 countries in Europe, the Americas, Asia and South Pacific, the Middle East, and Africa. Mortality risks were estimated for the total WMH population with data on chronic diseases, using a "risk engine" based on data from a Dutch cohort study. These estimated mortality risks were compared for persons with neither major depression nor an anxiety disorder, major depression only, an anxiety disorder only, and both major depression and an anxiety disorder. These analyses were repeated for the developed and developing countries separately.

24.2. APPROACH

24.2.1. Study Population and Psychiatric Diagnoses

The analyses reported here employ data from Belgium, France, Germany, Italy, the Netherlands, Spain, Colombia, Mexico, the United States, Japan, Beijing, Shanghai, New Zealand, Lebanon, Israel, Nigeria, and South Africa. Diagnoses of major depression and anxiety disorder (generalized anxiety disorder, social phobia, posttraumatic stress disorder, or panic disorder/agoraphobia) were made using Composite International Diagnostic Interview (CIDI) data. In this chapter we refer to anxiety disorder and major depression as common mental disorders. To obtain mutually exclusive categories, respondents were classified as having neither major depression nor anxiety disorder, major depression only, anxiety disorder only, or both major depression and anxiety disorder. The latter category was referred to as comorbid anxiety disorder and major depression.

24.2.2. Risk Engine – Development and Application to the WMH Data

Because the WMH Surveys were cross-sectional without follow-up data on mortality, we estimated mortality risks based on data from an external follow-up study among 40,856 unselected persons from a Dutch population: the Prevention of Renal and Vascular End Stage Disease (PREVEND) study (Hillege et al. 2002). Using data from this study, we developed a risk engine that estimates the probability of dying within the next 8 years as a function of age, gender, smoking during the past 5 years, and a history of myocardial infarction, diabetes mellitus, or hypertension.

These characteristics were chosen on content grounds (i.e., their predictive value for mortality) and because they were available in the WMH Surveys. The risk engine was based on a statistical multivariable model that accounted for the varying time from the baseline measurements of the participants' characteristics to the end of the PREVEND study, or in case a person deceased, time to death. This model was estimated using a Cox proportional hazards regression analysis. Complete data were available for 40,056 persons. For validation of the model, a 20% random "take-out" sample of size 8,018 was drawn first. The model was developed in the remaining derivation data set consisting of 32,038 subjects.

The six characteristics mentioned previously were the predictor variables and death was the outcome variable. We did not plan to reduce the number of predictor variables in the risk engine because all predictors were established determinants of mortality. This procedure minimizes bias in the estimation of the predictor coefficients (Harrell, Lee, & Mark 1996). Since the increase in mortality with age was, on graphical inspection, less steep among female than male subjects, we also entered a variable accounting for the interaction between age and gender. The hazard ratios obtained from the Cox proportional hazards models denote the relative risk of 8-year mortality. The risk engine was constructed using the regression coefficients for each predictor variable from the model (Spijker et al. 2006). As a final step, the risk engine was tested for its predictive accuracy in the "take-out" sample.

For each respondent in the WMH Surveys older than 50 years, the values for the six predictors were subsequently entered into the risk engine to obtain an estimated 8-year mortality risk. The predictor smoking entered into the engine concerned current smoking. The presence of the chronic diseases used to feed the risk engine was determined as part of a series of questions about the lifetime presence of chronic conditions adapted from the U.S. Health Interview Survey. Respondents were asked, "Did a medical doctor or other health professional ever tell you that you had been diagnosed with myocardial infarction?" This question was also asked for diabetes and hypertension.

24.2.3. Data Analysis

The associations of the common mental disorders with smoking and chronic disease were quantified as odds ratios that can be interpreted as measures of relative risk. Subsequent analyses were carried out using multiple linear regression models. After adjustment for age, gender, and educational status, the absolute predicted incremental 8-year mortality risk was compared for respondents with major depression only, anxiety disorder only, and comorbid anxiety disorder and major depression. The increments were expressed as absolute differences with the predicted mortality risk in the reference category, that is, respondents with neither major depression nor anxiety disorder. In addition, we calculated the incremental predicted mortality in respondents with common mental disorders as a percentage increase relative to the risk in the reference category. In these analyses, the mortality risks in the reference category for respondents from the developing countries were standardized to the age and gender distribution of the developed countries. We compared all results between developing and developed countries.

24.3. FINDINGS

Demographic characteristics for the total group ($N = 13,808$) of WMH respondents older than 50 years from developing and developed countries were generally similar (Table 24.1). However, the proportion that had completed secondary education was roughly twice as high in the developed as in the developing countries. The majority of respondents with a common mental disorder were female; in those without these disorders 54% of respondents were female. This figure was identical to that for the total PREVEND population in which the engine was developed.

The prevalence of cardiovascular risk factors among those without a common mental disorder is provided in Table 24.2. There were no material differences in risk factor prevalence rates between respondents from the developing and developed countries. The figures were quite divergent from the rates among respondents from the PREVEND study, however. In the latter study, 42.2% were smokers during the past 5 years, 3.3% reported myocardial infarction, 2.6% reported diabetes, and 29.1% reported hypertension.

Table 24.3 shows the association of common mental disorders with smoking and chronic cardiovascular diseases as measured by odds ratios. The associations with smoking were modest, particularly for the developing countries. Remarkably, in both developing and developed countries, only anxiety disorder was correlated with diabetes. Common mental disorders, either solitary or comorbid, were associated with a higher likelihood of cardiovascular disease, except for hypertension in the developed countries. The odds ratio for myocardial infarction in the developed countries just missed statistical significance.

In the derivation data set from the PREVEND study, there were 1,713 deaths during a median follow-up period of 7.2 years. The observed 8-year mortality was 5.8%. As expected, the results of the Cox proportional hazards models showed that all preselected predictors were significantly related to 8-year mortality. The interaction between age and gender was statistically significant and

Table 24.1. Demographic characteristics of the study population (N = 13,808) according to the presence of common mental disorders and economic development of country of residence

Characteristic	No common mental disorder	Major depression[a]	Anxiety disorder[b]	Comorbid anxiety and major depression
Developing countries				
Number	3,035	312	164	151
Female gender (%; SE)	53.9 (1.2)	66.0 (3.8)	65.2 (4.9)	76.6 (4.7)
Age (mean; SE)	61.0 (0.2)	62.7 (0.8)	60.9 (0.92)	61.5 (1.0)
Completed secondary education (%; SE)	26.7 (1.2)	32.4 (3.6)	29.1 (5.1)	28.7 (5.0)
Developed countries				
Number	8,605	551	634	356
Female gender (%; SE)	53.0 (0.8)	65.5 (2.6)	66.7 (2.3)	69.5 (3.1)
Age (mean; SE)	65.1 (0.2)	62.5 (0.6)	60.6 (0.4)	60.4 (0.6)
Completed secondary education (%; SE)	55.4 (0.8)	55.7 (2.8)	64.3 (2.3)	56.6 (3.2)

[a] Without anxiety disorder present.
[b] Without major depression present.

indicated that the increase in mortality with age was less steep in female than in male subjects. The mean predicted 8-year mortality risk from the model was 5.6%. The risk engine that was constructed on the basis of these analyses validated well in the take-out sample and was subsequently applied to the predictor data from the WMH Surveys.

Table 24.4 shows the absolute additional risk of dying in the following 8 years attributable to the association of common mental disorders with smoking and chronic disease. The percentages denote the 8-year risk of dying in addition to the risk in persons with neither depression nor an anxiety disorder, after adjusting for age, gender, and educational status. The general pattern was that of an absolute increment of almost 1% in the presence of a single common mental disorder with a somewhat larger effect of anxiety compared to depression, and the largest increment for comorbid anxiety disorder and major depression with an addition of an ample 1.2%. These patterns were not essentially different between developing and developed countries. The standardized predicted 8-year mortality risks in persons with neither major depression nor an anxiety disorder in the developing and developed countries were 10.31 and 10.37%, respectively. When we expressed the incremental mortality risk associated with common mental disorders as a percentage increase relative to the risk in persons with neither disorder, the figures were around 8–9% for the solitary common mental disorders and 12% for respondents with comorbid anxiety disorder and major depression (Figure 24.1). As evident from the lower limits of the 95% confidence intervals that

Table 24.2. Prevalence of cardiovascular risk factors in the study population by economic development of the country of residence

Risk factor	Developing countries	Developed countries
Current smoking	19.1 (1.0)	16.9 (0.5)
Diabetes	9.5 (0.7)	11.9 (0.5)
Myocardial infarction	7.1 (0.6)	7.1 (0.4)
Hypertension	31.1 (1.1)	35.3 (0.7)

Note: Values are percentages (SE).

Table 24.3. Common mental disorders associated with smoking and chronic disease by economic development of country of residence

Risk factor	Major depression[a]	Anxiety disorder[b]	Comorbid anxiety and major depression
Developing countries			
Current smoking	1.4 (1.0–2.1)	1.0 (0.5–2.0)	1.1 (0.5–2.1)
Diabetes	1.0 (0.6–1.7)	2.1 (1.3–3.5)	0.9 (0.5–1.7)
Myocardial infarction	3.4 (2.4–4.9)	2.8 (1.6–5.0)	7.7 (4.6–12.7)
Hypertension	1.5 (1.1–2.1)	2.5 (1.6–4.0)	2.8 (1.8–4.3)
Developed countries			
Current smoking	1.4 (1.0–1.8)	1.2 (0.9–1.5)	1.7 (1.3–2.3)
Diabetes	1.2 (0.9–1.8)	1.4 (1.1–1.9)	1.2 (0.8–1.7)
Myocardial infarction	1.6 (0.9–2.6)	1.9 (1.3–2.6)	2.0 (1.3–3.1)
Hypertension	1.6 (1.32.0)	1.7 (1.4–2.2)	1.1 (0.9–1.4)

Note: Values are odds ratios (95% confidence interval) adjusted for age, gender, and educational status. Reference category is neither anxiety nor major depression.

[a] Without anxiety disorder present.
[b] Without major depression present.

were close to zero, results were just statistically significant or approximating statistical significance.

24.4. DISCUSSION

In the present study we quantified the predicted incremental mortality linked to common mental disorders through their associations with smoking, diabetes, and cardiovascular disease in persons older than 50 years, using data from populations of developed and developing countries in the WMH Surveys. The estimates of mortality attributable to these risk factors were obtained by linking them to mortality using data from a cohort external to the WMH Surveys.

We found that the impact of a major depression or an anxiety disorder attributable to its association with smoking, a history of diabetes, myocardial infarction, or hypertension was a 8–9% higher 8-year predicted mortality risk for a solitary common mental disorder and a 12% higher risk for comorbid anxiety disorder and major depression, compared to none of these disorders. These

Table 24.4. Absolute increments in 8-year mortality (95% confidence interval) predicted from cardiovascular risk factors and cardiovascular disease history according to the presence of common mental disorders, by economic development of country of residence

Common mental disorder	Developing countries	Developed countries
Major depression[a]	0.85 (−0.13; 1.83)	0.77 (−0.23; 1.76)
Anxiety disorder[b]	0.98 (−0.08; 2.03)	0.86 (0.20; 1.52)
Comorbid anxiety and major depression	1.20 (0.14; 2.26)	1.28 (0.39; 2.16)

Note: Values are percentages adjusted for age, gender, and educational status. Reference category is neither anxiety nor major depression.

[a] Without anxiety disorder present.
[b] Without major depression present.

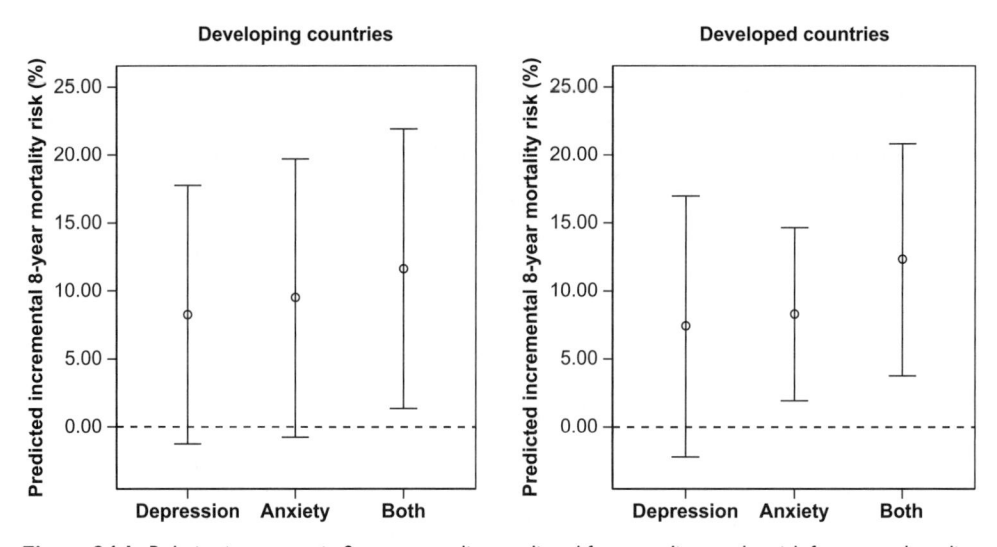

Figure 24.1. Relative increment in 8-year mortality predicted from cardiovascular risk factors and cardiovascular disease history according to the presence of common mental disorders, by economic development of country of residence. Values are percentages increase relative to the predicted 8-year mortality in persons with neither disorder, standardized to the age and gender distribution of the developed countries. Error bars represent 95% confidence intervals.

percentages were similar in developing and developed countries.

24.4.1. Implications

Our findings point to the clinical relevance of the unfavorable cardiovascular risk profile in major depression and anxiety disorders, in particular when they are comorbid. The increased risk of mortality in common mental disorders is not a new finding (Bruce et al. 1994), neither is the observation that it is partially caused by their association with smoking, diabetes, and cardiovascular disease (Thomas et al. 2004). The particular contribution of the present study is that on a global scale, it yielded an estimate of the amount of mortality that can be attributed to the association of common mental disorders with mortality risk factors that are, in principle, amenable to intervention. These results suggest the importance of greater attention to cardiovascular risk reduction among persons with mood and/or anxiety disorders.

The size of the absolute increase in mortality attributable to the association of major depression and anxiety disorders with smoking and chronic diseases may seem small. To get a feeling for the impact it may be useful to compare these mortality increments to the rates of suicide attributable to major depression. According to a recent review, the annual risk of suicide in patients with major depression varies substantially between studies, but in the two largest cohorts it was around 0.22% per year (Zonda & Groza 2000). Given a suicide rate of around 15 per 100,000 per year in the general population of the United States (Hirschfeld & Russell 1997), at least 0.2% per year can be attributed to major depression. Averaged over the 8-year period in our mortality predictions, the absolute mortality increments for major depression in our study were an ample 0.1% annually. This comparison indicates that the mortality impact of the increased prevalence of smoking, a history of diabetes, myocardial infarction, or hypertension in persons with major depression is in the order of magnitude of 50% of the suicide rate due to this mental disorder. It must be stressed that in addition to the increased risk of mortality through the association of common mental disorders with smoking, diabetes, and cardiovascular disease, they may increase mortality via other mechanisms (Amaddeo et al. 2007).

A substantial effect on ischemic heart disease mortality, independently of known risk factors, has been shown repeatedly for depression (Surtees et al. 2008; Thomas et al. 2004). The picture is less clear for anxiety. A recently conducted thorough cohort study did not show an independent effect of anxiety on all-cause mortality, while a substantial effect from depression was found (Mykletun et al. 2007). However, in the Framingham Offspring Study, a modest, though statistically significant, effect of anxiety on mortality was observed while adjusting for established risk factors (Eaker et al. 2005). The consequence of the evidence for an independent positive effect of common mental disorders on mortality is that the total added mortality risk caused by these disorders, at least by depression, is likely larger than the estimates we report here.

The effects we demonstrated were stronger for comorbid anxiety and depression than for each of these mental disorders alone, which is in accordance with previous studies (Scott et al. 2007; Stordal et al. 2003). An interesting explanation is that these disorders, when comorbid, form a different class of more severe mental problems than when they are "pure" disorders (Alonso et al. 2004; de Graaf et al. 2002). From that perspective, it is understandable that in this category the excess mortality was largest.

There were no differences in predicted mortality due to smoking and chronic cardiovascular disease between developed and developing countries. If true, this may eventually lead to higher mortality attributable to common mental disorders in the developing than in the developed world because the prevalence of one of the strongest risk factors for cardiovascular disease and diabetes, that is, obesity, is an increasing problem at least in Africa and Asia (McCurry 2007; Rguibi & Belahsen 2007).

24.4.2. Limitations

Some limitations that apply to this particular study need to be discussed. The concept of impact includes causality and therefore it is assumed in the present study that the common mental disorders are the causes of an unfavorable cardiovascular profile and therefore precede them. The direction of the relationship between common mental disorders and smoking, diabetes, myocardial infarction, and hypertension is unclear however, as anxiety and depression may result from poor cardiovascular health (Evans et al. 2005). Therefore, it does not follow that treatment or prevention of major depression and anxiety disorders will lead to reductions in cardiovascular risk related mortality.

We used self-report of smoking and chronic cardiovascular disease that may have resulted some error in documentation. We consider these errors unlikely to have biased the results, however (Ormel et al. 2007). Regarding the comparison between developed and developing countries, it is of note that there seem to be no marked ethnic differences in the accuracy of self-reports of diabetes and hypertension in populations at an increased risk of cardiovascular disease (El Fakiri, Bruijnzeels, & Hoes 2007).

24.5 CONCLUSION

Both in the developed and developing world, common mental disorders are associated with an 8–12% excess mortality risk through their association with smoking, diabetes, a history of myocardial infarction, and hypertension.

For major depression, this excess corresponds to approximately 50% of the mortality risk from suicide due to this disorder. These findings point to the need for more clinical and research attention altering the cardiovascular risk profile among patients with anxiety or depression.

REFERENCES

Alonso, J., Angermeyer, M. C., Bernert, S., Bruffaerts, R., Brugha, T. S., Bryson, H., de Girolamo, G., Graaf, R., Demyttenaere, K., Gasquet, I., Haro, J. M., Katz, S. J., Kessler, R. C., Kovess, V., Lépine, J. P., Ormel, J., Polidori, G., Russo, L. J., Vilagut, G., Almansa, J., Arbabzadeh-Bouchez, S., Autonell, J., Bernal, M., Buist-Bouwman, M. A., Codony, M., Domingo-Salvany, A., Ferrer, M., Joo, S. S., Martínez-Alonso, M., Matschinger, H., Mazzi, F., Morgan, Z., Morosini, P., Palacín, C., Romera, B., Taub, N., Vollebergh, W. A., & ESEMeD/MHEDEA 2000 Investigators, European Study of the Epidemiology of Mental Disorders (ESEMeD) Project. (2004). 12-Month comorbidity patterns and associated factors in Europe: Results from the European Study of the Epidemiology of Mental Disorders (ESEMeD) project. *Acta Psychiatrica Scandinavica*, **420**, 28–37.

Amaddeo, F., Barbui, C., Perini, G., Biggeri, A., & Tansella, M. (2007). Avoidable mortality of psychiatric patients in an area with a community-based system of mental health care. *Acta Psychiatrica Scandinavica*, **115**, 320–5.

Bruce, M. L., Leaf, P. J., Rozal, G. P., Florio, L., & Hoff, R. A. (1994). Psychiatric status and 9-year mortality data in the New Haven Epidemiologic Catchment Area Study. *American Journal of Psychiatry*, **151**, 716–21.

de Graaf, R., Bijl, R. V., Smit, F., Vollebergh, W. A., & Spijker, J. (2002). Risk factors for 12-month comorbidity of mood, anxiety, and substance use disorders: Findings from the Netherlands Mental Health Survey and Incidence Study. *American Journal of Psychiatry*, **159**, 620–9.

Eaker, E. D., Sullivan, L. M., Kelly-Hayes, M., D'Agostino, R. B., Sr., & Benjamin, E. J. (2005). Tension and anxiety and the prediction of the 10-year incidence of coronary heart disease, atrial fibrillation, and total mortality: The Framingham Offspring Study. *Psychosomatic Medicine*, **67**, 692–6.

El Fakiri, F., Bruijnzeels, M. A., & Hoes, A. W. (2007). No evidence for marked ethnic differences in accuracy of self-reported diabetes, hypertension, and hypercholesterolemia. *Journal of Clinical Epidemiology*, **60**, 1271–9.

Evans, D. L., Charney, D. S., Lewis, L., Golden, R. N., Gorman, J. M., Krishnan, K. R. R., Nemeroff, C. B., Bremner, J. D., Carney, R. M., Coyne, J. C., Delong, M. R., Frasure-Smith, N., Glassman, A. H., Gold, P. W., Grant, I., Gwyther, L., Ironson, G., Johnson, R. L., Kanner, A. M., Katon, W. J., Kaufmann, P. G., Keefe, F. J., Ketter, T., Laughren, T. P., Leserman, J., Lyketsos, C. G., McDonald, W. M., McEwen, B. S., Miller, A. H., Musselman, D., O'Connor, C., Petitto, J. M., Pollock, B. G., Robinson, R. G., Roose, S. P., Rowland, J., Sheline, Y., Sheps, D. S., Simon, G., Spiegel, D., Stunkard, A., Sunderland, T., Tibbits, J., & Valvo, W. J. (2005). Mood disorders in the medically ill: Scientific review and recommendations. *Biological Psychiatry*, **58**, 175–89.

Gu, Q., Burt, V. L., Paulose-Ram, R., Yoon, S., & Gillum, R. F. (2008). High blood pressure and cardiovascular disease mortality risk among U.S. adults: The Third National Health and Nutrition Examination Survey Mortality Follow-up Study. *Annals of Epidemiology*, **18**, 302–9.

Harrell, F. E., Jr., Lee, K. L., & Mark, D. B. (1996). Multivariable prognostic models: Issues in developing models, evaluating assumptions and adequacy, and measuring and reducing errors. *Statistics in Medicine*, **15**, 361–87.

Hillege, H. L., Fidler, V., Diercks, G. F., van Gilst, W. H., de Zeeuw, D., van Veldhuisen, D. J., Gans, R. O., Janssen, W. M., Grobbee, D. E., de Jong, P. E., & Prevention of Renal and Vascular End Stage Disease (PREVEND) Study Group. (2002). Urinary albumin excretion predicts cardiovascular and noncardiovascular mortality in general population. *Circulation*, **106**, 1777–82.

Hirschfeld. R. M., & Russell, J. M. (1997). Assessment and treatment of suicidal patients. *New England Journal of Medicine*, **337**, 910–15.

Kalman, D., Morissette, S. B., & George, T. P. (2005). Co-morbidity of smoking in patients with psychiatric and substance use disorders. *American Journal of Addiction*, **14**, 106–23.

Knol, M. J., Heerdink, E. R., Egberts, A. C., Geerlings, M. I., Gorter, K. J., Numans, M. E., Grobbee, D. E., Klungel, O. H., & Burger, H. (2007). Depressive symptoms in subjects with diagnosed and undiagnosed type 2 diabetes. *Psychosomatic Medicine*, **69**, 300–5.

Mathers, C. D., & Loncar, D. (2006). Projections of global mortality and burden of disease from 2002 to 2030. *PLoS Medicine*, **3**, 442.

McCurry, J. (2007). Japan battles with obesity. *Lancet*, **369**, 451–2.

Meyer, C. M., Armenian, H. K., Eaton, W. W., & Ford, D. E. (2004). Incident hypertension associated with depression in the Baltimore Epidemiologic Catchment area follow-up study. *Journal of Affective Disorders*, **83**, 127–33.

Mykletun, A., Bjerkeset, O., Dewey, M., Prince, M., Overland, S., & Stewart, R. (2007). Anxiety, depression, and cause-specific mortality: The HUNT study. *Psychosomatic Medicine*, **69**, 323–31.

Ormel, J., Von Korff, M., Burger, H., Scott, K., Demyttenaere, K., Huang, Y. Q., Posada-Villa, J., Pierre Lepine, J., Angermeyer, M. C., Levinson, D., de Girolamo, G., Kawakami, N., Karam, E., Medina-Mora, M. E., Gureje, O., Williams, D., Haro, J. M., Bromet, E. J., Alonso, J., & Kessler, R. (2007). Mental disorders among persons with heart disease: Results from World Mental Health surveys. *General Hospital Psychiatry*, **29**, 325–34.

Penninx, B. W., Geerlings, S. W., Deeg, D. J., van Eijk, J. T., van Tilburg, W., & Beekman, A. T. (1999). Minor and major depression and the risk of death in older persons. *Archives of General Psychiatry*, **56**, 889–95.

Peto, R., Lopez, A. D., Boreham, J., Thun, M., & Heath, C., Jr. (1992). Mortality from tobacco in developed countries: Indirect estimation from national vital statistics. *Lancet*, **339**, 1268–78.

Rguibi, M., & Belahsen, R. (2007). Prevalence of obesity in Morocco. *Obesity Review*, **8**, 11–13.

Schulz, R., Drayer, R. A., & Rollman, B. L. (2002). Depression as a risk factor for non-suicide mortality in the elderly. *Biological Psychiatry*, **52**, 205–25.

Scott, K. M., Bruffaerts, R., Tsang, A., Ormel, J., Alonso, J., Angermeyer, M. C., Benjet, C., Bromet, E., de Girolamo, G., de Graaf, R., Gasquet, I., Gureje, O., Haro, J. M., He, Y., Kessler, R. C., Levinson, D., Mneimneh, Z. N., Oakley Browne, M. A., Posada-Villa, J., Stein, D. J., Takeshima, T., & Von Korff, M. (2007). Depression-anxiety relationships with chronic physical conditions: Results from the World Mental Health Surveys. *Journal of Affective Disorders*, **103**, 113–20.

Spijker, J., de Graaf, R., Ormel, J., Nolen, W. A., Grobbee, D. E., & Burger, H. (2006). The persistence of depression score. *Acta Psychiatrica Scandinavica*, **114**, 411–16.

Stordal, E., Bjelland, I., Dahl, A. A., & Mykletun, A. (2003). Anxiety and depression in individuals with somatic health problems. The Nord-Trondelag Health Study (HUNT). *Scandinavian Journal of Primary Health Care*, **21**, 136–41.

Surtees, P. G., Wainwright, N. W., Luben, R. N., Wareham, N. J., Bingham, S. A., & Khaw, K. T. (2008). Depression and ischemic heart disease mortality: Evidence from the EPIC-Norfolk United Kingdom Prospective Cohort Study. *American Journal of Psychiatry*, **165**, 515–23.

Thomas, A. J., Kalaria, R. N., & O'Brien, J. T. (2004). Depression and vascular disease: What is the relationship? *Journal of Affective Disorders*, **79**, 81–95.

Zonda, T., & Groza, J. (2000). The long-term outcome of a depressive population in a Hungarian material. *Journal of Affective Disorders*, **60**, 113–19.

PART FOUR

Implications

25 Research Implications

EVELYN J. BROMET AND MICHAEL R. VON KORFF

25.1. INTRODUCTION

This volume presents a comprehensive set of analyses designed to disentangle the complex web of associations between psychiatric disorders and physical conditions. Many findings are noteworthy. First and foremost, consistent with previous reports, depressive and anxiety disorders occurred with greater frequency among persons with diverse chronic physical diseases and chronic pain conditions, but the majority of persons with a chronic physical disease did not report anxiety or depression in the year preceding the interview. Second, early childhood adversities and early-onset depression and anxiety were independent, nonspecific risk factors for a variety of medical conditions. Third, the combined effects of comorbid mental and physical disorders on disability and impairment were greater than the sum of their parts. Fourth, and what is most unique and astonishing about the findings presented in this volume, the pattern of results was reasonably consistent across the diverse cultural settings in the developed and developing countries participating in the World Mental Health (WMH) Survey Initiative, in spite of intrinsic constraints when applying a common interview schedule and nomenclature in very different settings. The findings reported in this book suggest provocative links of childhood risk factors and early-onset psychiatric disorders to onset of physical conditions and subsequent associations of psychiatric disorders with social role disabilities in a variety of domains.

The foundation for this book, the WMH Surveys, is one of the few international studies to address both physical and mental health in the general population. Compared to previous international studies, the WMH Surveys had the broadest coverage with respect to countries, populations, and range of disorders. Because the surveys employed a cross-sectional design, the findings are best regarded as hypothesis generating. Not only do the results confirm previous findings from clinical populations and community studies, but these new results provide important extensions for the field of behavioral medicine. The limitations of the WMH Surveys are discussed throughout the book, as is the predominate focus on psychosocial factors. In this chapter, we consider how, in the context of epidemiologic field studies, we can further our understanding of the nature of the substantial overlap of physical and mental disorders, or mental–physical comorbidity. We begin with potential extensions of analyses of WMH Survey data and then consider new twists on field studies, particularly longitudinal research, and the collection of biological specimens to test genetic hypotheses.

25.2. EXTENDING ANALYSES OF PSYCHOSOCIAL RISK FACTORS IN THE WMH SURVEYS

This book represents a major step forward in research connecting childhood risk factors to adult-onset conditions. Felitti et al. (1998) showed in a retrospective study of

Health Maintenance Organization enrollees that early childhood adversities were associated with health risk behaviors and increased risk of physical disorders many years later. This book confirmed and extended this line of research to include a broader set of adverse childhood exposures, more carefully obtained diagnoses of depression and anxiety with onset before the age of 21, and onset of a variety of physical disorders. Most importantly, the research was conducted in diverse countries around the world. In some countries, such as Mexico and Colombia, the rates of family violence and physical abuse exceeded 20%. In all countries, death of a parent in childhood exceeded 10%. These early life experiences often co-occurred; the presence of multiple adversities appeared to be the most robust predictor of increased risk of adult onset of physical disorders. In this book, childhood adversities and early-onset mental disorders are referred to as "broad-spectrum risk factors" because they were associated with elevated risk for later medical morbidity for diverse physical conditions, as well as for psychiatric disorders. This suggests that childhood adversities may need to be considered, along with tobacco use, sedentary lifestyle, poor nutritional practices, and inadequate self-management of prodromal disease states (e.g., hypertension and metabolic syndrome), as risk factors that may increase risks of a wide range of adverse chronic disease outcomes. Since childhood adversities and early-onset mental disorders may also play a role in the development of high-risk health behaviors (e.g., tobacco use, sedentary lifestyle, and poor self-management), the relationships among these broad-spectrum risk factors are also of considerable interest.

One important next step to be taken in analyzing data from the WMH Surveys is to move "upstream" to understand the role of the larger environments in which these individual-level adversities took place. Epidemiologists are increasingly recognizing the importance of considering multiple levels in causal analyses, from the macrolevel to the individual level and, of course, the microbiological level. In the context of this survey, this analysis could take the form of considering individual deviations from local norms derived from aggregated, geographically clustered variables. Some countries may have some relevant census and small area indicators that could also be included. This would allow persons using WMH Survey data to place family adversities in the context of the larger injustices occurring to children in those regions. The hypothesis here is that negative incongruence (i.e., greater family adversities than the local norm) will be more strongly predictive of later physical and mental disorder and their co-occurrence.

Similarly, the WMH Surveys could pinpoint protective family and social variables that buffer the effects of childhood adversities for long-term health outcomes. Such buffering factors may have effects on the individual level (e.g., greater educational attainment) or on regional levels (e.g., stronger social insurance and safety net programs supporting child development on a community basis). By studying how such buffering factors interact with exposure to childhood adversities, it may be possible to better understand how specific positive early family experiences balance, or fail to cushion, the long-term effects of adverse exposures. One example of a protective factor is stability of a loving mother or maternal figure in childhood and adolescence. Having a mother who did not die or leave during childhood, for example, might serve as an indirect indicator of maternal stability, but the effect on health outcomes may depend on the presence of other childhood adversities that increase the risks of long-term adverse health outcomes.

Another important step that could be taken with WMH Survey data is to disaggregate depressive and anxiety disorders occurring under age 21 into childhood, early adolescent, and late adolescent onsets, and also to consider their duration, recurrence, and the emergence of other disorders in the same class during these critically important developmental phases. For example, if some childhood-onset anxiety disorders are of shorter duration and less likely to reoccur than late adolescent–onset anxiety disorders, they might be less predictive of the onset and consequences of physical disorders than other types of early life disorders or the same disorder occurring in late adolescence. Along with this step, it would be important to integrate early-onset physical disorder and health behaviors (childhood asthma; smoking and drug misuse before age 13) because these variables might increase the risk for late adolescent psychiatric disorder and because of their potential direct links to adult-onset medical conditions of various types and their impact on functional impairments. There may indeed be synergism between aspects of environmental exposures and early-onset mental disorders when considered from this perspective. From a life-span developmental perspective, it may be more important to understand the total exposure to and sequencing of diverse, interrelated risk factors than to estimate the effects of a single risk factor as if it were acting in isolation.

Many of the chapters found that an additive model best explained the relationships of early childhood risk factors and diagnosable mood and anxiety disorders with adult-onset physical health. Synergistic effects were not typical. Another way to explore the issue of synergism is to follow the approach developed by Kate Scott in Chapter 5 on mental–physical comorbidity and disability, in which the sample was divided into pure and comorbid disorders in developing and developed countries. Using this approach, it would be possible to contrast respondents with childhood adversities only, childhood depression and anxiety only, both, and neither while further specifying different ages when these overlaps occurred prior to age 21. Such a reexamination of the effects of these risk factors on adult-onset physical disorders might indeed uncover synergistic effects that were masked by the broad measurement approach used here. While these analyses would necessarily be hypothesis generating, not hypothesis confirming, such work could provide a valuable platform to guide the design of and hypotheses tested by future prospective studies.

Another important opportunity for investigation is to identify cohort members free of psychiatric and physical disorders before adulthood. This pool of respondents could be regarded as an "historical cohort" in which it would be possible to observe the onset of psychiatric and medical illness from the point of entry into the study. The extent to which early childhood risk factors predict onset of illness in adulthood, and the timing of these onsets, would provide some clues as to the temporal effects of the various exposures, or combinations of exposures. In effect, this would maximize the use of WMH Survey data for prospectively derived trajectory analyses, to the extent that we can determine when health risk behaviors begin (e.g., smoking and heavy drinking), when the diseases themselves were first diagnosed, and how best to characterize the intervening pathways. While this cannot take the place of tracing cohorts from birth (or before) to midlife, such analyses could open a window into the antecedents and evolution of these disorders as well as their consequences.

An important strength of the WMH Surveys is that assessment covered a wide range of medical and psychiatric disorders. Most previous studies have focused on specific endpoints (e.g., cardiovascular disease, respiratory disease, and substance abuse). But the dilemma when considering how to create a healthy subsample is that respondents had an opportunity to report on at least 30 different conditions, each of which has a different developmental course over the life span. Thus, the concept of a "healthy" subsample may need to be operationalized as it "did not yet develop the disorder of interest or related conditions." The implications of studying diverse conditions, including both mental and physical disorders, in a single cohort are potentially profound, offering substantive, methodological, and logistical advantages over conventional epidemiologic studies that focus on a single disease or a narrow range of health outcomes.

In considering the possibility of organizing epidemiologic research for a wide range of physical and mental disorders, the life-span developmental perspective articulated in this book provides a useful framework. A life-span perspective integrates early childhood risk factors, early/late adolescence risk factors, subsequent life course events (marital, work, and family events), health risk behaviors, and environmental stressors, and supports with onset of psychiatric and physical disorders, treatment experiences, and social role disabilities. Such models have been articulated that specify causal linkages and their contexts. These models typically consider progression, and feedback loops across antecedent variables, mediators and moderators, and health outcomes. The model articulated by McEwen, discussed in various chapters of this book, has served as the basis for numerous studies of the links between early life stressors, changes in health behaviors (self-medication through eating or drugs, smoking, and lack of regular exercise), and dysregulation of basic physiological processes that ultimately leads to adverse health outcomes. While a formal causal model is undoubtedly premature given the exploratory nature of the research reported in this volume, Figure 25.1 offers an intuitive, generic perspective that integrates findings presented here with future opportunities that may employ more elegant designs and more sophisticated measures of risk factors and health outcomes.

From a life-span perspective, individual development is an integral process from fetal development through old age and frailty. Development is influenced by genes and gene expression, health behaviors, and life course events that may have effects on both psychological and physiological function (e.g., "allostatic load"). Development takes place within an environmental context (physical and social) that influences exposure to adversities, to stressors and to supports, and to health care and preventive services. Along a life course trajectory, disease and disability also have their own developmental sequences. This life-span perspective suggests the potential value of considering how one developmental phase leads to the next, how different risk factors and disease states affect each other, and how developmental processes intrinsic to an individual are influenced by social and physical environments. An implication of a life-span perspective is that childhood adversities and early-onset mental disorders may not only increase risks of developing chronic physical conditions in adulthood, as suggested by analyses reported in this volume, but also affect adaptation to and management of chronic physical conditions after onset.

Even though the WMH Surveys were cross-sectional and relied entirely on self-report, they are of use in assessing the relative strength of risk factors and the associations of illness with disability across different populations. Country-specific variation in the magnitude of these effects, however, was beyond the scope of the analyses reported here. Various publications from WMH teams have examined country-specific relationships, and readers are advised to review them as well. The comparison of effects, while of great interest, will lead to uncertainties in their interpretation, as is true for comparative international research of

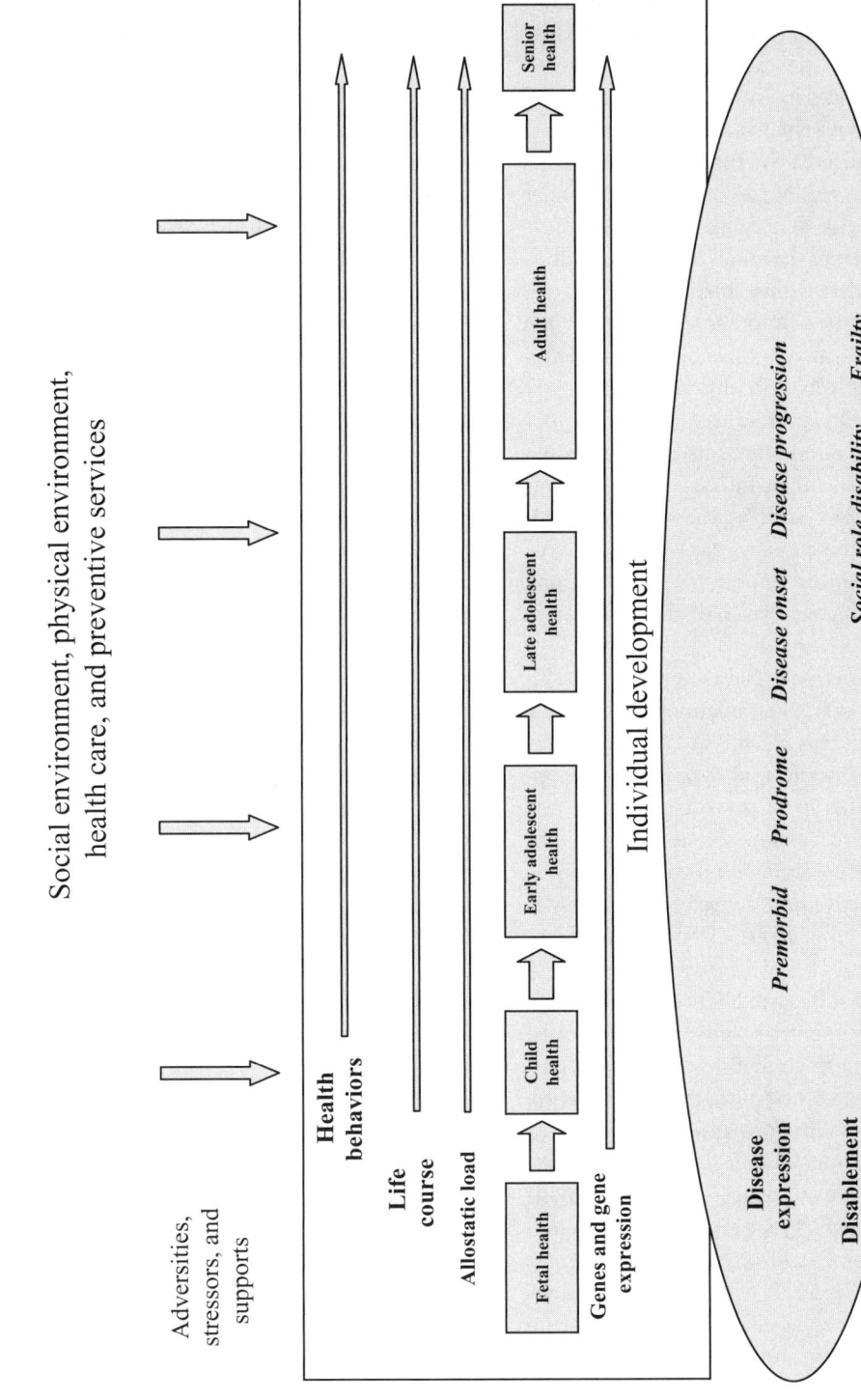

Figure 25.1. Chronic disease and disability life-span developmental perspective.

all types. There are, of course, vast differences in life expectancy and cause-specific mortality across the countries examined, along with cultural differences in symptom expression and medical and psychiatric service availability.

A fruitful area for future research, however, is to determine the circumstances under which the risk factors examined here have maximal versus minimal effects on adult-onset disorders within smaller regions of different countries. Another extension of the analyses presented in this volume is to determine under what circumstances effects are relatively more pronounced and when they are relatively minor. Circumstances that could be considered might include macroenvironmental factors, such as the level of development of the country, the level of congruence between the respondent's income, and the average income level, or familial characteristics.

Many different social factors could influence or modify these relationships. Indeed, a life-span approach, as illustrated in Figure 25.1, would lead to a more developmentally based approach to analyzing the risk and protective factors at different stages of the life cycle. Thus, even with the limits imposed by retrospective data collected by the WMH Surveys, an important next step might be to consider the onsets of disorder and health risk behaviors that occurred between ages 18 and 30. In many countries, this period marks the age at first marriage, first child, first loss of parent, first divorce, first job and perhaps first job loss, first episode of depression, onset of alcoholism, and many other life-altering events. These events may trigger a cascade of physiological processes that evolve into pathological, emotional, and physical conditions. As noted in Chapter 7, early adverse environments can shape behavioral responses and subsequent environmental exposures in a way that may increase risk of disease onset in adulthood. Events and decisions that occur in the decade of the twenties can be formative social experiences with dire (or positive) long-term consequences. While the life course perspective is best examined with prospective data, such as the follow-up of the Baltimore Epidemiologic Catchment Area surveys (Eaton 2006), the understanding of causal pathways can be enriched by thinking outside the box about how best to specify risk factors beyond those occurring in early childhood. Advanced methods of statistical modeling can be brought to bear on these questions. This is especially important given the findings in this volume that childhood adversities and early-onset mental disorders do not seem to have synergistic effects on risks of developing physical disorders, including nonspecific pain. And, not surprisingly, the level of risk explained by childhood adversities and early-onset mental disorders leaves plenty of room for other influential risk factors. Perhaps these adversities influence the life decisions and events that occur in the decade of the twenties, and this in turn influences later disorder.

Future WMH Survey analyses could also address protective factors that buffer environmental and individual risks more explicitly. Protective factors are not just the absence of risk factors. They include active variables such as religiosity, education, good dietary habits, and cohesion in the social environment. Such variables are often underdeveloped in health survey research. As a result, we know far less about their role in modifying the influences of early life risk factors than we ought to.

25.3. CONSIDERATIONS FOR NEW RESEARCH ENDEAVORS BEYOND THE WMH SURVEYS

All in all, the failure to include, concurrently, adequate measures of mental and physical health in epidemiologic surveys has been a showstopper for both psychiatric and chronic disease epidemiology. The basic approach of much of the mind–body literature, and a rate-limiting one as noted in this volume, is over-reliance on self-report measures of physical disease status. This is a limitation of many high-risk studies as well, as exemplified by the recent health surveys of veterans of the Gulf Wars (for review, see Institute of Medicine 2007). As we move forward in epidemiology, there is little doubt that cross-sectional and case-control designs involving general population samples and medical patients will continue to be implemented. They will always involve time and resource constraints as well as choices about what to address. In mental disorder epidemiology, should a wide range of emotional and substance-abuse problems be assessed or should the research focus on in-depth information on one or two conditions? In epidemiologic studies of physical disease, should a wide range of symptomatic conditions and diagnosable diseases be studied or should in-depth information on a specific disease be the focus?

The WMH Surveys, as noted in earlier chapters, chose to conduct detailed assessments of common mental disorders and a checklist of physical conditions. In some countries, respondents were also asked about less common psychiatric conditions and, for a subsample of respondents, greater details were obtained about one physical condition. How best to balance these options depends, of course, on the goals of the study. But increasing confidence in the self-report measures obtained in a study is an important first step. While self-report ascertainment of chronic physical disease status is far from perfect, imperfect data can yield new knowledge and suggest new hypotheses. A second step may be to employ high-quality case ascertainment of both physical and psychiatric disorders in the same research. If mental and physical disorders share common risk factors, and are themselves risk factors for one another, then perhaps we need large epidemiologic studies that assess a broader scope of physical and psychiatric morbidity than the typical studies that have focused on one specific disease, or a narrow class of disease.

Perhaps overidentification of researchers with specific diseases is part of the problem. This may have blinded researchers to the rapidly growing potential to study multiple diseases within a single, large cohort. Consider a future in which millions of individuals have information on key vital measures (weight and height, blood pressure, and glycemic control) and the occurrence and treatment of physical and psychological disorders recorded in an electronic medical record. In this not-too-distant future, it will be possible to collect longitudinal data from hundreds of thousands of volunteers on risk factors, life events, family history, symptomatic conditions, and social role disability at modest cost via the Internet, and to link that data to accumulating medical records data on medically diagnosed conditions. From volunteers enrolled through their health care systems, blood samples could be readily obtained via a standing laboratory order at each person's primary care clinic or DNA samples collected by sending a specimen collection kit through the mail. Organizing such a study is not a pipe dream as each of these techniques has been widely used in advanced health care systems in the United States and Europe. Rather, the limiting factors may be the traditional ways in which researchers conceive of and organize highly focused studies, along with funding agencies loath to fund research outside of their narrow disease-specific mandates. How much progress might be achieved over the next 20 years if a large consortium of researchers assembled relatively complete risk factor, developmental, environmental, and health outcome data on a cohort of, say, 1 million individuals with disease ascertainment achieved via electronic health record surveillance? With high-quality longitudinal data on a cohort with hundreds of thousands or millions of participants, it would become possible to investigate the development of disease from a life-span perspective in ways impossible with the smaller cohorts and more limited measurements that characterize most epidemiologic research today.

What kinds of research might be possible if we enlarged our ambitions regarding the size of cohort studies and broadened the scope of studies to a diverse set of physical and mental disorders? In schizophrenia research, considerable effort has gone into attempts to differentiate the premorbid period, the prodrome, the onset of first overt symptom, and the point at which the symptoms reached a diagnosable threshold. Except for a few prospective studies, this has been primarily done with careful retrospective interview methods. Within the WMH Surveys, it is possible to reconstruct the course of mental disorders with these concepts, but it is not possible to reconstruct the course of the chronic physical conditions to the same extent. Most adult-onset physical conditions do not begin at the point of diagnosis. To better understand "when the trajectories of disease risk begin," to borrow a phrase from Gilman (2007), it will be important for future studies to go beyond asking the age at diagnosis of medical conditions and begin to specify the nature and age of first symptom (or prodromal physical findings), the age when multiple symptoms began to cluster, and the duration of initial and subsequent episodes. Given that many chronic conditions are comorbid, this approach allows us to determine the timing of the onset of comorbid conditions and which ones precede the other in time. Although retrospective data will always contain restraints on validity, observational surveys could indeed provide better historical data on disease development if appropriate questions were asked. The result will be a better understanding of risk factor epidemiology more generally. In a large cohort, this kind of research could be extended from retrospective data collection to prospective, with detailed information collected on disease phases for participants sampled based on information gleaned from medical surveillance with electronic medical records.

In the United States and other industrialized countries, reliability studies have demonstrated reasonably good convergence between self-report and medical chart diagnoses. In other settings, whether or not there is convergence, there are serious questions about the validity of the clinical diagnoses themselves. For cross-national studies, going beyond self-report to include some basic medical tests will be important for subsequent evaluations of the cross-national differences. These measures could include automated blood pressure readings taken as part of the interview, blood tests to evaluate glycemic control, height and weight to assess body mass index, abdominal measure of girth, tests of respiratory capacity, and computer-administered tests of cognitive performance. Interviewers could also be trained to perform basic vision, hearing, and dental checks – areas that have received little attention in studies of mental–physical comorbidity but that have enormous influence on quality of life. In some cultures, breathalyzers to test for alcohol level might also be part of the package. As the salience of genetic analyses increases in future years, practical methods of collecting DNA samples (e.g., cheek swabs or Listerine rinses) could also be included. The general idea is that it is possible for lay interviewers to be trained to administer basic medical screening tests and for surveys to go beyond self-report with relative efficiency and accuracy. For the interviewers themselves, this experience is educational, and for the respondents, it is a sign that the study is serious and comprehensive. In the study of the nuclear disaster at Chernobyl, a two-stage study involving a home interview was followed by medical examination and blood tests at a clinic. The study provided free vision screening, which was a selling point that improved the response rate and enthusiasm for participation (Guey et al. 2008). However, as long as epidemiologic research on mental disorders and epidemiologic research on specific physical disorders are conceived and organized as separate endeavors, the opportunities to understand the shared determinants of physical and mental disorders will never be fully realized.

Beyond extending self-reports it is also possible to optimize data on current physical states, such as pain and depression. One such example is a telephone survey in which respondents were asked to list their activities over the prior 24 hours (e.g., shopping, housework, medical care, sports and exercise, telephone calls, etc.), and then three periods were selected in which respondents rated six different feelings and their level of pain (Krueger & Stone 2008). The results showed the utility of collecting time experience data with a relatively simple procedure. Another example is to assess severity of all current conditions. Given the important role of pain, for example, the inclusion of scales measuring pain severity (pain intensity and pain-related interference with activities), as was done for a subsample in some of the WMH Surveys, would allow the investigator to differentiate among conditions that cause more intense pain and greater disability within and across individuals, particularly as we begin to try to separate risk factors and disability effects of comorbid medical conditions. More importantly, current information has greater reliability and validity compared to retrospective reports for years prior to interview. We are now standing at the threshold of a new era in epidemiologic research, in which it will be possible to collect prospective data from extraordinarily large cohorts of participants with efficient linkage to information on disease outcomes from electronic medical records and to biological samples collected from volunteer participants. As we make this transition, embracing a life-span perspective to investigate and understand how physical and mental disorders develop (independently and in relationship to each other) has the potential to qualitatively advance understanding of the relationships between and among physical and mental disorders.

25.4. CONCLUSION

Future prospective studies of physical–mental comorbidity will no doubt be designed with multimethod measures and oversampling of high-risk groups. Cohort and panel studies, including future follow-ups of WMH Survey samples, will be invaluable resources for the field. No single study can address all questions well. The WMH Survey findings point to some important directions for future research regarding remote childhood exposures that were associated with adult onset of diverse physical diseases. These, in turn, influence quality-of-life outcomes. The universality of the WMH Survey results is both surprising and reassuring. Case-control designs, cohort studies, and ecoepidemiologic evaluations will pave the way for further integration of cumulative exposures beyond the individual and the family. New developments in basic science will hopefully point us to measures that we cannot foresee at the moment. These new developments will be particularly crucial for disentangling the risk factors and functional effects of diseases that often co-occur in nature, such as autoimmune disorders such as Sjogren's syndrome, lupus, and rheumatoid arthritis. The WMH Surveys, and cross-sectional surveys of the future, will help us to detect new patterns that will influence the design of future panel and intervention studies. Most importantly, this volume suggests that the rigorous application of a common methodology, as exemplified by the WMH Surveys, underscores the sense that we do indeed "live in a small world." Future analyses that are truly able to study the development of physical and mental disorders from a life-span perspective, taking a less linear approach, will doubtless suggest even more informative hypotheses about psychosocial contributions to the patterns of mental–physical comorbidity.

REFERENCES

Eaton, W. W. (2006). *Medical and Psychiatric Comorbidity over the Course of Life*. Washington, DC: American Psychiatric Publishing Inc.

Felitti, V. J., Anda, R. F., Nordenberg, D., Williamson, D. F., Spitz, A. M., Edwards, V., Koss, M. P., & Marks, J. S. (1998). Relationship of childhood abuse and household dysfunction to many of the leading causes of death in adults: The Adverse Childhood Experiences (ACE) study. *American Journal of Preventive Medicine*, **14**, 245–56.

Gilman, S. E. (2007). Invited commentary: The life course epidemiology of depression. *American Journal of Epidemiology*, **166**, 1134–7.

Guey, L. T., Bromet, E. J., Gluzman, S., Zakhozha, V., & Paniotto, V. (2008). Determinants of participation in a longitudinal two-stage study of the health consequences of the Chernobyl accident. *BMC Medical Research Methodology*, **8**, 8–27.

Institute of Medicine. (2007). *Gulf War and Health: Volume 6. Physiologic, Psychologic, and Psychosocial Effects of Deployment-Related Stress*. Washington, DC: Institute of Medicine.

Krueger, A. B., & Stone, A. A. (2008). Assessment of pain: A community-based diary survey in the USA. *Lancet*, **371**, 1519–25.

26 Clinical Implications

GREGORY E. SIMON

26.1. INTRODUCTION

Comorbidity of chronic physical conditions with common mental disorders is the norm across the life span. Even among young adults, more than half of those with a current anxiety or depressive disorder report at least one chronic physical disorder or pain condition. Among the elderly with anxiety or depressive disorders, co-occurrence of at least one chronic physical disorder is nearly universal.

Comorbidity of mental and physical disorders is not simply coincidence. Instead, this co-occurrence of mental and physical disorders reflects broad overlap of precursors, manifestations, and consequences.

Childhood adversity (including abuse or neglect, parental loss, parental psychiatric or substance-use disorder, family violence, or economic adversity) is consistently associated with development of anxiety or depressive disorder. It is more notable and unexpected that the same childhood risk factors are consistently and independently associated with development of a wide range of chronic pain conditions and chronic medical disorders (including diabetes, heart disease, asthma, and hypertension).

Daily functioning and economic productivity are strongly influenced by chronic illness, both chronic medical conditions and common mental disorders. Specific patterns of functional impairment may differ moderately between medical and mental disorders. But the effects of anxiety or depressive disorders on functional impairment and lost productivity are quite similar in magnitude to the effects of major chronic physical conditions such as diabetes, heart disease, or arthritis. Furthermore, mental disorders and physical disorders clearly have independent effects on disability and lost productivity. The apparent effects of anxiety and depression on functioning and economic productivity do not reflect the confounding influence of co-occurring medical illness.

26.2. IMPLICATIONS FOR ASSESSMENT AND DIAGNOSIS

Comorbidity research suggests that completely disentangling diagnosis of common mental disorders and chronic physical conditions is often difficult and ultimately fruitless. Traditional views (ensconced in the Diagnostic and Statistical Manual of Mental Disorders (DSM) and International Classification of Mental and Behavioural Disorders (ICD) systems) hold that any specific mental or physical symptom can and should be attributed to either a medical or a psychiatric condition, but not both (American Psychiatric Association 1994; World Health Organization 1992). For example, diagnostic criteria for mood and anxiety disorders call for excluding symptoms thought to be direct physiologic effects of a general medical disorder. For patients with comorbid mental disorders and physical illness, this distinction is rarely clear. For example, among patients with adult-onset diabetes, physical symptoms typically attributed to diabetes were more strongly associated with severity of co-occurring depression than they were with indicators of diabetes severity (Ludman et al. 2004). Additionally, diagnostic criteria for somatoform disorders call for including only symptoms that cannot be fully explained by a general medical condition (American Psychiatric Association 1994). For patients with comorbid mental disorder and physical illness, symptoms such as fatigue, sleep disturbance, or difficulty concentrating cannot be fully explained by either diagnosis.

Similarly, it is usually neither possible nor useful to determine whether an anxiety or depressive disorder is a "primary" condition or "secondary" to the effects of a general medical condition. As several of the chapters in this book clearly document, a wide variety of adverse experiences in early life are associated with later development of a wide range of common mental disorders and chronic physical conditions. If development of both depression and adult-onset diabetes are both linked to childhood adversity, it seems questionable to regard either diagnosis as primary – in terms of either temporal sequence or causal pathway. Furthermore, many of these conditions (such as anxiety disorders, depressive disorders, hypertension, diabetes, and heart disease) are defined by continua rather than dichotomies. Although we may define specific thresholds for diagnosis of diabetes or a depressive disorder, both blood sugar and depressive symptoms vary continuously – both across individuals and within individuals over time. One must question any determination that depression preceded diabetes (or diabetes preceded depression) based on when arbitrary diagnostic thresholds for either condition were crossed (or when crossing that threshold was first noticed).

26.3. IMPLICATIONS FOR CLINICAL MANAGEMENT

Available evidence also calls into question traditional efforts to recommend for or against treating anxiety or depressive disorders based on parsing of mental and physical conditions. It is true that co-occurring chronic medical conditions typically predict lower likelihood of recovery from anxiety or depression (Koike, Unutzer, & Wells 2002; Simon, Von Korff, & Lin 2005b; Unutzer et al. 2002). This finding, however, has often been misinterpreted as evidence that treatment of anxiety or depression is less beneficial for people with co-occurring chronic medical illness. The two questions "Does medical comorbidity predict poorer overall prognosis?" and "Does medical comorbidity predict less benefit from treatment?" are actually quite distinct. The second question has been most often studied with respect to treatment of depression, especially treatment with antidepressant medications. Available evidence suggests that clinical benefits of depression treatment are at least as great among those with chronic medical conditions as among those without (Katon et al. 2004; Koike et al. 2002; Unutzer et al. 2002). As discussed subsequently, the wider benefits of treatment (as measured by disability or work productivity) may actually be greater in those with co-occurring chronic medical conditions.

Comorbidity of mental and physical disorders does, however, have important implications for the process of treatment. The effects of comorbidity on the quality and effectiveness of health care flow in both directions.

First, the presence of a comorbid psychiatric disorder often interferes with effective care for chronic medical conditions. The core symptoms of depressive and anxiety disorders include discouragement, fatigue, impaired concentration, and loss of confidence. It is therefore not surprising that among people with chronic physical conditions, the presence of a common mental disorder is associated with poorer adherence to prescribed medical treatments, less effective self-management of medical conditions, and less favorable general health habits (Ciechanowski, Katon, & Russo 2000; DiMatteo, Lepper, & Croghan 2000; Lin et al. 2004). In addition, overt or covert biases of medical providers may lead to less aggressive treatment of chronic medical conditions in people with psychiatric disorders (Druss et al. 2000).

In a parallel way, the presence of a comorbid physical disorder can interfere with effective care for a depressive or anxiety disorder. Traditional biases may lead patients and providers to give greater attention or importance to physical disorders than to a mental health condition. Common symptoms of anxiety or depression (such as fatigue, anhedonia, and disturbed sleep) may be mistakenly attributed to a co-occurring physical condition. Or, these symptoms may be attributed to depression or anxiety, but interpreted as a normal or natural reaction to chronic medical illness. Or, limited time and competing demands may lead to medical problems receiving greater problem than co-occurring mental disorders (Williams 1998). In any case, the presence of a co-occurring physical disorder can contribute to nontreatment or undertreatment of an anxiety or depressive disorder.

Finally, research on the consequences of comorbidity underscores the importance of effective treatment and the potential consequences of undertreatment. As this book and earlier research (Von Korff et al. 2005a, 2005b, 2005c) document, the presence of a co-occurring anxiety or depressive disorder magnifies the effects of chronic medical illness on disability and lost work productivity. Parallel research documents a similar effect on health care costs. For any-level chronic medical morbidity, the addition of an anxiety or depressive disorder leads to a 50–100% increase in self-reported disability, work productivity lost to illness, and use of health care services. While the proportional impact of psychiatric morbidity on these measures of burden is similar among those with and without chronic medical illness, the absolute impact is dramatically larger in those with chronic medical illness. To illustrate, medical outpatients with a depressive disorder use approximately 75% more general medical services than those free of depression (Simon et al. 1995; Unutzer et al. 1997). This proportional difference is similar for those with and without chronic medical illness. But medical expenditures are relatively small for those with no chronic physical conditions, so the absolute increase in health care resource use is quite small. For those with multiple chronic physical conditions, health care costs are high. In this group, the 75% relative increase in those with depression results in a very large increase in absolute costs (Simon et al. 2005a; Unutzer et al. 1997).

26.4. IMPLICATIONS FOR PRIMARY CARE PROVIDERS

For primary care providers, the most important barriers to recognition and effective management of common mental disorders are similar to those for general medical conditions: high patient volume, brief visits, and competing demands.

Given the frequent overlap of mental and physical disorders, efforts to improve recognition of common mental disorders might focus first on patients with co-occurring conditions. Screening for depressive or anxiety disorders would have the greatest yield (in terms of both expected prevalence and expected public health benefit) in those with chronic medical conditions (Katon 2003). Absent a formal screening program, the presence of a chronic medical condition should increase a provider's suspicion regarding an anxiety or depressive disorder (rather than decrease suspicion because physical symptoms and disability are already "explained" by a medical condition).

Primary care providers should certainly expect that anxiety and depressive disorders will arrive wrapped in layers of somatic symptoms and chronic physical conditions (Simon et al. 1999). Rather than view somatic symptoms and medical diagnoses as a disguise to be removed, primary care providers might instead accept that these complex presentations are the norm. Efforts to completely disentangle common mental disorders from co-occurring physical disorders (based on patterns of symptoms, timing of onset, or apparent causal relationship) are not likely to prove useful.

A decision to offer or recommend treatment for an anxiety or depressive disorder should not be overly influenced by the presence of a chronic medical condition. Primary care providers should avoid falling into the "fallacy of good reasons." ("He has good reason to be depressed, so there's no point offering treatment.") When recommending treatment, providers should certainly emphasize the reciprocal relationship between mental and physical health: chronic illness contributes to depression and anxiety, *and* depression and anxiety make chronic illness more disabling and difficulty to manage.

But treatment for a depressive or anxiety disorder must often be adjusted or adapted to accommodate a co-occurring chronic medical condition. Selection of medication treatment might need to consider differences in adverse effects (e.g., weight gain and increased blood pressure) as well as potential for drug–drug interactions. And mental health treatment must respect the competing demands of managing a chronic physical condition – in both medication use and behavior change. If treatment for a mental health condition is perceived as an additional burden, then adherence to that treatment will certainly be poor.

26.5. IMPLICATIONS FOR MENTAL HEALTH PROVIDERS

Like primary care providers, mental health providers should not get too distracted by the effort to disentangle anxiety and depressive disorders from co-occurring chronic medical conditions. Mental health providers tend to overvalue questions regarding cause or etiology (hence the attention to the false dichotomy between "psychological" and "biological" depression). But disentangling mental and physical disorders based on cause or etiology will certainly have little value. As demonstrated in earlier chapters, etiologies of chronic physical conditions and common mental disorders appear to be completely entangled.

Mental health providers must also consider the need to adapt treatment of anxiety or depression to accommodate co-occurring medical conditions. As in primary care, prescribing of psychotropic medication may need to consider potential effects on weight, cholesterol, blood sugar, or blood pressure. Psychosocial or behavioral treatments should consider potential synergies between medical and mental health treatment. For example, behavioral treatment of depression in people with chronic illness might give greater attention to increasing physical activity and regulating sleep–wake cycles.

The overlap of mental and physical disorders should not, however, be seen as a call for the medicalization of mental health care. In fact, the epidemiologic data might be viewed as an equally strong argument for the "behavioralization" (if such a word exists) of general medical care.

REFERENCES

American Psychiatric Association. (1994). *Diagnostic and Statistical Manual of Mental Disorders, Fourth Edition (DSM-IV)*. Washington, DC: American Psychiatric Association.

Ciechanowski, P. S., Katon, W. J., & Russo, J. E. (2000). Depression and diabetes: Impact of depressive symptoms on adherence, function, and costs. *Archives of Internal Medicine*, **160**, 3278–85.

DiMatteo, M. R., Lepper, H. S., & Croghan, T. W. (2000). Depression is a risk factor for noncompliance with medical treatment: Meta-analysis of the effects of anxiety and depression on patient adherence. *Archives of Internal Medicine*, **160**, 2101–7.

Druss, B. G., Bradford, D. W., Rosenheck, R. A., Radford, M. J., & Krumholz, H. M. (2000). Mental disorders and use of cardiovascular procedures after myocardial infarction. *Journal of the American Medical Association*, **283**, 506–11.

Katon, W. J. (2003). Clinical and health services relationships between major depression, depressive symptoms, and general medical illness. *Biological Psychiatry*, **54**, 216–26.

Katon, W. J., Von Korff, M., Lin, E. H., Simon, G., Ludman, E., Russo, J., Ciechanowski, P., Walker, E., & Bush, T. (2004). The Pathways Study: A randomized trial of collaborative care in patients with diabetes and depression. *Archives of General Psychiatry*, **61**, 1042–9.

Koike, A. K., Unutzer, J., & Wells, K. B. (2002). Improving the care for depression in patients with comorbid medical illness. *American Journal of Psychiatry*, **159**, 1738–45.

Lin, E. H., Katon, W., Von Korff, M., Rutter, C., Simon, G. E., Oliver, M., Ciechanowski, P., Ludman, E. J., Bush, T., & Young, B. (2004). Relationship of depression and diabetes self-care, medication adherence, and preventive care. *Diabetes Care*, **27**, 2154–60.

Ludman, E. J., Katon, W., Russo, J., Von Korff, M., Simon, G., Ciechanowski, P., Lin, E., Bush, T., Walker, E., & Young, B. (2004). Depression and diabetes symptom burden. *General Hospital Psychiatry*, **26**, 430–6.

Simon, G., Ormel, J., VonKorff, M., & Barlow, W. (1995). Health care costs associated with depressive and anxiety disorders in primary care. *American Journal of Psychiatry*, **152**, 352–7.

Simon, G. E., Katon, W. J., Lin, E. H., Ludman, E., VonKorff, M., Ciechanowski, P., & Young, B. A. (2005a). Diabetes complications and depression as predictors of health service costs. *General Hospital Psychiatry*, **27**, 344–51.

Simon, G. E., Von Korff, M., & Lin, E. (2005b). Clinical and functional outcomes of depression treatment in patients with and without chronic medical illness. *Psychological Medicine*, **35**, 271–9.

Simon, G. E., VonKorff, M., Piccinelli, M., Fullerton, C., & Ormel, J. (1999). An international study of the relation between somatic symptoms and depression. *New England Journal of Medicine*, **341**, 1329–35.

Unutzer, J., Katon, W., Callahan, C. M., Williams, J. W., Jr., Hunkeler, E., Harpole, L., Hoffing, M., Della Penna, R. D., Noel, P. H., Lin, E. H., Arean, P. A., Hegel, M. T., Tang, L., Belin, T. R., Oishi, S., & Langston, C. (2002). Collaborative care management of late-life depression in the primary care setting: A randomized controlled trial. *Journal of the American Medical Association*, **288**, 2836–45.

Unutzer, J., Patrick, D. L., Simon, G., Grembowski, D., Walker, E., Rutter, C., & Katon, W. (1997). Depressive symptoms and the cost of health services in HMO patients aged 65 years and older. A 4-year prospective study. *Journal of the American Medical Association*, **277**, 1618–23.

Von Korff, M., Crane, P., Lane, M., Miglioretti, D. L., Simon, G., Saunders, K., Stang, P., Brandenburg, N., & Kessler, R. (2005a). Chronic spinal pain and physical-mental comorbidity in the United States: Results from the national comorbidity survey replication. *Pain*, **113**, 331–9.

Von Korff, M., Katon, W., Lin, E. H., Simon, G., Ciechanowski, P., Ludman, E., Oliver, M., Rutter, C., & Young, B. (2005b). Work disability among individuals with diabetes. *Diabetes Care*, **28**, 1326–32.

Von Korff, M., Katon, W., Lin, E. H., Simon, G., Ludman, E., Oliver, M., Ciechanowski, P., Rutter, C., & Bush, T. (2005c). Potentially modifiable factors associated with disability among people with diabetes. *Psychosomatic Medicine*, **67**, 233–40.

Williams, J. W., Jr. (1998). Competing demands: Does care for depression fit in primary care? *Journal of General Internal Medicine*, **13**, 137–9.

World Health Organization. (1992). *The ICD-10 Classification of Mental and Behavioural Disorders. Clinical Descriptions and Diagnostic Guidelines*. Geneva, Switzerland: World Health Organization.

27 Policy Implications

SERGIO AGUILAR-GAXIOLA

27.1. INTRODUCTION

In contrast with the increase in life expectancy experienced by most countries worldwide during the twenty-first century (see Chapter 2), there is a population group that has not benefited from the overall life expectancy gains. In fact, people with serious mental illness are experiencing astounding rates of premature death due to co-occurring chronic disease conditions. Recent studies estimate that persons with serious mental illness can expect to live 25 fewer years than the general population (Parks et al. 2006). Nearly half comorbid chronic physical diseases in persons with serious psychiatric disorders are missed (Koran et al. 1989; Koranyi 1979). Their increased morbidity and mortality are largely due to treatable medical conditions. These conditions are also preventable by modifying common risk factors such as smoking, unhealthy diet, physical inactivity, obesity, harmful use of alcohol and drugs, and inadequate access to medical care (Parks et al. 2006). These startling premature death rates underscore the importance of studying and gaining a better understanding of the extent and consequences of medical comorbidity among persons with mental illness.

Developed and developing countries alike now face common challenges in responding to the need to prevent chronic disease and care for persons with chronic conditions. Yet the resources available to meet these challenges differ markedly between developed and developing countries. Most developing countries have limitations in health care facilities and professionals available to manage the large and growing numbers of persons with chronic illness. As developing countries improve their health care services, they have unique opportunities to develop effective and efficient health care systems designed and staffed to optimize chronic disease management care. In contrast, developed countries have well-established health care systems developed predominately to manage acute presenting problems. Despite substantial investments in health care services in developed countries, the performance of their traditional health care systems in managing chronic disease remains far from optimal (Wagner, Austin, & Von Korff 1996).

In developing innovative approaches to reducing the burden of chronic physical and mental disorders, population-based data on the extent and distribution of physical and mental disorders are critically important. Large survey data sets are particularly useful in analyzing population data for policy input and decision making (Frank & Glied 2006). Using population-based, cross-national epidemiological data from both developed and developing countries, this volume adds to the scientific knowledge of the comorbidity of chronic disease conditions and mental illness. This chapter summarizes key findings from this volume, identifies and provides an overview of several components of policy development, and presents implications for public policy needed to promote better health and well-being of persons with mental illness who have coexisting chronic disease conditions. This chapter also considers policy implications germane to both developed and developing countries as they grapple with the challenges of comorbid chronic physical and psychological disorders in their populations. In considering policy implications, life-span developmental and systems perspectives are highly relevant.

Summary of findings

1. Associations between mental disorders and physical conditions:
    a. The co-occurrence of physical disease and mental disorders is common in both developed and developing countries.
    b. Mood and anxiety disorders are associated with increased risks of both chronic physical diseases and chronic pain conditions.
    c. The large majority of persons affected by chronic pain or with chronic physical diseases do *not* have a comorbid mental disorder.
2. Age patterning of mental disorders and chronic physical conditions:
    a. Depression and anxiety disorders declined with age.
    b. Chronic physical diseases and chronic pain conditions increased with age.
3. Associations of risk factors with the co-occurrence of chronic physical conditions and mental disorders:
    a. Both childhood adversities and early-onset mood and anxiety disorders may increase risks of a broad spectrum of chronic physical diseases and chronic pain conditions. Childhood adversities include physical abuse, sexual abuse, neglect, parental death, parental divorce, other parental loss, parental mental disorder, parental substance use, parental criminal behavior, family violence, and family economic adversity.
4. Consequences of mental–physical comorbidity for people's functional disability, labor force participation, health-related stigma, use of health care services, and mortality:
    a. Consequences of comorbid mental disorders for the health and well-being of persons with chronic physical conditions are significant in both developed and developing countries worldwide.
5. Relationships between physical disorders and mental disorders are multifaceted and develop over the life span:
    a. Childhood adversities may increase risks of early-onset mental disorders, while both childhood adversities and early-onset mental disorder may increase risks of a range of physical diseases in later life.

These findings provide the basis for policy development and may serve as a launching pad for consideration of broader and ultimately more cost-effective strategies to control chronic physical disease and psychological illness.

27.2. POLICY DEVELOPMENT

Vision

To achieve improved-quality mental health and a high standard of care for all through the provision of integrated, comprehensive, equitable, culturally and linguistically appropriate, and accessible community-based mental health care for all, regardless of class, race/ethnicity, status, and political affiliation. Services will uphold and protect the human rights of people with mental disorders and co-occurring chronic disease conditions. The

Table 27.1. Values and principles

Values	Principles
Mental health is an integral part of physical health	Mental health care should be integrated with holistic general health care.
	All health personnel should be trained to detect mental disorders, provide basic assessment and treatment, and refer to specialist mental health services when necessary.
Community-based care	Mental health care should be provided in the community where people live whenever possible.
	Communities and families should take an active role in the care of people with mental disorders.
Quality	Mental health care should be safe, equitable, effective, efficient, timely, and patient centered.
	Services should be provided according to established protocols.
Intersectoral collaboration	Mental health care cuts across traditional sectors and includes health, welfare, justice, education, housing, communities, and NGOs. These sectors therefore need to collaborate for improved mental health care of the population.
Respect for local culture and language	The culture, language, beliefs, and traditions of people with mental disorders should be respected.
	Traditional healers should be involved in mental health care.
Protection of vulnerable groups	The mental health needs and rights of vulnerable groups should be upheld, including those of women, children, adolescents, the elderly, refugees, and displaced persons.
Human rights	People with mental disorders should enjoy full human rights, including the right to appropriate health care and freedom from stigma in society.

value and principles that motivate this vision statement are summarized in Table 27.1.

Objectives

1. Foster awareness of the importance of the co-occurrence, age patterning, risk factors, and consequences of physical disease and mental disorders.
2. Improve access to health care of people with mental illness.
3. Improve the coordination and integration of mental health and physical health care in persons with mental disorders.
4. Design and implement comprehensive, well-coordinated, and integrated and efficient mental health systems that cover promotion, prevention, treatment, and rehabilitation and recovery.
5. Ensure the delivery of high-quality, evidence-based interventions for mental health promotion, prevention, treatment, and rehabilitation.
6. Address the need for a diverse and culturally and linguistically competent workforce, effective in addressing comorbid mental and physical conditions.
7. Empower and support people with mental health problems and their families to be actively engaged in this process.
8. Ensure the inclusion of children, adolescents, and the elderly's mental health and well-being as priorities.

Policy Implications

9. Expand community-based mental health services so that they become accessible to all people in need.

10. Foster intersectoral linkages, coordination, and integration and incorporate multisectoral and multidisciplinary approaches in promotion, prevention, treatment, and rehabilitation activities.

Areas for Action Identified as Priorities

1. Societal investments in disease prevention and health promotion.
2. Organization of health care services.
3. Human resources development and training.

Implications for these three priority areas follow.

27.2.1. Implications for Societal Investments in Disease Prevention and Health Promotion

A critically important question for both developed and developing countries is the extent and nature of health benefits likely to result from investments in health care services relative to investments in educational, environmental, and economic development. The Ottawa Charter for Health Promotion observed:

> the fundamental conditions and resources for health care: peace, shelter, education, food, income, a stable eco-system, sustainable resources, social justice and equity. Improvement in health requires a secure foundation in these basic prerequisites... The prerequisites and prospects for health cannot be ensured by the health sector alone... Professional and social groups and health personnel have a major responsibility to mediate between differing interests in society for the pursuit of health. (First International Conference on Health Promotion 1986)

Balancing investments in different sectors of society (e.g., health care, education, income maintenance for the elderly and the disabled, environmental protection, and economic development) in ways that optimize health outcomes requires a broad understanding of the determinants of health outcomes in the population at large across the life span.

The possibility that childhood adversities and early-onset mental disorders increase risks of developing a spectrum of adverse health outcomes has significant implications for disease prevention and health promotion strategies. Investment in educational services and community services and supports that strengthen the ability of families to raise healthy, happy children may reduce deleterious, long-term effects of childhood psychosocial stressors. Furthermore, given that mental disorders and physical condition are strongly associated at early ages and the uncertainty of which one is a risk for the other, children and adolescents diagnosed with physical disorders in primary health care clinics should be assessed for early signs of mental disorders and vice versa, given that physical and psychiatric comorbidity exist in children and adolescents with psychiatric disorders (Spady et al. 2005). In addition, early intervention programs (for both physical and mental health) should be available for these high-risk children in a normative environment such as school-based health programs.

Further research is needed to determine whether, and to what extent, childhood adversities have long-term effects on chronic disease risks and whether interventions to prevent or buffer childhood adversities can reduce risks of health consequences. As more is learned about the health implications of childhood adversities and promotion of optimal child development, a broad perspective should be taken on the kinds of societal investments that might prevent chronic physical and psychological conditions in adulthood. Too often, investments to improve health care services are evaluated only with respect to alternative investments within the health care sector, not to educational, economic, or social safety net investments that have potentially significant health benefits.

Further research is also needed to determine which comes first, mental illness or physical disease, or whether they develop "hand in hand." More focus needs to be on studies of children starting before typical onsets. Since anxiety age of onset can be very young (e.g., 6 years), studies need to focus on ages 6 through 25. Most of the studies have examined only adults 18 years or older. It is unclear whether educational, economic, and environmental improvements are more effective than improving mental and physical health care in health settings for children. Quality mental health care for children is not common for many common mental disorders, such as depression. We need to improve mental health services for children in settings where they spend most of their time (e.g., school-based therapy for anxiety or depressive disorders).

Improving population health requires evidence-based efforts across all sectors of society. For example, Australia's strategic framework for preventing chronic disease (National Public Health Partnership 2001) identifies a broad range of health promotion strategies including promotion of an active lifestyle, tobacco control, healthy eating, safe alcohol use and substance-abuse prevention, promotion of sexual health, immunizations, injury prevention, and environmental health. The research presented in this volume suggests that steps taken to promote health development over the full human life span can potentially benefit both physical and mental health. The results of the World Mental Health Surveys on risk factors for mental–physical comorbidity suggest taking a broad perspective on the kinds of societal investments that may be effective in preventing chronic physical and psychological disorders and in optimizing health outcomes when chronic conditions cannot be prevented.

The pattern that chronic physical diseases and chronic pain conditions increase as people age, especially after age 65, but that mental disorders decline after midlife suggest that most resources for studying and addressing the comorbid pattern need to be spent on the young (e.g., ages 6 through 30), and we need to better understand consequences of poor physical health among older adults (age >65 years). Children and young people and the elderly are particularly at risk from social, psychological, biological, and environmental factors. Given their vulnerability and needs, young and older people should be a high priority for activities related to the prevention and promotion of mental health and care of mental health problems. The World Health Organization notes, "Supporting the mental health of children and adolescents should be seen as a strategic investment which may create many long-term benefits for individuals, societies and health systems" (WHO European Ministerial Conference on Mental Health 2005).

Scott (see Chapter 6) reports fewer mental health problems for older adults (mental disorders decline as chronic disease conditions increases). But, is this really the case? Or, perhaps older adults (e.g., out of workforce and inactive in social life, etc.) do not do well with Diagnostic and Statistical Manual for Mental Disorders (DSM) (International Classification of Mental and Behavioural Disorders (ICD)) mental health case-ascertainment instruments. More resources are needed to study mental health problems of those 65 years and older and the causes of their poor mental health. Do those 65 years or older need to be assessed differently from those younger? What are the mental health implications of significant chronic diseases in this population?

The delivery of services of our mental health care systems is primarily focused on middle-aged persons (age 25–65). We need to do a better job at both ends of the developmental span spectrum: young and old.

27.2.2. Implications for the Organization of Health Care Services

Within health care systems, frontline responsibility for prevention and management of chronic illness lies with the primary health care service. The Declaration of Alma-Ata by the International Conference on Primary Health Care (1978) concluded that

> primary health care is essential health care based on practical, scientifically sound and socially acceptable methods and technology made universally accessible to individuals and families in the community through their full participation and at a cost that the community and country can afford to maintain at every stage of their development in the spirit of self-reliance and self-determination. It forms an integral part both of the country's health system of which it is the central function and main focus, and of the overall social and economic development of the community.

The World Mental Health Surveys have shown that in both developed and developing countries, common psychological disorders are often accompanied by chronic physical conditions, including both common chronic physical diseases (e.g., diabetes, asthma, hypertension, and heart disease) and chronic pain conditions (e.g., arthritis, back pain, and headache). In both developed and developing countries, primary health care is the setting in which common mental disorders are most likely to be recognized and treated. The fact that depressive and anxiety disorders often occur within the context of comorbid chronic physical conditions emphasizes the central role that providers of primary health care play in efforts to improve overall health outcomes of both physical and psychological disorders.

As the demographic transition unfolds, with increasing prevalence of chronic physical (in older age groups) and psychological disorders (in younger age groups), the capabilities and resources of primary health care are being tested and strained in developed and developing countries alike. The unique role of primary health care is to assume responsibility for a broad range of health care needs of the populations they serve, integrating and coordinating care across disparate health problems of individual patients. Since people with chronic physical conditions seek health care more often and in primary health care settings, their comorbid physical conditions may increase the likelihood of psychological disorder being detected and treated across multiple visits, even if it reduced the chances of recognition and treatment on any particular health care visit. It is the primary health care physician's responsibility to ensure continuity of care across time and to help patients prioritize and integrate their care if they are afflicted by several different conditions (e.g., diabetes, depression, and chronic back pain). All too often, primary health care physicians are asked to ensure continuity and integration of care for complex patients with limited resources and within systems of care not adequately designed for the tasks they are now being asked to perform. Inadequate health care systems can lead not only to less-than-optimal health care for chronically ill patients, but also to demoralization and burnout of primary health care workers.

The advanced, or patient-centered, "Medical Home" is an integrated system for comprehensive care model that has the potential to reinvigorate the delivery of primary health care and to better define the resources and capabilities now needed to deliver effective primary health care (Sia et al. 2004). The American College of Physicians (2006) identified the attributes of the patient-centered medical home as follows:

> Attributes of the advanced medical home include promotion of continuous healing relationships through delivery of care in a variety of settings according to the needs of the patient and skills of the medical provider. Physicians are once again partners in coordinating and facilitating care to help patients navigate the complex and often confusing health care system by providing guidance, insight and advice that is informative and specific to patients' needs.... Rather than being a "gatekeeper" who restricts patient access to services, a personal physician leverages the key attributes of the advanced medical home to coordinate, and facilitate the care of patients, and is directly accountable to each patient.

The "Medical Home" concept is not new. It was first articulated by the American Academy of Pediatrics in 1967 (American Academy of Pediatrics 1967, 2002). The current resurgence of interest in the original concept of the Medical Home has been reconceived as an integrated delivery system for children and youth with special health care needs. The Medical Home practice is identified by the following characteristics:

- Comprehensiveness
- Continuity
- Coordination
- Compassion
- Cultural effectiveness
- Family centeredness

Interest and support for the Medical Home concept has gained considerable support in the last few years. It has been enhanced and endorsed by the several U.S. organizations such as the American College of Physicians, American Academy of Family Physicians, American Academy of Pediatrics, American Osteopathic Association, and the National Association of Pediatric Nurse Practitioners.

If the care of chronically ill patients is to be adequately managed in primary health care settings, then communication and coordination barriers between primary health care and consultative specialists (both medical and mental health specialists) need to be eliminated. In both developing and developed countries, specialists typically practice in hospitals or other care settings isolated from primary health care practice. As a result, communication and coordination between primary health care physicians and consultative specialists is less than optimal. As e-mail, voice mail, and shared electronic medical records become more widely used in the delivery of health care in developed countries, there are new opportunities to reduce the communication and collaboration barriers between primary health care physicians and consultative specialists (Katon et al. 2001). In developed countries, greater use of efficient communication tools to increase collaboration between primary health care physicians and consultative specialists is sometimes stymied by long-standing practice patterns, medical norms, and/or physician reimbursement practices. As health care systems in developing countries evolve, they have the potential to prevent some of these barriers to communication and collaboration among professionals.

While the issue of better coordination and integration of mental health and physical health care in persons with mental disorders is relevant to the overall organizational transformation of health care systems in both developed and developing countries, the integration of effort on the part of the public agencies responsible for child, family, adult, and elderly mental health – child welfare, special education, primary health care, mental health, juvenile or criminal justice, and substance abuse – is of particular relevance to vulnerable populations including the poor, uninsured, elderly, abused women, refugees, displaced persons, or otherwise disadvantaged individuals and families (World Health Organization

2001). These agencies are often their only source of support and therefore integrated agency efforts must be made. Thus, fostering intersectoral links between the mental health and other sectors is of critical importance for the effective delivery of services for those with comorbid physical and psychological conditions.

In the case of children and adolescents, primary health care may not be the best first line of mental health care. One good alternative is to turn to schools as the entry point for health care, given that a great proportion of children in both developed and developing countries attend school. It may be ideal to have different first-line modes of health care delivery at different ages. At a minimum, three age groups should be considered: young (25 years or so), adult (20–64 years), and older adult (65 or older). In the United States, the age group of 65 years or older gets lots of physical health care (e.g., lots of physician visits), but not very much mental health care. But perhaps the elderly do not appear to need much mental health care, given that depression and anxiety disorders decline with age – it is not clear. Or maybe they do, and just are not being properly assessed. Adults need special attention because of disability and high costs associated with mental–physical comorbidity (see Chapters 19–21).

The results of the World Mental Health Surveys indicate that about half the adult population is affected by a chronic physical disease, a chronic pain condition, and/or a common psychological disorder. The sheer numbers of persons who are affected by chronic conditions means that health care services need to be organized as a vehicle for delivering effective interventions on a mass basis while striving to achieve the personalized care that patients desire. The scope of the problem, and the constraints on resources that can be devoted to health care, will require innovative new approaches if the potential of health care services to improve population health is to be fully achieved.

27.2.3. Implications for Human Resource Development and Training

As health care services change to meet the rising tide of chronic physical and psychological illness, traditional methods of training health care professionals will need to give way to new approaches. Still for many countries in both developed and developing countries, general practitioners (GPs) and other primary health care staff continued to be the point of entry and main source of help for common mental health problems. Mental health problems, however, often remain undetected in people receiving services from GPs and treatment is not always adequate when they are identified (WHO European Ministerial Conference on Mental Health 2005). Providers of primary health care services need to be trained in best-evidence and practice-based promising practices tailored to the target populations and develop capacity and competence to detect and treat people with mental health problems in the community, supported by a network with specialist mental health services. Fortunately, increasingly more physicians and allied health professionals are being trained to recognize and treat common mental disorders as well as physical disorders. In contrast, it is unusual for mental health workers to receive training in the implications of comorbid chronic physical conditions for the management of depressive, anxiety, or substance-abuse disorders. It may be time for the cult of specialization to give way to more holistic approaches to health care in which health care professionals are trained to improve the overall health outcomes of their patients, rather than manage specific disorders. The following recommendations for mental health workers endorsed by the U.S. National Association of State Mental Health

Program Directors Medical Directors Council provide a glimpse of where the field is moving toward: (1) screen for comorbid conditions such as obesity, diabetes, and high blood pressure; (2) routinely assess treatment outcomes (physical as well as mental health); and (3) routinely share clinical information with other providers (primary and specialty health care providers as well as mental health providers) (Parks et al. 2006).

27.3. CONCLUSIONS

The demographic transition confronts society in general and health care services in particular, with chronic illness being common in the population at large. This is now true in both developed and developing countries. New strategies for educating, supporting, and empowering individuals and families are needed, which prevent chronic disease when possible and maximize the ability of individuals with chronic illness to live full and productive lives when chronic disease cannot be prevented. The legacy health care systems of both developed and developing countries need to be reorganized to optimize the abilities to improve population health, focusing on the challenges of managing chronic conditions. In addition, the working practices of primary health care providers and mental health care workers need to be modernized and new staff roles and responsibilities, requiring changes in values and attitudes, knowledge, and skills, need to be taught and supported in order to offer effective and efficient care. These challenges are more complex than the traditional public health agendas of immunization, ensuring sanitary and healthful food and water and improving general living conditions. Given the scope of chronic physical and psychological illness in the populations of both developed and developing countries, the health challenges of the twenty-first century may require rethinking how health is sustained and illness managed on a population basis. While health care services need to change to meet these challenges, the scope and nature of the problems of preventing and caring for chronic illness require viewing these as challenges that face all individuals and all sectors of society in both developed and developing countries.

REFERENCES

American Academy of Pediatrics. (1967). Council on Pediatric Practice. Pediatric Records and a "Medical Home." In *Standards of Child Care*, p. 22. Evanston, IL: American Academy of Pediatrics.

American Academy of Pediatrics. (2002). Medical home initiatives for children with special healthcare needs advisory committee. Policy statement: The "medical home." *Pediatrics*, **110**, 184–6.

American College of Physicians. (2006). The advanced medical home: A patient-centered, physician-guided model of health care. Retrieved June 4, 2008, from http://www.acponline.org/advocacy/where_we_stand/policy/adv_med.pdf.

First International Conference on Health Promotion. (1986). Ottawa charter for health promotion. *Canadian Journal of Public Health*, **77**, 425–30.

Frank, R. G., & Glied, S. (2006). Changes in mental health financing since 1971: implications for policymakers and patients. *Health Affairs*, **25**, 601–13.

International Conference on Primary Health Care. (1978). Declaration of Alma-Ata. Retrieved June 9, 2008, from http://www.who.int/hpr/NPH/docs/declaration_almata.pdf.

Katon, W., Von Korff, M., Lin, E., & Simon, G. (2001). Rethinking practitioner roles in chronic illness: The specialist, primary care physician and the practice nurse. *General Hospital Psychiatry*, **23**, 138–44.

Koran, L. M., Sox, H. C., Marion, I., Moltzen, S., Sox, C. H., Kraemer, H. C., Imai, K., Kelsey, T. G., Rose Jr., T. G., & Levin, L. C. (1989). Medical evaluation of psychiatric patients. *Archives of General Psychiatry*, **46**, 733–40.

Koranyi, E. A. (1979). Morbidity and rate of undiagnosed physical illnesses in a psychiatric clinic population. *Archives of General Psychiatry*, **36**, 414–19.

National Public Health Partnership. (2001). Preventing chronic disease: A strategic framework. Retrieved June 5, 2008, from http://www.dhs.vic.gov.au/nphp/publications/strategies/chrondis-bgpaper.pdf.

Parks, J., Svendsen, D., Singer, P., & Foti, M. E. (2006). Morbidity and mortality in people with serious mental illness. Retrieved April 8, 2009, from http://www.nasmhpd.org/general_files/publications/med_directors_pubs/Technical%20Report%20on%20Morbidity%20and%20Mortaility%20-%20Final%2011-06.pdf.

Sia, C., Tonniges, T. F., Osterhus, E., & Taba, S. (2004). History of the advanced medical home concept. *Pediatrics*, **113**, 1473–8.

Spady, D. W., Schopflocher, D. P., Svenson, L. W., & Thompson, A. H. (2005). Medical and psychiatric comorbidity and health care use among children 6 to 17 years old. *Archives of Pediatrics & Adolescent Medicine*, **159**, 231–7.

Wagner. E. H., Austin, B. T., & Von Korff, M. (1996). Organizing care for patients with chronic illness. *The Milbank Quarterly*, **74**, 511–44.

World Health Organization. (2001). *Mental Health: New Understanding, New Hope*. Ginebra: World Health Organization.

WHO European Ministerial Conference on Mental Health. (2005). *Mental Health Action Plan for Europe: Facing the Challenges, Building Solution*. Ginebra: World Health Organization.

Index

AAFP. *See* American Academy of Family Physicians
AAP. *See* American Academy of Pediatrics
ACE. *See* Adverse Childhood Experiences study
ACP. *See* American College of Physicians
additive model of comorbidity, 230
adrenocorticotropic hormone (ACTH), 98
adult obesity, childhood adversities
   anxiety, depressive disorders, 169–170
   associations, 167
   BMI, 165, 166
   childhood adversities
   clinical care, prevention
   dose–response relationship
   early-onset mood/anxiety disorders, 168, 169
   mental disorders, childhood adversities prevalence, 166–167
   multiple childhood adversities and obesity
   multivariate logistic regression analysis, 166
   obesity causes, 165
   obesity health risks, 165
   obesity prevalence, 165
   obesity sample characteristics, 167
   PTSD
   recall bias
   research, 165–166
   study aims, 166
   weight, height bias
adult-onset asthma, psychosocial predictors
   adversity and mental disorder, 113–115
   AOO, 109, 115, 116
   asthma severity, 116
   ATS, 110
   childhood adversity, immune system function and, 113–114
   childhood adversity and, 108–109, 112–113
   childhood adversity and mental disorder, 110
   differential recall, 110–111
   disorder, adversity prevalence, 111–112
   early-onset mental disorders, 113–115
   ECRHS, 110–117
   etiology, 108
   mood-congruent recall bias, 116
   NCHS, 110
   psychosocial factors, 108
   study approach, 109–110
   study findings, 113–115
   study limitations, 115–117
   underrecall, 116
adult-onset diabetes, psychosocial factors
   ACE study, 137
   allostatic load, 139–140
   AOO adult diabetes, 140
   approach, 137
   childhood adversity, 139–141
   Cox proportional hazards models, 137
   diabetes mellitus, 136
   diabetes prevalence rates, 137
   early-onset mental disorder, 137–139
   etiologic role, 137
   family economic adversity, 141
   HPA axis–mediated sensitivity, 139–140
   Kaplan–Meier curves, 137
   metabolic syndrome, 136–137
   multiple childhood adversities, 138–139
   prevalence, 136
   self-report limitations, 140–141
   stress, 136
   type 2 diabetes, 136
adult-onset spinal pain, childhood adversities
   childhood abuse and mental disorders, 154–155
   Cox proportional hazards models, 155
   depressive disorders, 154
   dose–response relationship, 161
   early-onset mental disorder, 159, 160–162
   effect of, 156–157
   Kaplan–Meier curves, 155
   mental disorders and, 155–156, 160
   past research, 155
   predictors, 160–161
   Raphael, 161
   recall bias, 162
   self-report, 162
   severity, 162
   sexual, physical abuse, 161

adult-onset spinal pain (cont.)
  specific adversities, 157
  study approach, 155
  study limitations
Adverse Childhood Experiences (ACE) study, 137
age of onset (AOO), 109, 115
age patterns
  age prevalence, 87–88
  CES-D, 84
  chronic physical conditions, 85, 86–87
  comorbidity, 89
  depression manifestation, 90–91
  depressive/anxiety disorder decrease, 91
  diagnostic criteria, older persons, 85
  disability, 92
  DSM-IV, 84
  effects of age, 88
  global, 92
  mental, physical condition groups, 87
  mental disorder and increasing age, 84
  mental disorder comorbidity, 89, 91
  mental disorder status, 86
  odds ratios, 86–87
  organic exclusion criteria, 90
  physical, pain condition comorbidity, 85–86
  sampling limitations, 89–90
  scale measures, 84–85
  self-report limitations, 91–92
AIMS. See Arthritis Impact Measurement Scale
alcohol abuse
  asthma and, 57
  spinal pain and, 56
allostasis, 3
allostatic load
  adult-onset diabetes, 139–140
  arthritis, 144–145
  hypertension, 134
  mental–physical comorbidity, 102–103
  mental–physical condition with disability, 235
  physical, psychological morbidity, 3–4
American Academy of Family Physicians (AAFP), 308
American Academy of Pediatrics (AAP), 308
American College of Physicians (ACP), 308
American Osteopathic Association (AOA), 308
American Thoracic Society (ATS), 110
analytic methods
  childhood stressors, adult physical disorders, 43–44
  complex sample design, 43
  Cox proportional hazards models, 43
  hazard ratios, 43
  Kaplan–Meier curves, 43
  odds ratios, 43
  pooled odds ratio, 43
  weights, 42–43
antecedent model, mental disorder to physical condition, 97–99
anxiety, depressive disorders
  chronic pain, 24–25, 26
  chronic physical disease, 19–20
  prevalence, 17–18
AOA. See American Osteopathic Association
AOO. See age of onset
APA. See American Academy of Pediatrics
Aristotle, 2
arthritis, psychosocial predictors
  adult-onset arthritis, increased risk, 152
  allostatic load, 144–145
  arthritis prevalence, 144
  arthritis risk factors, 144
  childhood psychosocial stressors, 151–152
  chronic psychosocial stressors, 145
  comorbid depressive illness, 144
  Cox proportional hazards models, 145
  early-onset mood/anxiety disorder, 146, 148–150, 151
  future research, 152
  Kaplan–Meier curves, 145–146
  mood/anxiety disorder prevalence, 148
  multiple childhood adversities, 146–147, 150–151
  prospective studies, 151
  psychosocial stressors, risk, 145
  research limitations, 151
  sample population childhood adversities, 146
  specific disorders, adult-onset arthritis, 150
  study approach, 145–146
Arthritis Impact Measurement Scale (AIMS), 198
ASP. See International Association for the Study of Pain
Asthma. See also adult-onset asthma, psychosocial predictors
  alcohol abuse, 57
  mental disorder, 54–55, 56
ATS. See American Thoracic Society

bidirectionality, 99–100, 236
biological vulnerability, 101
body mass index (BMI), 165

CAPI. See computer-assisted personal interviews
Centre for Epidemiologic Studies Depression Scale (CES-D), 84

Index

childhood adversity
  adult-onset asthma. *See also* adult-onset asthma, psychosocial predictors
    AOO, 109, 115, 116
    association, 113
    asthma severity, 116
    differential recall, 110–111
    effect, 112–113
    immune system function, 113–114
    mental disorders and, 110
    mood-congruent recall bias, 116
    predictors, 113, 115–117
    relationship, 108–109
  mental disorder and heart disease
    associations, 120–121, 124, 126
    Cox proportional hazards models, 121
    depression, role of, 125
    frequency and distribution of adversities, 121, 122
    heart disease, 121–124
    independent associations, 125
    Kaplan–Meier curves, 121
    life-years lost, 120
    mechanistic pathways, 125
    onset, mental disorder and heart disease, 121, 122
    previous studies, 120
    research, clinical practice implications, 125–126
    sexual, physical abuse, 125–126
    shared risk factors, 120
    study approach, 121
    study limitations, 124–125
    study population, 121
  underrecall, 116. *See also* later hypertension
    allostatic load, 134
    associations, 132–133
    Cox proportional hazards models, 128
    dose–response relationship, 133
    early-onset depression/anxiety disorders, 129–130, 131
    hypertension by age, 129, 131
    hypertension etiology, 128
    Kaplan–Meier curves, 128–129
    lack of research, 128
    psychobiological mechanisms, 133–134
    sample characteristics, 129
    self-reports, 129, 130
    specific adversities, 130–132
    study approach, 128–129
childhood family adversities
  clinical implications, 297

  family economic adversity, 49–50
  neglect, 48
  parental criminal behavior, 49
  parental death, divorce, loss, 48–49
  parental mental illness, 49
  parental substance-use disorder, 49
  physical abuse, 48
  sexual abuse, 48
  survey methods, 42
children and youth with special health care needs (CYSHCN), 308
chronic illness self-regulation
  catastrophizing, 197–198
  fear-avoidance, 197–198
  management, 196–197
  self-regulatory model, 198
chronic obstructive pulmonary disease (COPD), 199
chronic pain, 24
  age-specific, 25
  anxiety disorder and, 24–25, 26
  ASP, 22
  comorbid conditions, 27
  defined, 22, 26–27
  depressive/anxiety disorders, 25
  gender-specific, 24, 25–26
  pain assessment, 23
  physical, psychological features, 22
  physical conditions, 35–37
  prevalence, 22, 23–24
  survey methods, 35–37
chronic pain and medical conditions
  mental disorder prevalence, 52
  odds ratios, 52–53
  pattern, mental–physical comorbidity, 52–54
  physical conditions, 52
chronic pain mechanisms, 4
chronic physical disease
  age-specific prevalence, 19
  age-standardized crude prevalence, 18
  anxiety disorders, and, 19–20
  common diseases, 19
  developed, developing countries, 18–19
  elderly, 15–16
  global burden, challenges, 15–17, 20
  health care costs, 16–17
  per capita income, 16
  prevalence
CIDH. *See* International Classification of Impairments, Disabilities, and Handicaps
CIDI. *See* WHO Composite International Diagnostic Interview

clinical implications
  childhood adversity, 297
  comorbid treatment, 298–299
  comorbidity norm, 297
  functional impairment, 297
  mental health providers, 300
  primary care providers, 299–300
  traditional treatment, 298
cognitive–behavioral therapy, 195, 200–201
collaborative care program, 200
comorbid treatment, 298–299
computer-assisted personal interviews (CAPI)
consequence model, physical condition to mental disorder, 99
consequences, mental–physical comorbidity
  AIMS, 198
  antidepressant medications, 195
  behavioral interventions, 202
  broad-spectrum risk factors, 193
  catastrophizing, 197–198
  chronic illness management, 193–194, 196–197
  cognitive–behavioral therapy, 195, 200–201
  collaborative care program, 200
  COPD, 199
  Dartmouth Co-Op Charts, 198
  depression treatment, 200–203
  disability, 198
  fear-avoidance, 197–198
  Groningen Social Disabilities Schedule, 198
  health care use, psychological illness, 201
  ICF, 198
  impairment, 198
  internalization, psychological disorders, 202
  Medical Outcomes Survey SF-36, 198
  pain–psychological disorder relationship, 195–196
  participation, 198
  pathogenesis, physical disease, 203
  physical impairment, 199
  physiologic outcomes and mortality, 202–203
  positing mechanisms, 196
  postonset disease outcome, 193
  psychological distress, physical symptoms, 194–195
  psychological impairment, 194, 199
  self-regulatory model, 198
  Sickness Impact Profile, 198
  somatosensory amplification, 196
  treatment, 195
  usual care program, 200
COPD. See chronic obstructive pulmonary disease
CYSHCN. See children and youth with special health care needs

DALYs. See disability-adjusted life-years
Dartmouth Co-Op Charts, 198
depression/anxiety disorders and headache, childhood adversity
  additional predictors, 175
  association, specific adversities, 178–180
  childhood adversity predisposition, 180–181
  comorbidity support, 176–178
  Cox proportional hazards models, 175
  data limitations, 176
  demographics, 175
  DSM-IV axis-I disorders, 180
  early-onset depression/anxiety disorders, 176, 179
  headache–mental disorder comorbidity, 174
  independent associations, 181
  independent predictors, 175
  Kaplan–Meier curves, 175
  loss of parents, 175–176
  multiple childhood adversities, 176, 180
  NCHS, 175
  psychosocial development, 174
  research limitations, 174–175
  sexual, physical abuse, 180
  specific adversity distribution, by country, 177
depression manifestation with age, 90–91
depressive and anxiety disorders
  aging and, 91
  chronic pain, 24–25, 26
  chronic physical disease, 19–20
  prevalence, 17–18
Descartes, René, 2
development of mental–physical comorbidity
  allostatic load, 102–103
  antecedent model, mental disorder to physical condition, 97–99
  behavioral pathways, 98–99
  bidirectionality, 99–100
  biological pathways, 99
  biological vulnerability, 101
  consequence model, physical condition to mental disorder, 99
  developmental plasticity, 100–101
  dysregulation, stress systems, 97–98
  early-life risk factors, 103
  HPA axis response, 97
  illness representation, 99
  latency model, 101
  pathways, cumulative effects, 101–102
  risk factors, 97
  shared determinants, life-span perspective, 100
  stress responsiveness, critical periods, 101

Index

diabetes. *See also* adult-onset diabetes, psychosocial factors
  mellitus, 136
  mental disorder and, 56–57
  prevalence rates, 137
  self-reports, 37–38
  type 2, 136
Diagnostic and Statistical Manual of Mental Disorders, Fourth Edition (DSM-IV), 35
  age patterns, 84
  measurement methods, 42
  mental disorders, headache, childhood adversity, 180
  mental–physical comorbidity pattern, 52
differential item functioning (DIF), 247
disability, pure versus comorbid mental–physical conditions
  chronic conditions, 239, 240
  communication problems, 247–248
  data analysis, 240
  DIF, 247
  disability attribution, 247
  disability days, 241–247
  disability measures, 239
  mobility problems, 247–248
  participant characteristics, 241
  participants
    comorbid conditions, 241
    pure conditions, 241
  prototypic chronic conditions, 240
  pure versus comorbid conditions, 240, 241
  pure versus comorbid prevalence, 248
  WMH WHODAS, 239–240
  World Mental Health Survey Initiative, 239
disability-adjusted life-years (DALYs), 210
disability and treatment, mental and physical disorders
  activity limitations, 223
  aggregate disability estimates, 222
  assessment, 212
  bidirectional effects, 224–225
  burden, 210
  cancer prevalence estimates, 221
  chronic pain disorder disability, 214
  CIDI, 211
  condition-specific disability, 210–211
  condition-specific measurement, 222
  DALYs, 210
  disability comparisons, 225–226
  disability self-report scales, 222
  disorder-specific disability, 216, 217
  DSM-IV mental disorders, 211
  health care, 210, 225
  ICF, 223
  ICIDH, 223
  major depression disorder disability, 222–223
  Mann–Whitney tests, 214
  measurement limitations, 221
  mental disorder assessment, 211–212
  mental disorder disability, 214
  mental–physical disability, 218
  mental–physical disorder pairs, 214–218
  musculoskeletal disorder disability, 222–223
  physical disorder assessment, 211
  physical disorder prevalence estimates, 221–222
  PPGHC, 210
  residual disability, 225
  sampling limitations, 218–221
  SDS scales, 212–213
  self-reported disorder prevalence and treatment, 213–214
  severe mental–physical disability, 218
  social role performance, 224
  statistical analysis, 213
  study approach, 211
  treatment implications, 224
DSM-IV. *See Diagnostic and Statistical Manual of Mental Disorders, Fourth Edition*
Dubos, Rene, 5

ecological perspectives, 5–6
epidemiologic map, 1–2
European Community Respiratory Health Survey (ECRHS), 110–117

fear-avoidance, 197
functional disability
  AIMS, 198
  COPD, 199
  Dartmouth Co-Op Charts, 198
  depression treatment, 200–201
  disability, 198–199
  Groningen Social Disabilities Schedule, 198
  ICF, 198
  impairment, defined, 198
  Medical Outcomes Survey SF-36, 198
  participation, 198
  physical impairment, 199
  psychological impairment, 199, 200
  Sickness Impact Profile, 198

global burden, chronic physical disease, 15–17
Goffman, E., 256
Groningen Social Disabilities Schedule, 198
gross domestic product (GDP), 16–17

headache and depression, 54–55, 56
headache and depression–anxiety disorders, childhood adversity
  additional predictors, 175
  childhood adversity predisposition, 180–181
  comorbidity support, 176–178
  Cox proportional hazards models, 175
  data limitations, 176
  demographics, 175
  DSM-IV axis-I disorders, 180
  early-onset depression/anxiety disorders, 176, 179
  headache–mental disorder comorbidity, 174
  independent associations, 181
  Kaplan–Meier curves, 175
  loss of parents, 175–176
  multiple childhood adversities, 176, 180
  NCHS, 175
  psychosocial development, 174
  research limitations, 174–175
  sexual, physical abuse, 180
  specific adversity association, 178–180
  specific adversity distribution, by country, 177
health care
  AAFP, 308
  ACP, 308
  AOA, 308
  APA, 308
  behavioral interventions, 202
  communication, coordination, 308
  costs, 16–17
  CYSHCN, 308
  Declaration of Alma-Ata by the International Conference on Primary Health Care (1978), 307
  depression treatment, 201–202
  implications, 7
  intersectoral links, 308–309
  Medical Home, 307–308
  NAPNAP, 308
  primary health care, 307
  psychological illness, 201
  schools, 309
heart disease. *See also* heart disease, psychosocial factors
  mental–physical comorbidity pattern, 56, 57
  self-report, 38
  sexual physical abuse, 125–126
host–agent environment, 5–6
hypothalamic–pituitary–adrenocortical (HPA) axis
  abuse, 101

  adult-onset diabetes, 139–140
  dysregulation, 97–98, 101

interactional model of comorbidity, 230
internalization, psychological disorders, 202
International Association for the Study of Pain (ASP), 22
International Classification of Functioning, Disability, and Health (ICF), 198, 223
International Classification of Impairments, Disabilities, and Handicaps (CIDH), 223
International Classification of Mental and Behavioural Disorders (ICD-10), 35

joint association, mental–physical condition with disability
  additive model of comorbidity, 230–231
  allostatic load, 235
  analysis methods, 232
  bidirectional relationship, 236
  disability, 231–232
  disability prevalence, country-specific, 232–234
  impact, 230
  interactional model of comorbidity, 230–231
  linear regression, 231
  logistic regression, 231, 232
  mental disorder status, 231
  pooled estimates, 234
  shared pathophysiology, 235
  study limitations, 236
  synergistic effect, comorbidity, 235, 236–237
  treatment indications, 236
  WMH WHODAS, 231, 232

labor force, unemployment, mental–physical comorbidity
  challenges, 249
  comorbid, noncomorbid comparison rates, 251–252
  gender-specific comparison rates, 252–253
  health-related effects, 249
  implications, 249–250
  labor force participation rates, 251
  labor force reduction, 253, 254
  logistic regression models, 250
  multivariate analyses, 253
  odds ratios, 250
  psychological status, 254
  study approach, 250
  unemployment rate, 251
  unemployment risk, 253
  work productivity, 253–254
  World Mental Health Survey Initiative, 250

Index

life-span perspectives, 4–6
linear regression, 231
logistic regression, 43, 231
longevity, 1–2

MCS. *See* mental component score
measurement methods
   childhood family adversities, 42
   CIDI v. 34–35
   DSM-IV, 42
   ICD-10, 35
   SDS, 41–42
Medical Outcomes Survey SF-36, 198
mental component score (MCS), 258
mental health providers, 300
mental–physical comorbidity, predicted mortality
   cardiovascular risk, 280, 281–282
   comorbid anxiety, depression, 281
   Cox proportional hazards models, 276, 277
   data analysis, 277
   developed, developing countries, 281
   impact, 280–281
   independent effect, mental disorders, 281
   mental disorders, smoking, chronic disease, 277
   mortality risk, depression
   predicted incremental mortality, 279–280
   PREVEND, 276
   risk engine, 275–277
   study limitations, 281
   study population, psychiatric diagnoses, 276
mental–physical comorbidity development
   allostatic load, 102–103
   antecedent model, mental disorder to physical condition, 97–99
   behavioral pathways, 98–99
   bidirectionality, 99–100
   biological pathways, 99
   biological vulnerability, 101
   consequence model, physical condition to mental disorder, 99
   developmental plasticity, 100–101
   dysregulation, stress systems, 97–98
   early-life risk factors, 103
   HPA axis response, 97, 101
   illness representation, 99
   latency model, 101
   pathways, cumulative effects, 101–102
   risk factors, 97
   shared determinants, life-span perspective, 100
   stress responsiveness, critical periods, 101
mind–body duality, 2–3

NASMHPD. *See* U.S. National Association of State Mental Health Program Directors
National Association of Pediatric Nurse Practitioners (NAPNAP), 308
National Comorbidity Survey – Replication, 154
National Health Interview Survey (NHIS), 35
NCHS. *See* U.S. National Health Interview Survey

Obesity. *See also* adult obesity, childhood adversities
   BMI, 165
   causes, 165
   health risks, 165
   mental disorder and, 56, 57

pain assessment, chronic pain, 23
paper-and-pencil (PAPI) interviews, 30
pattern and nature, mental–physical comorbidity
   alcohol abuse and asthma, 57
   alcohol abuse and spinal pain, 56
   arthritis and depression, 54–55
   association, disorders, 57–59
   asthma and mental disorder, 54–55, 56
   bidirectional relationship, 59
   chronic pain and medical conditions, 52–54
   diabetes and mental disorder, 56–57
   headache and depression, 54–55, 56
   heart disease and mental disorder, 56, 57
   management outcome, 58
   mental and chronic physical disorder, 51–52
   mental disorder status, 52
   obesity and mental disorder, 56, 57
   prevalences, by disorder, 55
   research attention, 58
   shared origin, 59
   spinal pain and depression, 54–56
PCS. *See* physical component score
perceived stigma, mental–physical comorbidity
   activity limitation, 264
   analyses, 259
   chronic physical conditions, 258
   comorbid versus noncomorbid, 262–264
   differential prevalence, 264–265
   health-related stigmatization, 256
   help-seeking behavior, 259
   impact, 258–259, 264
   MCS, 258
   measurement, 256–258
   mental disorder, 261–262, 264
   mental disorders, chronic conditions, 258
   mental–physical disorder, 259–261
   PCS, 258
   prevalence, 259

perceived stigma (*cont.*)
   professionals, 257
   research implications, 265
   social limitation index, 258
   stigma, defined, 256
   study limitations, 257–258
   WHODAS-II, 257
   WLD, 258
   WMH Survey Initiative, 257
physical and psychological morbidity
   allostasis, 3
   allostatic load, 3–4
   bidirectional links, 3
   chronic pain mechanisms, 4
physical comorbidity, major depression treatment
   care provision, 268–269
   chronic physical disease, 272
   depression comorbidity, 268
   depression detection, 273
   major depression criteria, 269
   multivariate analyses, 270–272
   study approach, 269–270
   treated depression comorbidity cases, 271
   treated major depression cases, 270, 271
   treatment, developing countries, 272
   treatment influences, 272
physical component score (PCS), 258
physical conditions
   chronic, 35–37
   life activities, 41
   NHIS, 35
   self-reports, 37–38
   WHODAS-II, 38–41
Plato, 2
policy implications, 7–8
   AAFP, 308
   ACP, 308
   age patterning, mental–physical conditions, 303
   AOA, 308
   APA, 308
   associations, mental–physical conditions, 303
   challenges, 310
   childhood adversities, early-onset mental disorder, 305
   communication, coordination, 308
   comorbidity consequences, 303
   CYSHCN, 308
   Declaration of Alma-Ata by the International Conference on Primary Health Care (1978), 307
   health benefits, 305
   health care services, 302
   intersectoral links, 308–309
   Medical Home, 307–308
   mental health services
      children, 306
      elderly, 306–307
   NAPNAP, 308
   NASMHPD, 309–310
   physical–mental disorder relationship, 303
   policy development, 303–305
   population-based data, 302–303
   population health, 306
   premature death rates, 302
   primary health care, 307
   risk factor associations, 303
   schools, 309
population perspectives, 5–6
posttraumatic stress disorder (PTSD)
PPGHC. *See* psychological problems in primary health care
Prevention of Renal and Vascular End-Stage Disease (PREVEND), 276
primary care providers, 299–300
psychological problems in primary health care (PPGHC), 210
PTSD. *See* posttraumatic stress disorder
pure versus comorbid chronic conditions, 240

Raphael, K. G., 161
research implications, 7–8
   assessment, 289–290
   childhood adversity buffering factors, 288
   childhood risk factors, adult-onset conditions, 287–288
   cohort study size, 294
   country-specific variation, 290–292
   data analyses, 288
   data optimization, 295
   epidemiological surveys, 292–293
   future prospective studies, 295–296
   historical cohort, 289
   international study, 287
   interrelated risk factor exposure, 288–289
   life-span developmental perspective, 290
   overidentification, 293–294
   protective factors, 292
   psychiatric disorder, physical conditions, 287
   reliability studies, 294–295
   risk factor circumstance, 292
   self-report ascertainment, 293
   social factors, 292
   synergistic effects, 289
   WMH Survey Initiative, 287
   WMH Surveys, 287

Index

SAM. *See* sympathetic–adrenal–medullary axis
sampling methods
  country-specific adaptations, 33
  final sampling frames, 33
  multistage probability, 33–34
  target population, 33
  two-part sampling, 34
SCID. *See* Structured Clinical Interview for DSM-IV
self-report(s)
  adult-onset diabetes, psychosocial factors, 140–141
  adult-onset spinal pain, childhood adversities, 162
  age patterns, 91–92
  arthritis, 38
  childhood adversity, later hypertension, 129, 130
  chronic disorders, 37
  diabetes, 37–38
  diagnostic data, 38
  heart disease, 38
  limitations, 44
  physical conditions, 37–38
  research implications, 293
  survey methods, 37–38, 44
  WMH Surveys, 293
sexual abuse
  adult-onset spinal pain, 161
  childhood family adversities, 48
  mental disorder and heart disease, 125–126
Sickness Impact Profile, 198
societal investment, disease prevention
  childhood adversities, early-onset mental disorder, 305
  health benefits, 305
  mental health services
    children, 306
    elderly, 306–307
  population health, 306
somatosensory amplification, 196
spinal pain. *See also* adult-onset spinal pain, childhood adversities
  alcohol abuse, 56
  childhood adversity and mental disorders, 154–155
  depression, 54–56
  predictors, 160–161
Structured Clinical Interview for DSM-IV (SCID), 35
survey methods
  analytic, 31
  childhood family adversities, 39, 42
  chronic pain, 35–37
  chronic physical conditions, 37
  CIDI, 31, 34–35
  content, 30
  data collection mode, 30
  data coordination, 29
  informed consent, 31
  interview verification, 31
  interviewer payment, 30–31
  interviewer training, 30
  life activities, 41
  measurement, 31
  pretesting, 30
  sampling, 30, 31, 33
  SDS, 41–42
  self-reports, 37–38, 44
  study design, 31–33
  survey administration, 30
  translation, 31
  two-part sampling, 34
  WHO regions, 31–33
  WHODAS-II, 38–41
  WMH Survey Initiative, 29
  WMHS sample design, 32
sympathetic–adrenal–medullary (SAM) axis, 97–98
symptom burden
  antidepressant medications, 195
  cognitive–behavioral therapy, 195
  pain–psychological disorder relationship, 195–196
  positing mechanisms, 196
  psychological distress, physical symptoms, 194–195
  somatosensory amplification, 196

type 2 diabetes, 136

unemployment, labor force, mental–physical comorbidity
  challenges, 249
  comorbid, noncomorbid comparison rates, 251–252
  gender-specific comparison rates, 252–253
  health-related effects, 249
  implications, 249–250
  labor force participation rates, 251
  labor force reduction, 253, 254
  logistic regression models, 250
  multivariate analyses, 253
  odds ratios, 250
  psychological status, 254

unemployment, labor force (*cont.*)
　study approach, 250
　unemployment rate, 251
　unemployment risk, 253
　work productivity, 253–254
　World Mental Health Survey Initiative, 250
U.S. National Association of State Mental Health Program Directors (NASMHPD), 309–310
U.S. National Health Interview Survey (NCHS), 110
usual care program, 200

WHO. *See* World Health Organization
WHO Composite International Diagnostic Interview (CIDI), 31, 85, 211
WHO Composite International Diagnostic Interview (CIDI v.)
　measurement methods, 34–35
　mental disorder diagnoses, 35
　mental–physical comorbidity, 35
　modifications, 34–35
WHODAS-II. *See* World Health Organization Disability Assessment Schedule – II
WLD. *See* work lost days index
WMH. *See* World Mental Health Survey Initiative
WMH Surveys. *See* World Mental Health Surveys
women, depression, chronic pain
　anxiety disorder and chronic pain risk, 183
　association, 188–189
　causality, pain and depression, 188
　chronic pain, medical conditions, 188
　depression
　　anxiety disorder and gender effect, 186–187
　　anxiety disorder occurrence, 188
　　anxiety disorder prevalence, 184–187, 188
　developed and developing countries, 188
　shared mechanism, 189
　shared origin, 189
　study approach, 183–184
work lost days (WLD) index, 258
World Health Organization Disability Assessment Schedule – II (WHODAS-II), 38–41, 231, 239
World Health Organization (WHO), 223
World Mental Health (WMH) Survey Initiative, 287
World Mental Health (WMH) Surveys
　assessment, 289–290
　buffering factors, childhood adversities, 288
　childhood risk factors, adult-onset conditions, 287–288
　cohort study size, 294
　country-specific variation, 290–292
　data analyses, 288
　data optimization, 295
　epidemiological surveys, 292–293
　future prospective studies, 295–296
　historical cohort, 289
　international study, 287
　interrelated risk factor exposure, 288–289
　life-span developmental perspective, 290
　overidentification, 293–294
　protective factors, 292
　risk factor circumstance, 292
　self-report ascertainment, 293
　social factors, 292
　synergistic effects, 289